✓ W9-BXQ-608

COMPETENCIES *and* STRATEGIES *for*

Speech-Language Pathology Assistants

Susan M. Moore

Lynea D. Pearson

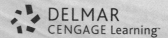
TOURO COLLEGE LIBRARY
Kings Highway **WITHDRAWN**

DELMAR
CENGAGE Learning™

Australia • Brazil • Japan • Korea • Mexico • Singapore • Spain • United Kingdom • United States

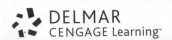

MW

Competencies and Strategies for Speech-Language Pathology Assistants
Susan M. Moore, Lynea D. Pearson

Executive Director, Health Care Business Unit: William Brottmiller

Executive Editor: Cathy L. Esperti

Developmental Editor: Juliet Byington

Executive Marketing Manager: Dawn F. Gerrain

Channel Manager: Jennifer McAvey

Editorial Assistant: Maria D'Angelico

Executive Production Manager: Karen Leet

Art/Design Coordinator: Connie Lundberg-Watkins

Project Editor: Shelley Esposito

Production Editor: John Mickelbank

© 2003 Delmar, Cengage Learning

ALL RIGHTS RESERVED. No part of this work covered by the copyright herein may be reproduced, transmitted, stored or used in any form or by any means graphic, electronic, or mechanical, including but not limited to photocopying, recording, scanning, digitizing, taping, Web distribution, information networks, or information storage and retrieval systems, except as permitted under Section 107 or 108 of the 1976 United States Copyright Act, without the prior written permission of the publisher.

For product information and technology assistance, contact us at
Cengage Learning Customer & Sales Support, 1-800-354-9706

For permission to use material from this text or product,
submit all requests online at **www.cengage.com/permissions**
Further permissions questions can be emailed to
permissionrequest@cengage.com

Library of Congress Control Number: 2002007947

ISBN-13: 978-0-7693-0248-5

ISBN-10: 0-7693-0248-3

Delmar
Executive Woods
5 Maxwell Drive
Clifton Park, NY 12065
USA

Cengage Learning is a leading provider of customized learning solutions with office locations around the globe, including Singapore, the United Kingdom, Australia, Mexico, Brazil, and Japan. Locate your local office at **international.cengage.com/region**

Cengage Learning products are represented in Canada by Nelson Education, Ltd.

For your course and learning solutions, visit **delmar.cengage.com**

Visit our corporate website at **www.cengage.com**

Notice to the Reader
Publisher does not warrant or guarantee any of the products described herein or perform any independent analysis in connection with any of the product information contained herein. Publisher does not assume, and expressly disclaims, any obligation to obtain and include information other than that provided to it by the manufacturer. The reader is expressly warned to consider and adopt all safety precautions that might be indicated by the activities described herein and to avoid all potential hazards. By following the instructions contained herein, the reader willingly assumes all risks in connection with such instructions. The publisher makes no representations or warranties of any kind, including but not limited to, the warranties of fitness for particular purpose or merchantability, nor are any such representations implied with respect to the material set forth herein, and the publisher takes no responsibility with respect to such material. The publisher shall not be liable for any special, consequential, or exemplary damages resulting, in whole or part, from the readers' use of, or reliance upon, this material.

Printed in Canada
3 4 5 6 7 11 10 09 08

5/26/09

Contents

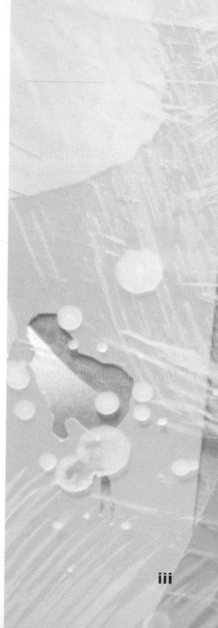

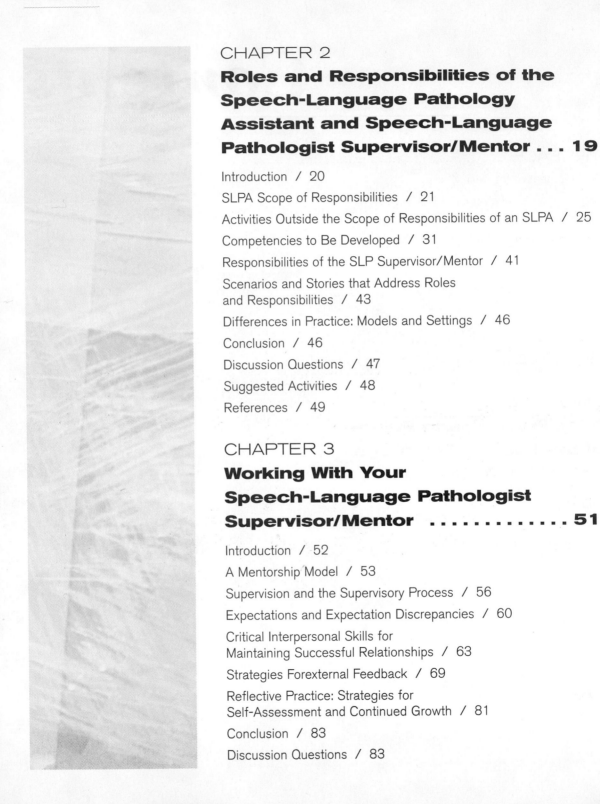

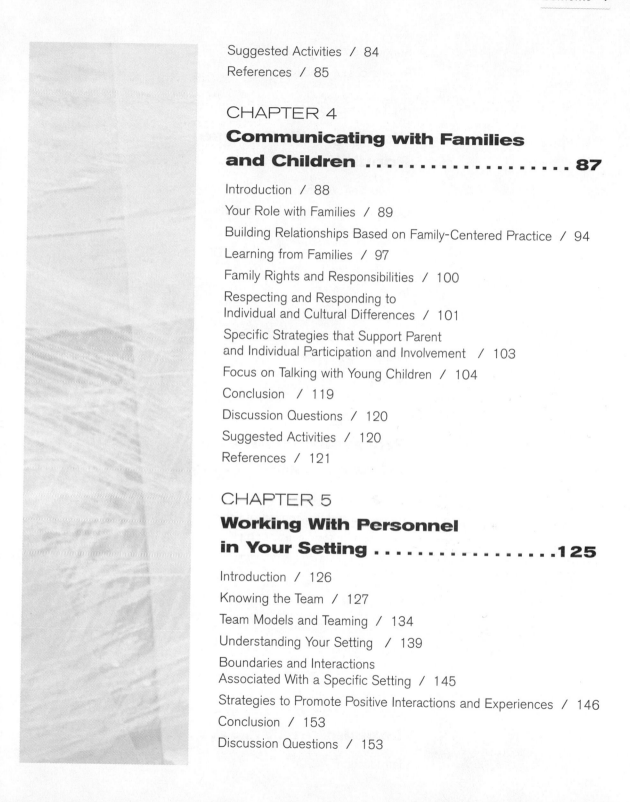

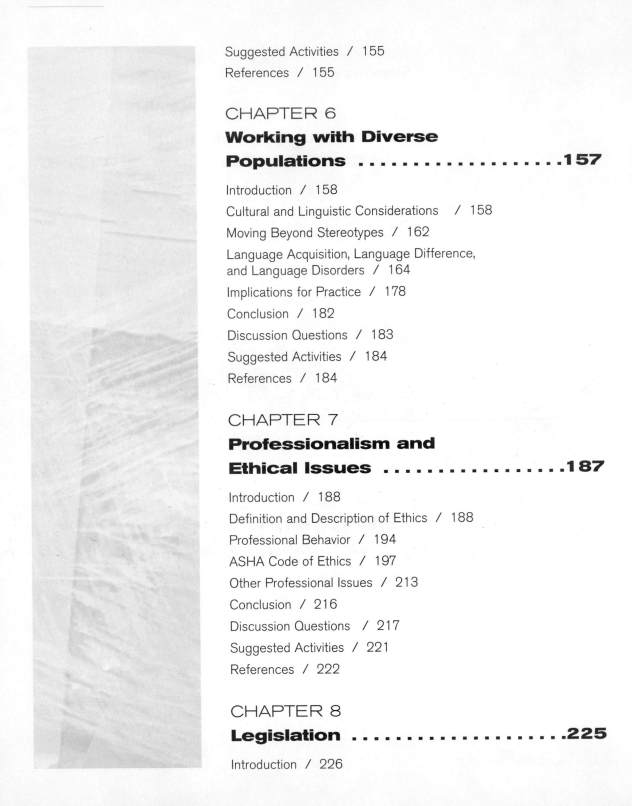

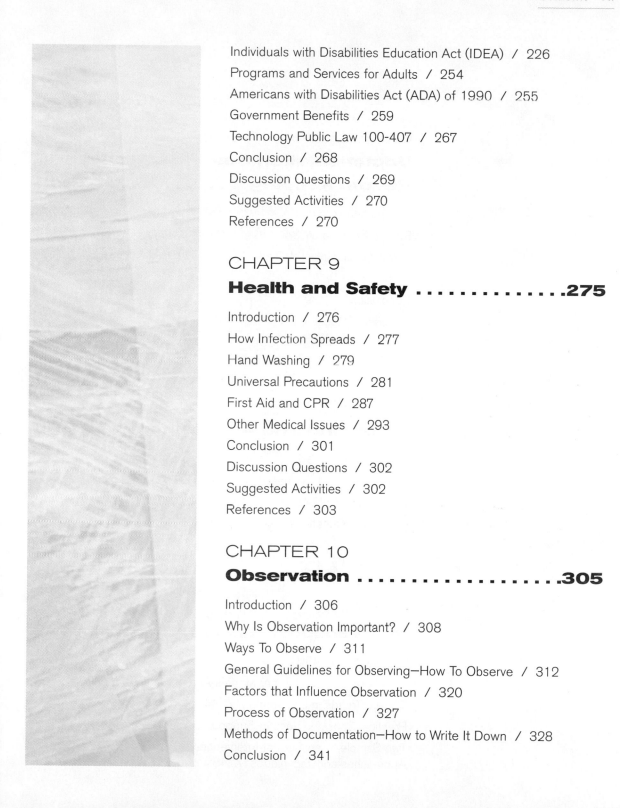

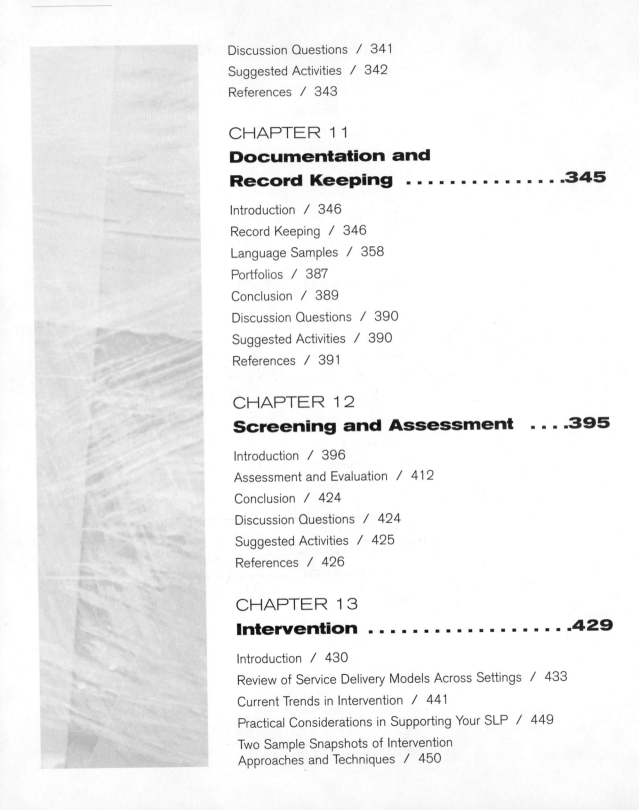

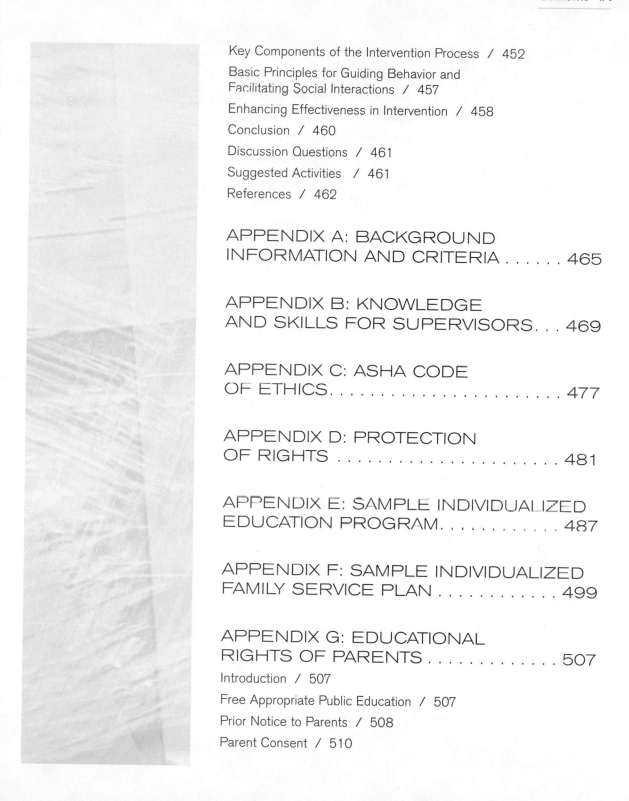

Preface

The profession of speech-language pathology is entering a new decade and a new century. Many challenges and opportunities are emerging as professionals work together to truly make a difference in the lives of individuals with speech, language, hearing, or communication differences and disorders. One of the most significant changes is the increasing reliance on speech-language pathology assistants (SLPAs) to support speech-language pathologists (SLPs) in their work with individuals with communication challenges. SLPAs have a significant role to play in this work as delivery of service models change and as cost-effective ways of extending services without jeopardizing quality are discovered and implemented. Quality preparation of SLPAs can only result in better, more intensive services and supports to those who need them. Thus, this text focuses on the importance of relationships—relationships with individuals receiving speech-language pathology services, with the families of those individuals, and with the supervising SLP—as the foundation for SLPA training and development. At the same time, the concrete skills and knowledge needed for a successful career as a speech-language pathology assistant are comprehensively covered. Although licensure and educational requirements for SLPAs vary from state to state, the competencies and strategies for speech-language pathology assistants covered in this text are fundamental to the successful development of support skills. This text serves as a strong foundation to what is sure to be a rewarding and fulfilling career as an SLPA.

DEVELOPMENT OF THE TEXT

It has been an exciting journey for us as authors to put together this text, which we feel will be invaluable to anyone preparing to become an SLPA. The journey began as we worked together, along with our colleague, Nan Eller, MA CCC, to

develop an educational curriculum for an AA level SLPA program at a local community college. As we approached this task, we discovered the need for a comprehensive text that could be used in an SLPA personnel preparation program at several levels. We were disheartened at finding very few resources available that dealt with SLPA preparation in a comprehensive and useful way. So we persevered in writing this comprehensive text, including the salient information critical to the preparation of successful SLPAs. We asked ourselves many questions during this process: What do future SLPAs need to know? How do we share the most meaningful and helpful information that will promote successful employment across a variety of settings? How do we communicate the importance of this position, and how can it be the beginning of a truly rewarding experience? How do we synopsize key concepts while at the same time provide suggestions for resources for in-depth exploration and ongoing learning? ASHA's implementation of an SLPA certification program underscores the importance of developing a comprehensive and timely resource such as this text to enhance the quality of preparation materials available to those providing educational programs for SLPAs. We have explained the ASHA model in depth and included materials for the student as well as the supervisor regarding roles, responsibilities and implications for practice. We wrote and rewrote and filtered down the information into what we believe is a rich resource for developing SLPAs.

ORGANIZATION AND FEATURES OF THIS TEXT

This text includes many special features, and to get the maximum benefit from each, we offer a few helpful hints. First, we know that the number of acronyms (SLP, SLPA, IEP, IFSP) in speech-language pathology, medicine, and education can be overwhelming. We suggest that you begin your own list of the most commonly used terms and acronyms, consult the text's glossary frequently, and never be afraid to ask the meaning of a term and how it can be used. This will help you to become comfortable with the multitude of new

terms, labels, and concepts that are used in speech-language pathology and related disciplines.

Second, the information is organized in each chapter to facilitate your learning. Brief overviews and key concepts are offered as a starting point in each chapter. These features allow the user to focus in on the most important concepts of each chapter and are a great tool for chapter review. Follow-up questions for discussion and suggested activities are listed at the end of each chapter to further your in-depth preparation as an SLPA. Although these are ideal tools for use in class with your peers, they also provide activities and topics for consideration that can be done independently to really bring the chapter concepts home. Observing, asking questions, reading, and reflecting on new learning will serve you well as you prepare for responsibilities as an SLPA. The more experience you have during your preparation, the more confidence you will have in seeking employment as an SLPA, and the more enjoyable and rewarding you will find your work.

Finally, throughout the text there are numerous boxed sidelights containing case studies, interesting facts, and helpful hints that further illustrate the concepts discussed in the main text. Some sidelights contain stories about individuals' personal experiences to help you see in greater detail what exactly the scope of professional responsibility is for SLPAs. Others highlight individuals receiving services for communication disorders to help developing SLPAs see the impact their work can have on these individuals and their families. Balancing out these case studies and personal experiences are sidelights containing additional resources and bulleted lists of key information. Look to this feature to augment and highlight key competencies and strategies for success in speech-language pathology assisting.

This text introduces you to key concepts and terms that provide the foundation for best practices in assessment and intervention with individuals receiving services from an SLP. It provides resources you can use as you complete your SLPA training, as well as useful tools and strategies to facilitate continued growth and development once you are employed as an SLPA. This text provides you with an understanding of the importance of the relationships you will develop with your SLP supervisor and the individuals with whom you will

work. We wish you the best in your chosen path as an SLPA and sincerely hope that this text facilitates your learning and preparation for this role. Better yet, may your journey also lead to many rewarding interactions with individuals who will benefit from your services.

Susan M. Moore
Lynea D. Pearson

Acknowledgments

To my family, Chris, Elissa, and, especially, Bob, for always being there with understanding and support. I would also like to thank the University-LEA Consortia members for their input and model of excellence in training of SLPAs. A special thank you to Morna Clement, who modeled the way. And to Brenda Dowell, for her ongoing support and patience with me during another one of my projects.

Susan M. Moore

To my husband, Scott, and my children, Hannah and John, who provided neverending support and understanding during this project. Couldn't have done it without you. Hannah, your determination to overcome your disabilities is inspiring. Keep it up!

A special thank you to those who helped with resources and support: Sheila Goetz, Kathy Tucker, Linda Brewer, Mara Kuczun, Bette Hadler, and Renee Heldman. Also thanks to those who graciously allowed us to include their pictures.

Lynea D. Pearson

We would both like to recognize the efforts and express our appreciation to Nan Eller. Thank you for your idea, many hours of work, research, and contributions to Chapter 12.

A very special thank you to our editor, Juliet Byington, from Delmar Cengage Learning. Her patience and support and holding of the candle while we burned it at both ends is so very much appreciated.

About the Authors

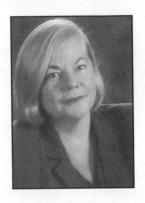

Susan M. Moore, JD, MA, CCC-SLP is Director of Clinical Education and Services at the University of Colorado, Boulder, in the Department of Speech, Language, and Hearing Sciences. She also holds a teaching faculty appointment in the School of Education at the University of Colorado, Denver, where she teaches coursework in early childhood special education. She is an ASHA Fellow. Her experience as the Project Director for a University-LEA Partnership Program designed to prepare SLPAs to join the workforce in Colorado and as team leader for writing a curriculum for SLPA training in a community college uniquely qualifies her to author this book. She has over 25 years' experience teaching and has implemented several personnel development programs in the state of Colorado.

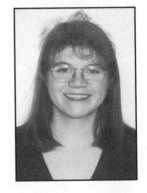

Lynea D. Pearson, MA, CCC-SLP is the mother of a 7-year-old daughter who has significant disabilities. She also is the Low Incidence Disability Grant Coordinator at the University of Colorado, Boulder. She supervises speech-language pathology graduate students in their clinical studies and provides specialized training in AAC and assistive technology. Before joining the University of Colorado, she worked in both school and hospital settings. She was part of a team that developed and wrote the curriculum for a proposal for an SLPA program in Colorado. She received her bachelor's and master's degrees from University of Colorado, Boulder, in speech-language pathology.

To the Reader

LETTER FROM A SPEECH-LANGUAGE PATHOLOGY ASSISTANT

Dear Colleague,

I began working as a speech-language assistant while I was working on my undergraduate degree. The job sort of "fell into my lap" during my senior year. I came across the advertisement while looking through job listings in an employment newspaper. Once I read the advertisement, I became very excited. It was just the job that I was looking for. I was excited about this position for several reasons. One, I really needed a job. Two, it was a job that would have me working in the exact area that I had been studying for the past several years. And three, I would finally get an idea of what it was truly like to work in the area of speech and language disorders in children. Most importantly, I hoped that I would receive reassurance that I had chosen the right career path for myself. As it turned out, I had. Working as a speech-language assistant was one of my most enjoyed jobs. My position consisted of carrying out therapy plans designed by the speech-language pathologist (my supervisor). I worked with children between the ages of preschool and 8th grade who had various abilities. It was very rewarding to work with these children. They really taught me a lot, not only about speech and language but also about life. Not only did I affect their lives, they truly affected mine. During the three years that I worked in this position, I watched many children change and grow. That I think was the most rewarding part.

I was allowed my own creative freedom (under the approval of my supervisor) but I wanted to be responsible for more. I decided to continue my education and obtained a master's degree. Now the experiences I had working as a speech-language assistant and my educational experiences

helped me to be the best professional that I can be. So with that, I wish all you aspiring speech-language assistants the best of luck. I hope to see you around!

Sincerely,
Morna Clement

CHAPTER 1

Past, Present, and Future of the Speech-Language Pathology Assistant

Key Concepts

There are many individuals in this country who need support and services given identified speech, language, or communication challenges.

◼

The speech-language pathology assistant (SLPA) is not a new concept. SLPAs are one level of support personnel who work with individuals with communication challenges under the direct supervision and guidance of appropriately certified and credentialed speech-language pathologists (SLPs).

◼

Specific information regarding the ASHA model of credentialing SLPAs can be found on the ASHA Web site at http://www.professional.asha.org

◼

Differences in credentialing requirements and procedures may vary depending on the state in which you are seeking employment. It is thus important to investigate the specific policy and procedures of your state when seeking a credential as an SLPA.

◼

Overview

◼

History of the Speech-Language Pathology Assistant

◼

Current Status: ASHA's Position

◼

State Level Requirements and Regulation

◼

Future Directions

◼

Opportunities and Challenges

Key Concepts continued

Appropriate training and credentialing are critical to the successful use of an SLPA and ensure quality of service is maintained for the individual with speech, language, or hearing challenges.

■

There are many opportunities and positive incentives for people who become employed as SLPAs, including a rich and rewarding experience of working with individuals who need your help and potential access to a career ladder that can lead to many exciting directions.

INTRODUCTION

You have decided to become an SLPA. Congratulations! This is an important role in the effort to meet the needs of children and adults with communication challenges. You will become part of a team, under the supervision of your licensed or certified SLP and work with people who need assistance and help. Many people are needed to provide quality services to individuals who are challenged by communication. You will be one of these individuals. The children and adults you work with will benefit from your support as they strive to improve or learn new ways of communicating and functioning in their lives.

DEFINING THE SLPA

SLPAs are considered to be one level of support personnel in speech-language pathology. Support personnel are individuals who perform tasks as prescribed, directed, and supervised by ASHA-certified SLPs. There are different levels of support personnel based on the types of training (on-the-job, academic) and the scope of their assigned responsibilities. Aides, for example, have a different, usually narrower, training base and a more limited scope of responsibilities relative to SLPAs. Many states use different terminology to refer to support personnel in speech-language pathology (e.g., communication aides, paraprofessionals, or service extenders). It is important that you become familiar with the terms and types of credentialing used in your state for SLPAs. Visit the ASHA Web site for more information about definitions, categories, and state regulations regarding the work of SLPAs at http://www.professional.asha.org.

It is exciting to be part of the effort in a hospital or rehabilitation center to work with a team, including your supervising SLP, to make a difference in helping individuals recover and relearn communication skills. You may work with many individuals because they have experienced such conditions as **aphasia** associated with strokes, **Parkinson's disease**, head injury, and other communication disorders associated with varying medical or health-related conditions. You will work in a team effort to help these people recover and learn ways of communicating to maintain their quality of life. You could choose to work in school systems with young children with identified disabilities or older students with language and learning disabilities. This is critical to their learning in school and their success in becoming competent communicators with those around them. You may have the opportunity to work with children who are deaf or hard of hearing, where you might learn another language such as **American Sign Language** (ASL). You may also have the opportunity to work with young nonspeaking children who are learning language and another mode of "talking" with their **augmentative alternative communication** (AAC) devices. Perhaps you will work with young adults who have suffered head injuries and need assistance in regaining their communication abilities. There are many opportunities to work with young children and families, school-age children and adolescents, adults and others in programs that serve a wide spectrum of individuals with communication issues and concerns.

HELPFUL HINT

You may want to visit the glossary of this text frequently to clarify new and different terms. For example, it is important to remember that individuals with communication challenges may be referred to in several different ways, depending on the setting or context for services. If you obtain employment in a hospital or nursing home, the individuals you work with will most likely be referred to as **patients**. Children and adults who receive services in outpatient settings such as clinics or private practices may be called **clients**. In a school setting the individuals receiving services are most commonly referred to as **students**. Throughout this text you may see these terms used interchangeably, depending on the term most commonly used to refer to individuals in a certain context. Do not be confused by this change in terms because all may be used appropriately, depending on the context for service delivery.

One in 10 Americans has a communication problem because of an undetected hearing loss, a stuttering problem, a **stroke**, a head injury, a language disorder, or some other disorder or problem that interferes with speech, language, or hearing. Thus, there are many people in the United States with identified communication challenges associated with different conditions or developmental delays. As an SLPA, you will be a major player in the effort to assist their growth, development, and academic learning. As you take on this exciting and rewarding career, it is important that you understand the role you play and how your supervising SLP will direct and support your work as an integral member in this team effort. You have chosen a challenging, but rewarding path that requires you to learn a great deal of new information and acquire many skills. However, the critical piece of your work will be about establishing relationships with people. Your interpersonal skills will help you be successful. If you enjoy working with and supporting others, you have chosen a much needed and satisfying role, because you will make a difference for people.

SIDELIGHT: *Tim's Story*

Tim was beginning his core requirements for an associate's degree in a 2-year program at Arapahoe Community College when his brother was in a horrific car accident. His brother was badly hurt and was in the hospital recuperating for 2 months and then was transferred to a specialized rehabilitation center. He was there for an intensive treatment program that took several months to complete. He needed Tim's help and support because their Dad had been killed in the accident and their mother was working full time to pay the bills. Tim spent many hours with his brother and also learned about the many professionals who played a role in his brother's recovery. He continued to volunteer at the rehabilitation center even after his brother was discharged. He was impressed not only with the level of care but also with the "team" that worked tirelessly to ensure each patient got what he needed. It was because of this experience that Tim decided to transfer into the SLPA program at school that would allow him to finish his associate's degree and also to begin to gain knowledge about disabilities, especially the communication needs of individuals he was volunteering with. He was enjoying the relationships he was establishing with both the patients and the professionals at the center. He was excited about a career working with people, especially people who needed help and had difficulty communicating.

The rehabilitation center agreed to hire him as an aide as he continued his SLPA program because they valued his ability and interest in the patients. He began to work with several patients who had had strokes. He transported them from their rooms to the speech-language sessions and often had the opportunity to "sit in" and help them in group sessions as they tried to practice their speech and share their stories. One thing was for sure, these individuals often regained their sense of humor, and Tim found he could use humor and laughter to communicate even if the patients could not remember the "right word." He learned a great deal from just observing and "trailing" the SLPs in the rehabilitation center. He was especially impressed by their patience and willingness to listen to their patients even though they were often struggling to say what was on their mind. Tim loved helping patients with practice sessions on the computers because it gave him additional time to interact with them and be supportive.

Tim enjoyed his position and realized he had made a good decision about his future direction as an SLPA. He was excited about the opportunities of being an SLPA would bring him and knew that he would probably continue to learn as he worked. He even thought of one day finishing his BA degree at Metropolitan State College and go on from there. (*Note*: Tim eventually completed his program to become an SLPA and continued his employment at the rehabilitation center. After working for 2 years as an SLPA, he started back to school to finish his 4-year degree. He then applied for a traineeship and was accepted at the university program to complete his MA degree as an SLP. Now he is working in a private practice with young children and their families and completing continuing education coursework because he wants to work as a developmental specialist with premature babies and their families in a neonatal intensive care unit.)

SIDELIGHT: *Sylvia's Story*

Sylvia is the mother of two children who attended the neighborhood elementary school in her community. She often volunteered in their classrooms and was sometimes asked to work with one little boy who had difficulty talking and learning. She especially enjoyed the relationship she had established with this little boy and his communication specialist (SLP). She learned a great deal about how children learn to talk and what was preventing this little boy from succeeding in school. Her brother had had trouble in school, and she had always thought that he could have been more successful in school if only someone had taken the time to understand his learning difficulties and why he was having problems reading. The SLP talked with her about becoming an SLPA and beginning a course of study at the local community college. The SLP encouraged Sylvia to learn more about communication and disorders and how she could be hired to work with students and support the work of an SLP. Sylvia decided to enroll in classes while her children were at school. She was interested in finding a position that would allow her to be at home when her young children were home but that would also allow her to work with other children who needed support. This was something she could do and be close to home and on the same school schedule as her children. She was excited to learn that an SLPA program would provide her with the knowledge and skills she needed to help children. Sylvia was eager to work with young children and looked forward to the rewarding relationships she could develop while helping children who were having difficulty communicating and learning (Figure 1-1).

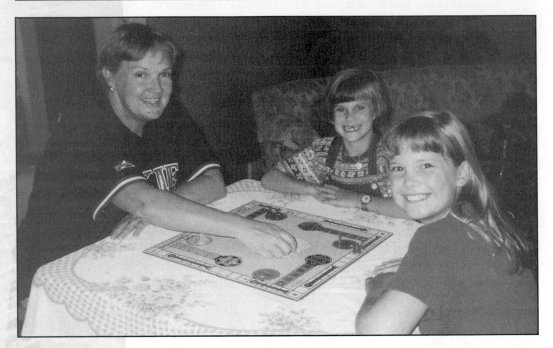

Figure 1-1 An SLPA at work

HISTORY OF THE SPEECH-LANGUAGE PATHOLOGY ASSISTANT

Many individuals think that the use of support personnel, specifically SLPAs, is a relatively new development. Actually, SLPAs have been used and regulated by many states since the 1970s. The American Speech-Language-Hearing Association (ASHA) has had guidelines for the use of support personnel since 1969, followed by subsequent revisions in 1988, 1995, and again in 2000. ASHA has developed guidelines for use of SLPAs as noted in Figure 1-2. The attention to the use of assistants has increased in many other professions (such as occupational therapy, physical therapy, and education) as professionals attempt to expand services to individuals across many settings that need support (French, 1993). Another reason for recent developments regarding use of support personnel is the need to contain costs in health care and education.

WHAT IS ASHA?

The **American Speech-Language-Hearing Association (ASHA)** is the professional, scientific, and credentialing, national association for more that 103,000 audiologists, speech-language pathologists, and speech-language and hearing scientists. ASHA's mission is to ensure that all people with speech, language, and hearing disorders have access to quality services to help them communicate more effectively. You can find out about ASHA by linking with http://www.asha.org.

Recently, ASHA has begun to implement a plan for national **registration** of SLPAs as well as approve programs offering training for this role. This initiative has become increasingly needed as ASHA views its role to ensure that speech-language pathology services provided to the public are of the highest quality and that SLPs continue to be responsible for maintaining that quality of service.

CURRENT STATUS: ASHA'S POSITION

As noted, in November 1996, approval of a strategic plan was brought forward to the legislative council, the policy approving board of the association. The Council of Professional Standards in Speech-Language Pathology and Audiology was charged by the legislative council to develop and administer a credentialing process for assistants in speech-language pathology. The resulting document was approved in September 2000 and revised again in April

■ ASHA Committee on Supportive Personnel. (1981, March). Guidelines for the employment and utilization of supportive personnel. *ASHA, 23*,165–169.

■ Utilization and employment of speech-language pathology supportive personnel with underserved populations. (1988, November). *ASHA, 30*, 55–56.

■ ASHA policy regarding support personnel. (1994, March). *ASHA, 36*(Suppl. 13), 24.

■ Training, credentialing, use, and supervision of support personnel in speech-language pathology. (1995). *ASHA, 37*(Suppl. 14), 221.

■ Guidelines for the training, credentialing, use, and supervision of speech-language pathology assistants. (1996, Spring) *ASHA, 38*(Suppl. 16), 21–34.

Note: In November 2000, ASHA approved the following documents. Implementation of these criteria and development of the policies and procedures for registration of assistants and approval of training programs is currently under way.

■ Criteria for approval of associate degree technical training programs for speech-language pathology assistants (approved by the Council of Academic Accreditation, October 2000; revised April 2001) Effective January 1, 2002.

■ Background information and criteria for the registration of speech-language pathology assistants (approved by the Council on Professional Standards, September 2000). Effective January 1, 2003.

See http://www.professional.asha.org for additional updates of information and resources.

Figure 1-2 Timetable of ASHA guidelines

2001. This document describes the minimum criteria and competencies for the approval of individuals to become registered nationally as SLPAs through ASHA. The Council of Academic Accreditation (CAA) of ASHA links these criteria for approval of technical training programs. It is important to become familiar with this information, *Background*

RESPONSIBILITIES FOR SLPAS

The following is a list of SLPA responsibilities taken from *Background Information and Criteria for the Registration of Speech-Language Assistants* (ASHA, October 2000, p. 2).

- Assist the SLP with speech-language and hearing screenings (without interpretation).
- Follow documented treatment plans or protocols developed by the supervising SLP.
- Document patient/client performance (e.g., tallying data for the SLP to use; preparing charts, records, and graphs) and report this information to the supervising SLP.
- Assist the SLP during assessment of patients/clients
- Assist with informal documentation as directed by the SLP.
- Assist with duties such as preparing materials and scheduling activities as directed by the SLP.
- Collect data for quality improvement.
- Perform checks and maintenance of equipment.
- Support the SLP in research project, in-service training, and public relations programs.
- Assist with departmental operations (scheduling, record keeping).
- Exhibit compliance with regulations, reimbursement requirements, and other responsibilities associated with the assistant position.

Information and Criteria for Registration of SLP Assistants (ASHA, October 2000) if you are interested in the national registration process through ASHA as a credentialing option for your work as an SLPA. These criteria will be effective as of January 2003.

It is also important to note that as of January 2001, ASHA reported that there were 26 known operational associate's degree programs for SLPAs and that 48 additional institutions were considering developing a program in this area. Some of the programs have explored distance learning options and collaborations between community programs and institutions of higher education. According to ASHA, "the curriculum guidelines were designed to provide technical training that leads to the fulfillment of the specified job responsibilities, core technical skills, and workplace behaviors"(ASHA, 2000, p. 1).

The responsibilities of the SLPA are specified and provide that the training, supervision, documentation, and planning are appropriate. Many tasks may be delegated to the assistant, including assisting with screening (excluding interpretation of results) and working with individuals directly by following treatment plans developed by the supervising SLP. The SLPA may also be involved in documentation and record keeping, working with and maintaining equipment, supporting the SLP in research projects, assisting with departmental operations, and collecting data for quality management. Additional information regarding suggested guidelines and use of SLPAs with sample tools and forms can be found in several ASHA publications (ASHA, 1997, 1998).

STATE LEVEL REQUIREMENTS AND REGULATION

State laws vary and may differ significantly from the ASHA criteria for credentialing and practice. It is important to become aware of the applicable state law for the state in which you may be seeking employment. Specific educational requirements and tasks permitted by assistants in a particular state may be different from those delineated by ASHA's credentialing process. It is also important to know that as of this writing, there are a few states, such as New York, that do not permit the use of support personnel. In the states that do, agencies (licensure boards) currently regulate support personnel and have training requirements that range from a high school diploma to a baccalaureate degree and graduate school hours, as well as a range in the requirements for supervision of SLPAs. In addition to state regulatory agencies, state departments of education may also credential support personnel to work solely in public schools to support the services provided by a qualified SLP (for example, Kentucky). The most common title for support personnel seems to be that of an assistant. It is interesting to note that in several states, there are levels or tiers of support personnel in which each level has its own educational requirements, title, and specified level of authorized responsibilities. It is also notable that in at least seven states, some level of *continuing education* is a requirement for support personnel.

In order to ensure quality of care to consumers, most states have stipulated one or more supervision requirements. Some states limit the number of support personnel that one licensed SLP or audiologist may supervise. For example, the SLP may not be able to complete her responsibilities and supervise more than two SLPAs at one time. This makes sense given the need and desire for supervision and mentorship. Some states specifically prescribe the amount of direct and indirect supervision that a supervisor must provide to the SLPA. There are even some states that specify what activities and tasks may or may not be performed by the SLPA versus others that simply provide a general statement to the effect that the support personnel are the responsibility of the licensed SLP and should be appropriately supervised given her individual education and experience.

It is thus very important to investigate the state law or regulations or guidelines governing the agency or district you might want to seek employment with. Now is the time to discover what your work with individuals with communication challenges might be like. It may be helpful to discuss the specific requirements, or lack thereof, that apply in your state with your instructor and investigate what, if any, state regulations or requirements you might encounter as you seek employment. If you have not done so already, it would be worth your time and effort to arrange an observation in a community facility or public school setting that employs support personnel and specifically SLPAs. This is where you will be able to find out about the specifics of the position. Let your interest areas guide you but not limit your exposure to various work settings. If you know you definitely want to work with children in a public school setting, take the time to visit and talk with SLPs and SLPAs, who can guide your thinking. As part of your training, you will most likely be involved in a practica or field placement experience; however, now is the time to investigate options across settings so you can request or target specific competencies and experiences you want to have as part of your educational program.

Sample Comparisons Across States

It is interesting to consider how much the role and educational requirements for SLPAs can differ across the United

States. California has specific licensure laws and regulations that are applicable to the SLPA. Regulations align with ASHA and govern the practice of an SLPA across various settings. The Iowa Administrative Code (Frelinger, 1992, p. 52) requires a minimum of a high school education as the required qualification for a "communication aide," and further stipulates that special education support aides may be employed to provide assistance to professionals in special education. The rules also require these paraprofessionals to work under the supervision of professional staff that is appropriately authorized to provide direct services in the same area that the paraprofessional provides assistive services. In New Mexico, state licensure law regulates the practice of the SLPA. SLPAs must have a BA-level degree and be enrolled in a graduate program working toward their master's degree. This is inconsistent with the current ASHA position regarding use of SLPAs, yet functions as a career ladder to encourage recruitment into the profession.

Then there are states like New York that do not recognize the need for SLPAs and prohibit their use through licensure laws. You might ask why? As the role and function of SLPAs has evolved over time, it has done so because the need is great for qualified providers to work with individuals with communication challenges associated with related conditions or problems. However, there has also been a great deal of concern that this would result in a lowering of the established standards of the profession and interfere with the ability of the qualified professional (SLP) in meeting the needs of this population. Thus, the SLPA, although trained at a certain level, needs to be supervised by a qualified or licensed SLP in order to maintain quality of service and support. Many SLP professionals are concerned that the introduction of the SLPA threatens their job security, and in some instances pose a threat, because it could increase their caseloads and responsibilities. However, others see the SLPA as an extender of services that can address the needs for quality of care and thus in no way should or can replace the professional expertise and skills of the practicing SLP.

In Colorado, another model has developed for training "extenders of service" in the public schools. Colorado is a "nonregulation state." There is no licensure beyond that

required to work in the public schools with a master's level of education in speech-language pathology. This has developed given the ongoing shortage of qualified SLPs, credentialed with an MA degree through the Colorado Department of Education, to work in school-based settings. Three university programs and several participating school districts have developed consortia to train SLPAs at the BA level to work in public school settings. This pilot training program has been funded by the Colorado Department of Education as one strategy to develop a "stepping stone" or career lattice wherein individuals can enter and exit the personnel preparation system at several points or "steps" in a career plan. It allows for extenders of service without increasing caseload size and promotes a mentorship model of personnel preparation. The trainee (potential SLPA) works side by side with the supervising SLP/mentor in a practica or field-based experience. Trainees develop competency in their role as an SLPA while also taking additional coursework that adds to their knowledge and skill base.

Information found on the ASHA Web site indicates that there are now 31 states that officially regulate the use of support personnel. Of these 31, there are 8 states (Illinois, Kentucky, Louisiana, New Mexico, Ohio, Oregon, South Carolina, Texas) that regulate support personnel through licensure and 23 that regulate support personnel through registration. In several states, support personnel are not directly regulated; however, licensed SLPs who use support personnel are required to observe specific supervisory guidelines. It is important to note that these data continually change given the increased attention and practice in use of support personnel. It thus makes sense for you to investigate the regulations that apply in your own state. Change is rapid and updates are necessary.

FUTURE DIRECTIONS

What does the future hold for SLPAs? As you can see, the SLPA position is here to stay despite variations in the training, regulations, and use from state to state. There is now a national credentialing body, ASHA, that offers a national registry or registration process to ensure basic knowledge and

competencies are developed for those seeking this role. ASHA has also made recent changes in the **ASHA Code of Ethics** (ASHA, 2001), explained in depth in subsequent chapters, to promote adherence to practices that reflect quality of care for all consumers. There are a number of complexities, such as inconsistencies across states in credentialing procedures and acceptance and funding of SLPAs by local school districts. Yet, there are many opportunities for developing programs that extend services to children and adults with communication challenges and their families through the use of trained and qualified SLPAs.

OPPORTUNITIES AND CHALLENGES

Appropriate training and supervision is critical to the successful use of a practicing SLPA. You have chosen to learn the basic information needed to develop competencies in this position. One might predict the continued growth of training programs for this purpose as well as an increase in the use of distance learning opportunities so that knowledge and skills can be acquired and maintained in a timely and cost-effective way. This may prove critical to ensuring adequate access to training programs, especially for individuals from rural areas who do not have ready access to training in their community. Development of these programs will be critical to ongoing access to continuing education opportunities because the SLPA's scope of responsibilities will most likely evolve as new approaches are developed and practices in management of specific challenges change. The scope of practice in speech-language pathology is ever changing as theory translates into practice and newly developed technology affects preferred practice patterns. This will certainly affect what you do as an SLPA and how you will do it. It is thus critical that even if you choose to work as an SLPA for many years, there will be a need for you to participate in continuing education as the field introduces new ways of facilitating and enhancing the communication function of those individuals needing support and care. This may happen at an in-service level or you may choose to take continuing educa-

tion courses through community college or university programs. This will also ensure your ability to fulfill your responsibility as an SLPA and reap the rewards of your work with children and adults needing your assistance.

Other opportunities and challenges to consider in the future may involve the working conditions and pay for this position. For example, the working conditions of schools and changes in the landscape of health care contain both incentives and disincentives for support personnel. As noted for Sylvia, the school schedule is desirable, because she wants to spend time with her children when they are home from school. Yet, she feels she has something to contribute and her work is valued and respected by her supervising SLP. She has a positive relationship with her supervisor and enjoys her work with children. Often, as in Sylvia's situation, support personnel are valued and treated as critical team members in recognition of the important work they do.

Despite these positive incentives, disincentives may exist. Concern about "burnout," a condition that results from prolonged distress (Fimian, 1988), sometimes can affect the work of support personnel (Frith & Mims, 1985; Logue, 1993). Distress can be related to dissatisfaction with working conditions, poor relationships with supervising SLPs, prolonged work with difficult students, or patients, hectic schedules, or too little time to complete assigned tasks. Other factors might include the lack of respect from team members, supervisors, students or patients themselves, low salaries, no employer-paid benefits, and lack of appropriate supervision. It has been reported in the literature (French, 1993) that the average annual salary of a paraprofessional is about one third of the average teacher or professional salary. Remember that SLPAs represent one category of more than 400,000 paraprofessionals employed just in educational settings (Pickett, 1994). In the future, the overall numbers of paraprofessional positions it is expected to continue to grow as they probably have since this report from 1994. Thus, one can expect SLPA positions to also increase in number. It is also important to note that two other professions (occupational therapy and physical therapy) that use assistant-level positions have successfully established a salary wage range considerably higher on average than that of the typical paraprofessional in a school-based setting. This

bodes well for the salary level of an SLPA. In summary, although use of SLPAs is not a new development, there is considerable attention being given now to the evolution of this role through establishment of training programs, credentialing processes, regulation, and guidelines that will have an impact on the future of the SLPA.

CONCLUSION

The opportunity to participate in a meaningful and important role as an SLPA leaves the door wide open for you to further your own growth, development, and education. It may be time to think about what you are going to do with this training. As noted many states are building career ladders or lattices in personnel preparation, with many points of entry and exit depending on training, education, experience, and desired work settings. Where does the SLPA training you are now receiving fit in your career plan? At this point, are you completing this course of study to gain the knowledge and skills you will need to work with a qualified, licensed, or certified SLP so that you can work in a public school setting? Are you hoping to work in a hospital, agency, or private practice? Will you be using this training as a stepping stone to gain direct experience in a job-related setting and then go on with your education? There are many opportunities associated with this course of study and you certainly do not have to make your final decisions now. You can take one step at a time as you work toward completing the course of study to become a qualified SLPA.

DISCUSSION QUESTIONS

1. What is an SLPA? Who does one work with in this position? What do you have to do to become one?
2. Why are SLPAs growing in number? Why has ASHA chosen to develop a credentialing process for this role?
3. What do you perceive the opportunities and challenges to be for an SLPA? Relate this to your personal goals and objectives.

4. Where do you think you would like to work as an SLPA? What settings interest you the most?

SUGGESTED ACTIVITIES

1. Have you had the opportunity to observe an SLP or SLPA in action? Arrange an appointment to observe an SLPA or SLP in a setting in your community that you are interested in. Shadow and talk with the SLP or SLPA about the position and learn who he provides services to and what he does in his practice and how he does it. You may want to arrange this observation or visit through your instructor. Consider exploring several settings, because there may be significant differences in the roles and responsibilities across agencies, rehabilitation centers, hospitals, and schools. Reflect on what you learned and discuss this with your instructor and peers. Listen to your peers' experiences and compare their experiences to your own.

2. Investigate your state requirements for credentialing and use of SLPAs. What policy and procedures apply? You may find some information through the state licensing board for speech-language pathologists or the Department of Education or the state professional association for SLPs. Many professional state associations have Web sites that you can visit to find out a great deal of information about the use of SLPAs in your state or another state of interest.

3. Visit the ASHA Web site (http://www.professional.asha.org) and look for updated information on the ASHA registration and credentialing process. Compare this information with what you have discovered in your exploration of your state's policy and regulations.

4. Reflect on your decision to become an SLPA. What are you looking for in a position? Will this enable you to follow your dreams and realize your possibilities? Are you well informed about your options? You may want to begin a journal or portfolio of your experiences, and keep a record of your questions and con-

cerns as you proceed with your training. Begin with a reflection of why you chose this path. Writing things down may be a helpful way to gather your thoughts and share your questions and concerns with your instructor or advisor as you develop your career goals and objectives.

REFERENCES

American Speech-Language-Hearing Association. (1997). Preparing and using speech-language pathology assistants, *ASHA*, 1–10.

American Speech-Language-Hearing Association. (1998). Practical tools and forms for supervising speech-language pathology assistants. *ASHA*, 1–10.

American Speech-Language-Hearing Association. (2000, October). *Background information and criteria for the registration of speech-language pathology assistants*. Retrieved March 2, 2002, from http://www.professional.asha.org/

American Speech-Language-Hearing Association. (2001). *Code of Ethics*. Retrieved March 2, 2002, from http://www.professional.asha.org/

Coufal, K. L., Steckelberg, A. L., & Vasa, S. (1991). Current trends in the training and utilization of paraprofessionals in speech-language programs: A report on an eleven-state survey. *Language, Speech & Hearing in the Schools, 22,*51–59.

Fimian, M. J. (1988). *Teacher stress inventory*. Brandon, VT: Clinical Psychology.

Frelinger, J. J. (1992, November). Support personnel. *ASHA, 34,*51–53.

French, N. K. (1993). Are community college training programs for paraeducators feasible? *Community College Journal of Research and Practice,17,*131–140.

French, N. K. (1997). Management of paraeducators. In A.L. Pickett & K. Gerlach (Eds.), *Supervising paraeducators in public school settings: A team approach* (pp. 91–169). Austin, TX: PRO-ED.

Frith, G. H., & Mims, A. (1985). Burnout among special education paraprofessionals. *Teaching Exceptional Children, 17,*225–227.

Logue, O. J. (1993, April). *Job satisfaction and retention variables of special education paraeducators*. Paper presented at the 12th Annual Conference on the Training and Employment of Paraprofessionals in Education and Rehabilitation, Seattle, WA.

Pickett, A. L. (1994). *Paraprofessionals in the education workforce*. Washington, DC: National Education Association.

CHAPTER 2

Roles and Responsibilities of the Speech-Language Pathology Assistant and Speech-Language Pathologist Supervisor/Mentor

Key Concepts

The speech-language pathology assistant (SLPA) and mentoring/supervising speech-language pathologist (SLP) have clearly delineated scopes of responsibilities consistent with guidelines set by the American Speech-Language-Hearing Association (ASHA).

■

Scopes of responsibilities for the SLP and SLPA also are referred to in the ASHA Code of Ethics (ASHA, 2001).

■

Variations in responsibilities may be associated with the specific type of delivery of service models—individual, group, or consultation—associated with each setting.

■

Specific competencies need to be developed so that the SLPA is appropriately prepared and understands the boundaries of the position.

Overview

■

SLPA Scope of Responsibilities

■

Activities Outside the Scope of Responsibilities of an SLPA

■

Competencies to Be Developed

■

Responsibilities of the SLP Supervisor/Mentor

■

Scenarios and Stories That Address Roles and Responsibilities

■

Differences in Practice: Models and Settings

INTRODUCTION

Now that you have decided to become a qualified SLPA and work with your supervisor, who is a licensed or certified SLP, you will be working with people who need assistance and help. You will learn about typical communication patterns and development, and about how these processes and abilities can be impaired. You will learn about disorders related to age, development, medical or health-related conditions, and developmental delays. You will work with a variety of individuals who demonstrate a wide range of communication abilities and differing severities of disability as it relates to communication. And of course you will be working with your supervisor and other team members, depending on the specific setting in which you are employed.

SIDELIGHT: *Who Is My Supervisor?*

Chris is a communication specialist with the local school district. She completed her undergraduate work in speech pathology and audiology at the local state university and went on for her master's degree in speech-language pathology, which took her an additional two years. While taking courses, she completed over 375 clock hours of direct work with a variety of individuals, including children and adults. She developed competencies in assessment and intervention practices, program planning, counseling, and report writing. She worked hard to become proficient in administration of over 30 different tests and protocols. Chris planned and implemented therapy programs for children with developmental disabilities and language and speech problems, and for individuals who stutter and those with hearing and voice problems. She also completed two full-time internships, one in the public school and another in a hospital setting, working with a wide range of children with language and learning disabilities and adults with aphasia or other conditions related to stroke and neurologic disease. She completed her comprehensive exams, graduated, and obtained a position in a public school setting for her clinical fellowship year. Then she obtained the certificate of clinical competence (CCC) from ASHA after passing the necessary national exam to demonstrate knowledge and proficiency to practice. Chris now works with students of all ages and their families. She has a caseload of approximately 50 students, although this varies depending on the number of evaluations she must do. Now that she has worked in the schools for 2 years and has taken some coursework about the supervisory process, she is ready to supervise an SLPA. Chris needs help to extend her services, especially to underrepresented populations that need more intensive services than she can provide on a weekly basis.

SLPA SCOPE OF RESPONSIBILITIES

What would you do if you were to obtain a position with Chris? As noted in Chapter 1, you may be asked to assist your supervising SLP in several ways. Provided that the training you receive is appropriate, the ASHA guidelines (2001) indicate that you may be asked to do the following:

- Assist Chris with speech-language and hearing screenings by following a specified screening protocol she had developed or by following one that is similar to those reviewed in Chapter 12 of this text. This calls for competency development in a number of areas such as accurate recording and appropriate presentation of stimuli. You may become well trained in standard screening procedures. However, Chris will determine what the results mean in relation to the functioning level, age, and abilities of the individual being screened. She will interpret the results.

- Follow documented treatment plans or protocols designed by Chris. This involves working directly with students in individual, group, or classroom sessions. In order to do this, you will need to understand the type of disorder of the individual you are working with and what goals and measurable objectives Chris has developed to demonstrate improvement in communication and function. You will need to understand and be able to implement a variety of approaches and activities with her help and guidance. You with be working with each person to practice new learning of skills. In most cases, your work will make a difference.

- Document the student's progress toward meeting established objectives as stated in the treatment plan, and report this information to Chris. This is critical for accountability. Chris needs this information not only to document progress, but also to help determine the next steps in the treatment plan. There are many ways to document progress, some of

which are described in Chapter 11 of this text. You will learn about these strategies, which may vary depending on your workplace setting and its policies or procedures.

■ Assist Chris during assessment of patients/clients or students. Again, you may be asked to help Chris in setting up equipment, gathering materials, collecting data strategies such as language samples or recording of conversational interactions, and in other informal ways. This will contribute significantly to the overall assessment process that is ongoing and necessary to successful programming of therapy for an individual.

■ Assist with responsibilities, such as preparing materials and scheduling activities, as directed by Chris. Your organizational and creative abilities, and maybe your computer skills, will come into play if you are asked to schedule or prepare data for presentations. Confidentiality is the cornerstone of your responsibility to the individuals you work with and applies when you are preparing charts and records and filing reports or other forms that include confidential information. Organization and preparation of materials are key to the successful implementation of therapeutic programs. You can play a key role in supporting Chris in daily documentation of progress; developing motivating, creative activities and materials for use in therapy; and assisting with those routine activities that keep things running smoothly.

■ Perform checks on the equipment that Chris uses in therapy and maintain it in good working order. This function is critical given the dependence on equipment for data collection or for use in therapy by the individual under treatment. You may need specific training and experience with certain types of equipment, such as dedicated communication devices, digital recorders, and visipitch programs, that may be particular to the setting or to the individuals you are working with.

■ Support Chris in research projects, in-service training, and public relations programs. This may prove

to be a very exciting part of your work because it may entail collecting data that supports a particular type of treatment and documents your successful implementation of a therapy plan. Working with Chris to organize and prepare in-service training for others or educational programs for families may prove rewarding and contribute to your own learning and skill development at the same time.

- Assist with departmental operations such as scheduling, record keeping, and safety and maintenance of supplies and equipment. This is an opportunity to learn the " ins and outs" of how the system works and to understand the need for organization and safety, which ensures your productivity as well as the quality of care for students. The specific "culture of your setting" may vary depending on the interaction of policies and procedures and how these are implemented for the individuals served. A hospital setting has a very different "culture" from a school-based setting. You will see differences in how scheduling is accomplished, the types of service delivery models used, how professionals interact with each other, and certainly the different types of equipment used given the variation in needs of the populations served in each setting.

- Collect data that document quality of care provided by Chris. Here is another opportunity to understand the methods of documenting satisfaction with services. You may also be asked to collect data that support the effectiveness of programs offered and implemented. Variations in how data are collected about quality of care will be evident across settings and often will depend on the types of disorders seen in the individuals served.

You will be expected to comply with regulations, reimbursement requirements, and guidelines for the SLPA's job responsibilities. Knowing the applicable rules and regulations that guide your behaviors and complying with the applicable set of guidelines specific to your job setting and state credentialing process are important aspects of your responsibilities as an SLPA. As noted, the ASHA Code of

Ethics (see Appendix C) speaks of the need for clarity in your responsibilities so that no misrepresentation of your role is possible. It is important to know that your supervising SLP is responsible for ensuring that she is practicing within the Code of Ethics (Revised 2001, pp. 1-185) as stated in the following rules:

- "Individuals (SLPs) shall not misrepresent the credentials of an assistant, technicians, or support personnel and shall inform those they serve professionally of the name and professional credentials of the persons providing services."

- "Individuals (SLPs) who hold the Certificates of Clinical Competence shall not delegate tasks that require unique skills, knowledge, and judgment that are within the scope of their profession to assistants, technicians, support personnel, or any nonprofessionals over whom they have supervisory responsibility. An individual (SLP) may delegate support services to assistants, technicians, support personnel, or any other persons only if an individual who holds the appropriate Certificate of Clinical Competence adequately supervises those services."

As you can see, the activities and tasks are varied and certainly not boring given the important work you will be doing. It can be a position that provides ongoing opportunities for new learning and may provide opportunities for experience in a multitude of areas. It is important to understand your responsibilities, because you will be held accountable for the successful completion of your assigned tasks and activities. It is also important to recognize that state law and regulation may expand on the responsibilities described above or may limit what you might be asked to do. You need to familiarize yourself with your state's regulations and practices so you know what to expect when you are offered a position as an SLPA. It is also important to understand not only what you might be asked to do in this position, but also what you cannot do, given your current level of training and experience. This makes sense because the ultimate responsibility for patient/client or student care and quality of services provided rests with the supervising SLP. As your supervisor, she is the one charged with the legal and ethical responsibility for services and treatment provided. You need to understand this relationship and how it will affect what you do and your own ethical responsibility to adhere to regulations and policies for practice.

SIDELIGHT: *A Day in the Life of an SLPA*

Marsha began her day at the rehabilitation center at 7:30 A.M. She was there on time to assist the SLP in preparing for the day's schedule of services. Her SLP was involved in an assessment all morning, and Marsha was there to observe and make sure the equipment that the team needed was in good working order. After the assessment, Marsha prepared the materials to use in the group she was working with after lunch. She particularly enjoyed working with this group of aphasic patients. It was an interesting group, and she had seen much progress in the patients' ability to communicate with each other over the past several weeks. She was improving her skills in documenting their progress. She had designed a chart so she could write comments and mark frequency of initiations beside each of their names. This way she would have some data to back up her impressions. Then Marsha was scheduled to work with Bill and then Gladys to practice with the computer programs their SLP has selected for them. After these sessions, her SLP wanted her to complete some paperwork and start scheduling the newer patients for a group program that was scheduled to begin next week. She ended her day by seeing one of her favorite patients, Mark. She implemented the practice activities that the SLP had suggested be added to the treatment plan. She was excited to see how Mark responded to the activities. After her last session, she was free to tidy up and prepare for another full day tomorrow.

ACTIVITIES OUTSIDE THE SCOPE OF RESPONSIBILITIES OF AN SLPA

ASHA Do's and Don'ts

Your work as an SLPA will involve many tasks. However, if the ASHA model (2001) is followed, your day with your SLP will look something like Marsha's day. Although you may be asked to assist your SLP in preparing for an assessment, you should not perform standardized or nonstandardized diagnostic tests, formal or informal evaluations, or interpret test

results. These responsibilities remain as tasks solely for the supervising SLP because they require extensive training and competency development beyond the training you will receive in your program at this level (ASHA, 2001).

It is important to remember that you cannot be asked to screen or diagnose patients/clients for feeding and swallowing disorders. Again, extensive knowledge of anatomy and physiology of both normal systems and their functions as well as the pathology of systems involved in swallowing and feeding is necessary. A great deal of specialized training and experience is needed to determine if a disorder exists. This is typically completed by an experienced SLP who has chosen to specialize in this area, in collaboration with an interdisciplinary team of professionals who have specific training and a great deal of knowledge and experience in this area.

You may not participate in parent conferences, case conferences, or on any interdisciplinary team without the presence of the SLP or other ASHA-certified SLP designated by the supervising SLP. This is for your protection as well as that of your SLP. When time is short and people want to move ahead, they sometimes may try and "bend the rules," thinking that your presence alone fulfills the necessary "letter of the law" at **individualized educational plan (IEP)** meetings, case staffing, or patient conferences. Remember, this is not acceptable and you should resist being placed in this position. If you participated in a parent or case conference without the appropriate supervision, it might be misconstrued as a misrepresentation of your position, which as noted is a violation of the ASHA Code of Ethics, and may endanger your standing with ASHA as a registered SLPA. It is critically important to keep clear what your role and responsibilities are in these situations to avoid misrepresentating your credentials and experience.

Counseling is an art as well as a science that requires knowledge of family systems, in-depth experience with a variety of disorders and situations, and a knowledge of potential options that the individual, the family, or both, may need to consider as they make decisions about care or about their child's educational program. Counseling is outside the scope of your responsibilities as an SLPA. This does not mean that your SLP does not value your role with a particu-

lar patient, client, or family. In fact, you may be requested to provide descriptions or explanations about what or how a patient/client or student is performing in therapy sessions. Your information can be an important contribution to the discussion and help the SLP to provide the patient/client, family, or both critical information, so that as consumers and family members, they can make an informed decision about a particular course of action or recommendation. Remember, all information is ultimately shared with the family by the supervising SLP, because she has the knowledge and expertise regarding the interpretation of the data you may have helped to collect or the analysis and implications of the behaviors you may have observed.

Remember, your responsibility is to carry out or implement the treatment plan designed by the SLP you are working with. Although you are not to develop the treatment plan or modify it in any way, you will need to collect data that help the SLP decide what to do in terms of "next steps" or changes in the program. It is important that you are not only supervised with the patients/clients/students you work with, but also that you "communicate" to your SLP what you know about these individuals and their participation in the treatment sessions. She can then accurately document what is happening and make modifications in the prescribed treatment program as necessary. This will help you learn more about new or alternative activities for intervention based on changes made by the SLP.

Access to supervision is critical. You need to be appropriately supervised when providing treatment. Again, this is a protection for all concerned that recognizes the need for supervision and monitoring of the patient or client's progress. Adherence to the boundaries of the SLPA and SLP in relation to their roles and responsibilities is required. This also includes the signing of any formal documents. Again, patient, client, or student care remains the responsibility of the supervising SLP, who signs all documents related to care. You may be asked to sign a document that verifies your attendance at a meeting, but this should also be co-signed by the supervising SLP attending the IEP or conference. Discuss the specific setting's policies and procedures in depth with your supervisor before any meetings in which you are asked

to participate. Be sure to ask your supervisor if there is any question about which types of documents you are allowed to sign so that you are not put in a position that could misrepresent your role and responsibilities.

Your SLP will select patients/clients for services. This function is related to assessment and evaluation decisions and recommendations and thus is not a responsibility of the SLPA. Many clients, patients, or students are recommended for service based on a complete assessment and evaluation of their communication abilities and functioning level. Specific criteria are used to determine eligibility and may vary across settings and policies of the agency or school district. These decisions are governed in public schools by criteria put forth in applicable legislative mandates such as the Individuals with Disabilities Act (IDEA). It is important that you become familiar with applicable mandates and policies, because this will aid your understanding of specific issues related to continuity and eligibility of care. However, decisions regarding who is on a caseload or who will receive services, how often, and for how long are influenced by a number of factors and remain in the scope of practice of your supervising SLP.

Any decision regarding **discharge** or changes in schedule is part of the SLP's responsibility. It is also her responsibility to interpret data collected through ongoing assessment and to determine if progress is sufficient to terminate services. The team sometimes makes decisions regarding termination of services. Participation in this type of decision making remains in the scope of practice of the supervising SLP.

You may not disclose clinical or confidential information either orally or in writing to anyone other than the supervising SLP. As noted in the introduction to this text, confidentiality is a critical cornerstone of practice for all professionals, including the SLPA. It is so important to safeguard the rights of patients/clients and students, and you play an important role in this regard. How would you feel if you were sitting in a local restaurant and heard people at the next table talking about your child or brother or father? It is critical that all aspects of professional conduct be followed, including avoidance of informal discussions about patients, clients, or students and their families in hallways, elevators, or other public places. You must also avoid discussions with

other personnel you may be working with. These discussions are held only with your supervising SLP.

Referrals for additional services are also made by your SLP. This function is associated with the evaluation and ongoing assessment decisions that remain in the purview of the supervising SLP. If parents or others ask your opinion about availability or recommendations for additional services, you need to refer these types of requests and discussions to your supervising SLP.

The ASHA Code of Ethics (2001) specifically states that you may not represent yourself as an SLP. You provide a valuable service and support for your SLP in the extension of services, but it is critically important for you to understand the boundaries of your role so that you do not end up in compromising situations that cause misunderstandings or require you to perform tasks beyond your level of expertise and training. This endangers quality of care and services provided to those you work with. Be clear and adhere to these boundaries. Request clarification if you are concerned about taking on a task or performing an activity that is outside your role and associated responsibilities.

Two other responsibilities mentioned by ASHA (2001) pertain to involvement in swallowing evaluation or treatment. Again, this is an area of practice demanding specialized skill and experience given the significant impact swallowing disorders can have on function and health of the individual. Thus this area of practice is reserved for those SLPs with the requisite training knowledge and skills.

For further description or reference to the current ASHA criteria, please see the ASHA Web site at http://www.professional.asha.org. It is important to note that this document also describes workplace behaviors of the SLPA and mentions the ability to build relationships as one of several key competency areas. Key competencies described also include the ability to:

- Relate to clients/patients in a supportive manner
- Follow supervisors' instructions
- Maintain confidentiality and other appropriate behaviors
- Communicate in oral and written form

■ Follow health and safety precautions

The ASHA criteria for voluntary national registration also stipulate that to qualify for registration, the applicant must have an associate's degree with a program course of study designed to prepare the individual to be an SLPA. All program graduates must be referred for registration by the program director of the associate degree technical training program attended by the SLPA. Remember that national registration through ASHA is a voluntary program and may not be required, depending upon the specific regulations of the state in which you are seeking employment. If you decide to apply for registration, you must have earned 60 semester hours of general studies and specific knowledge and skills for SLPAs at an accredited program through ASHA. Clinical observations and a minimum of 100 clock hours of supervised (at least 50% of time) field experience are also required, with a written verification of completion and evaluation of technical proficiency. This is ASHA's current model for training and credentialing of SLPAs.

Variations by State Regulation

It is very important to note that these guidelines may not be consistent with what is required by your state regulatory agency or licensure law. As noted, many states require a baccalaureate degree and additional training specific to the role and responsibilities of the SLPA. Other states may have limitations on roles and responsibilities and only require a high school diploma with "on-the-job" training. It is critical to understand these variations in requirements and the credentialing process. How you enter the personnel development "lattice" in your state may be very different from the model explained above. There are many ways to enter the system and many ways to continue your education and training to better meet the needs of individuals with communication challenges. However, there are several basic competencies that you will need to develop to be a valued and contributing addition to any employment setting that helps people with communication challenges.

COMPETENCIES TO BE DEVELOPED

There are several areas of competency that the SLPA needs to develop and demonstrate to fulfill the roles and responsibilities associated with the position. These areas are suggested in the 1996 Guidelines for the Training, Credentialing, Use, and Supervision of the SLPA (ASHA, 1996) as areas for assessment as part of a functional proficiency evaluation. This has been adapted for use in some programs as an evaluation of performance in field-based placements associated with training of SLPAs.

Competency Development: Personal Skills and Behaviors

Competencies involve a specific set of behaviors that can be demonstrated. Competencies and indicators that guide assessment of your performance include:

- Interpersonal skills as reflected in the demonstrated ability to:
  - Deal effectively with attitudes and behaviors of the client/patient/student
  - Use appropriate language (written and oral) in dealing with patients/clients
  - Deal effectively with supervisor
- Personal qualities such as:
  - Manages time effectively
  - Demonstrates appropriate conduct

What Do Personal Skills and Behaviors Look Like in Practice?

Your supervising SLP is interested in how you use appropriate forms of addressing clients, patients, family members, and others. For example, you would always address an adult patient using their appropriate title and last name (e.g., Mrs. Gonzalez, Dr. Anderson) unless specifically directed to do otherwise by the client or supervisor. Courtesy and respectful communication are expected in all situations, including phone calls, face-to-face interaction, and E-mail. Use of language appropriate to a person's developmental level, age, education level, communication style, communication ability, and appropriate responses to client, family, and others' emotional states or behaviors are critical competencies needed by the SLPA. Using professional terminology correctly and maintaining legible records, log notes, and written communication in a manner prescribed by your supervising SLP are expected. Your ability to organize and use time effectively, including punctuality, preparation, and timely documentation are competencies very much appreciated by your SLP supervisor. Again, your ability to maintain confidentiality and to recognize and respect boundaries within job responsibilities are critical to your success as an SLPA. Appropriate conduct also includes maintaining your personal appearance appropriate to your work setting. Specific dress codes may be part of the policy and practice at a particular setting, and variations will be noted depending on your function and tasks. As a female, it may be desired for you to wear pants when working on the floor with children, whereas more professional dress may be required for meetings with family members or in hospital practices. Always check with your SLP supervisor for the norms established for your place of employment.

SIDELIGHT: *Establishing Relationships*

Sheila was asked by her supervisor to work with a patient who had had a stroke. This gentleman had been an active and productive member of the medical profession before his stroke. It was important to this man and his family that he continue to be addressed as Dr. Peacock in all interactions, even though he had to give up his practice as a result of his communication challenges. It was critical for the SLPA to honor this request in order to establish a positive relationship with this patient.

Competency Development: Technical Skills

Another set of competencies involves technical-assistant skills. You will be assessed in this area based on your abilities, including:

- Maintains a facilitating and environment for assigned tasks
- Uses time effectively
- Selects, prepares, and presents materials effectively
- Maintains documentation
- Provides assistance to the SLP

SIDELIGHT: *Tim's Story*

Tim, an SLPA, was setting up for a practice session on the computer with an elderly patient. He thought that there was no need to change the chairs or rearrange the furniture to prepare for Mr. Garcia's session, which followed a play-based interaction session with a young child and her mother in the same room. Unfortunately, Mr. Garcia became quite agitated and confused and had difficulty concentrating on his work with the computer. He seemed very distracted by the number of toys for young children that were still out on the tables surrounding his work area. He kept indicating that he wanted to leave because he thought he was in the wrong room, and the session did not go well. As noted in Figure 2-1, planning is critical to the success of a session. What could Tim have done to better prepare for this session?

What Do Technical Skills Look Like in Practice?

Developing competencies in the above areas of technical assistance is part of your role as an SLPA. Knowing how to set up a room or environment for therapy sessions and interactions and organizing space may make a significant difference in how the session goes. Bringing an adult into a session that has been set up with toys for a child does not set a tone, or age appropriate environment, for an older individual. This may prove important to the success of the session. Another example may be misuse of materials that have been developed for young children with older children who have very different interests, even though they may be currently functioning at a lower level in terms of communication. Performing necessary tasks and activities without unnecessary distractions and in a timely manner will also make an impact on the quality of your work. Selecting and preparing materials that are appropriate, based on the treatment plan,

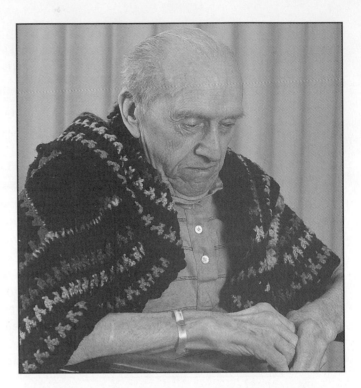

Figure 2-1 Developing SLPA competencies is important for building successful relationships. When a therapy session is not properly planned for, the patient can become frustrated, confused, or withdrawn.

age, culture, and interests of the client, is another competency and skill to be developed.

Knowing how to document implementation of treatment plans and protocols accurately and concisely as well as reporting patient, client, or student performance to your supervisor is another critical competency that affects the quality of services provided. The specifics of different ways to collect data appropriate to the individuals you are working with are explained in Chapter 11. However, your supervising SLP will also provide you with the formats she uses to collect accurate and timely documentation of what is happening in a session. You may be expected to prepare and

maintain working files and records in a manner prescribed by the supervising SLP and sign those documents once they are reviewed and co-signed by your supervisor. Accurate calculation of chronological age of the individual being served from the clinical records is very important, and if recorded in error, can make a huge difference in the interpretation done by your supervising SLP. Your supervising SLP relies on the accuracy of information when planning, implementing, and analyzing standardized tests. Accurate calculation of percentages, frequencies, and averages is also important to your supervising SLP in interpreting behaviors and performance during sessions and in determining progress and next steps. As you can see, accuracy in record keeping is an important competency to develop and can significantly make an impact on the quality of care you and your supervising SLP provide in any setting.

Competency Development: Screening

You may also be assessed in the area of screening. Screening may become a competency that you need to develop, depending on the type of position you obtain. Your competency in screening would be assessed based on your knowledge and use of a variety of screening tools and protocols; your ability to appropriately administer and score screening protocols; your management of screening and documentation; and your ability to accurately communicate results and all supplemental information to your supervisor.

What Does Screening Competency Look Like in Practice?

Training on screening procedures is covered in Chapter 12. As noted earlier, with regard to any type of documentation of behaviors, accuracy is critical so that reliable information is obtained. You will most likely be trained to use specific protocols used by your supervising SLP. These may include both formal and informal procedures for collecting information about the student, client, or patient. You should be checked on the reliability of your observations and recording of accurate information, both in your training program and in your setting, before you are asked to complete these activities. Being checked on accuracy and reliability means your scoring of specific types of behaviors should match that of your supervisor. You may also be asked to set up schedules so that screening activities proceed smoothly, and you may need to report any difficulty encountered in screening to your supervising SLP. An important aspect of this function is to again be prepared for any eventuality and organize screening materials ahead of time to ensure an effective process. As you develop a smooth working relationship with your supervising SLP, you will feel comfortable seeking guidance should any adaptation of the schedule or procedures be needed. You will also be asked to develop your ability to provide descriptive observations that contribute to screening results. As you become familiar with the population served, you will gain confidence in your ability to contribute to the success of screening procedures.

Experience and clear direction from your supervising SLP will enhance your competency development in this area. Accurate observation of targeted communicative behaviors is critical to the screening process. Chapter 10 covers observation. It will help you to distinguish what you are looking for and what is important about describing sig-

SIDELIGHT: *Taking the Initiative*

Michele was asked by her supervising SLP to gather the protocols necessary to screen a number of kindergarten-age children for speech and language development. She reviewed the protocols and what might be expected of her in terms of assisting her supervisor in scheduling the children to be seen. She actually enjoyed the process of trying to figure out how to schedule the children with the least interruption in their daily routine. She found out that the teacher thought free time was the best time to schedule the children. This way they would not miss the activity the teacher had prepared for the week. She knew that if she scheduled during recess, the children would resist. The teacher and her supervising SLP commented that her level of preparation and organization was certainly appreciated given the task to be accomplished. She then was able to organize all of the resulting information and learned a great deal from her SLP regarding the distinguishing behaviors that indicated some of the children would benefit from additional assessment to determine if they needed services.

nificant behaviors that the SLP deems important to her interpretation of results. Knowing what to look for will help you assist the SLP in providing a timely and cost-effective service that is productive in determining which, if any, individuals screened need further assessment of their speech, language, or hearing abilities. Remember that current ASHA criteria are clear on what types of screening you may participate in, and your supervising SLP will provide the appropriate information regarding screening procedures specific to your setting.

Competency Development: Intervention

Another competency area is providing direct treatment by following the plan designed by your SLP. You will be assessed on your intervention skills according to the following criteria:

- Performs tasks as outlined and instructed by the supervisor
- Demonstrates skill in managing behavior and treatment programs
- Demonstrates knowledge of treatment objectives and plan

What Does Intervention Competency Look Like in Practice?

As an SLPA you will learn about **Individual Educational Plans (IEPs)** in school settings that delineate the specific goals and objectives for a particular student receiving services from the SLP. In a rehabilitation program for adults, you may read or follow **SOAP notes**, which document the particular goals and objectives for the treatment of an individual seen in that setting. SOAP stands for subjective, objective, assessment, and plan. SOAP notes offer a format for recording subjective impressions of progress of the patient, followed by objective data collected during the session. The next part involves summarizing an assessment of current status followed by the planned activities for the next session. Regardless of the specific type of treatment plan used by your SLP, you will have clear direction and explicit instructions regarding what to do and how to do it with the patients, students, or clients seen in your setting. It is very important that you perform the tasks as outlined and instructed by your supervisor. Accurate and efficient implementation of the procedures planned by your supervisor guarantees that intervention is delivered in a way that will help the individual succeed. It will be up to you to use the constructive feedback from your supervisor for modifying the interactions with the patients, students or clients you see for intervention.

SIDELIGHT: *Beth—Working With Older Adults*

Beth loves working as an SLPA with the older adults in her setting. She receives explicit instructions from her SLP supervisor about how to implement the treatment plans for each of the patients she sees individually. She has worked with her SLP in designing creative activities that are of interest to these individuals and works with them in improving the intelligibility of their speech, as well as their use of language. Many of the patients also exhibit word retrieval or word-finding problems during conversation. She has learned multiple strategies to cue or prompt them to say the word they want to use. She really likes the opportunity to work in groups with these people and finds this to be a very rewarding part of her job. They may have partially lost their ability to speak or communicate but they certainly have not lost their sense of humor. She loves the banter and support they provide each other as they work hard to recover their language and speech abilities.

Competencies like managing **on-task** behavior, providing appropriate feedback and reinforcement specific to the individual's responses or performance, and consistently using the strategies outlined by your supervisor are very important for successful outcomes. Your ability to provide clear, concise directions or instructions to the individuals you work with that are appropriate to their age and ability level will make a significant difference in their ability to understand and get the most out of their session.

As you guide social interactions in small groups of children or adults you work with, you will have many opportunities to apply basic behavior modification and learning principles that you will read about in Chapter 13. It is important that you learn to apply these principles so that you can implement the intervention plan designed for each individual client, patient, or student, regardless of setting or specific population. It is also important to implement the designated intervention plan by working on the specified objectives or goals in the appropriate sequence as outlined by your supervising SLP. Many skills build one on the other so that the sequence of activities and tasks may be important to successful outcomes. For example, you may have a plan that directs you to first introduce new vocabulary to a child with specific language impairment by doing an experiential activity that involves use of the targeted vocabulary. You might then be asked to check for comprehension or understanding of the meaning of the words before you ask the student to use the words in describing the task that she did. There are many other examples of how the sequence of the activities or tasks may make a difference in how the individual responds. Thus, it is important to follow the plan as directed by your SLP so that objectives and goals are addressed as intended.

SIDELIGHT: *Jayne—Working With School-Age Children*

Sara, Charlie, and Jose were second-grade children seen for small group work outside of their classroom to improve their phonemic awareness skills in relation to their reading abilities. Jayne, an SLPA, was asked to implement a game to have them practice segmenting sounds in words and identify what sounds they heard in the beginning, middle, and end of the words and then match them to letter names. But Charlie was a classic "cut-up" and was easily distracted by Jose's antics. She felt the practice was not happening as planned, so she asked her SLP for ideas on how to set up the session so that the children would spend the time practicing as needed. The SLP came into the session and demonstrated how to anticipate Charlie's behaviors and set the stage for the activity by letting the children know the "rules of the game" in a nonpunitive way. Her SLP said it might help to begin with a listening activity such as reading a fun, rhyming book or using a song with rhyming words to get the children involved in the activity. She suggested ways to reinforce their practice and learning that were age-appropriate and fun. Jayne tried this and found it worked. The children were engaged in the session and had fun practicing what they needed to do to improve their language- and literacy-related behaviors.

You will learn a great deal about specific language and speech disorders and challenges in communication experienced by those you work with. You will be expected to develop competency in understanding these disorders and the specific needs of those who exhibit a particular type of disorder. This may seem overwhelming at times because you will learn a whole new vocabulary and need to understand and use terminology that at first may sound like a foreign language. However, it is critical for you to become familiar with certain conditions and disorders and to understand the behavioral as well as communication characteristics that are associated with each in order to fulfill your role as an SLPA. As you learn more about all aspects of speech, language, and communication, you will be better able to describe behaviors demonstrating knowledge of the individual's disorder and needs. You will be able to identify correct versus incorrect responses, and describe behaviors that demonstrate knowledge of the individuals' overall level of progress, which you will then be able to verbally report on and appropriately document for your supervising SLP.

Competency development in all of the skills described above will come with your reading of the materials in subsequent chapters of this text as well as in your field-based placement in a school or hospital. In this placement, you will gain experience as an SLPA. Use this opportunity to practice the skills described above so that you are prepared for your first position. As you proceed through your program, take the time to self-reflect on where you are regarding your competency development across the skill areas. Use your instructors and your field placement supervisor for guidance, and respond to their feedback regarding your demonstrated knowledge and skills. Continue to address those areas for growth that are identified in the feedback process by observing others in their work with individuals with communication disorders. Seek out experiences that help you to develop and enhance your knowledge and skill base in working with varied populations.

RESPONSIBILITIES OF THE SLP SUPERVISOR/MENTOR

Although you are currently learning about your responsibilities as an SLPA, you will not be on your own in actualizing your role. The Knowledge and Skills for Supervisors of Speech-Language Pathology Assistants (ASHA, 2001) is an official statement of the ASHA that outlines what you might expect from your SLP supervisor/mentor as you continue to develop as an SLPA. There are several areas listed regarding what you might expect of your supervisor, including:

1. Selecting and assigning appropriate patients/clients or students for you to work with who are consistent with your abilities and within the scope of responsibilities of your position

2. Determining the nature of the supervision that is appropriate for you, which includes determination of the amount of supervision required based on the needs of the individual receiving services, the service delivery setting, the task assigned, and your level of experience

3. Establishing and maintaining an effective relationship with you that involves understanding how to effectively communicate with you and supervise your work. This means understanding your learning style and facilitating a positive, supportive relationship that enhances your growth and development in this position

4. Directing you in following screening protocols specific to your setting, teaching you to administer and appropriately score the assigned screening tools, and instructing you on management and reporting of results without interpretation

5. Demonstrating and participating with you in the clinical process, including demonstration of preferred practices, effective ways of building relationships with individuals you work with, clinical strategies and techniques, and supporting your development of competencies needed in your role as an SLPA

6. Directing you in following the individualized plans that she has developed for each of the individuals you work with, including how to address specific goals and objectives, and how to properly document progress

7. Directing you in the maintenance of clinical records that adhere to guidelines for confidentiality and are specific to the setting and delivery of the service model used in intervention

8. Interacting with you and scheduling meetings with you on a consistent basis, which provides you with feedback and discusses your progress in developing as an SLPA

9. Providing feedback regarding your skills, which enhances your ability to self-evaluate your skills and document your own job performance

10. Working with you in developing your verbal reporting skills and any assigned written informal reporting that you may need to do as an SLPA

11. Helping you to effectively organize the environment, and select, prepare, and present materials that are appropriate to the age, interest, and ability level of individuals you work with in your setting

12. Sharing pertinent information with you regarding current ethical, legal, regulatory, and reimbursement aspects of professional practice specific to your employment as an SLPA

13. Modeling professional conduct, which includes maintaining ultimate responsibility for all care provided by you

14. Assuming responsibility for directing you in the implementation of any research procedures, in-service training, and public relations work you may do as part of your job as an SLPA

15. Training you with regard to use and maintenance of equipment and adherence to universal precautions as needed in your position as an SLPA

16. Teaching you the use of appropriate language (oral and written) when interacting with individuals you work with and others in your job setting

17. Documenting the supervision provided to you as an SLPA

You need to understand these aspects of your supervisor's/mentor's role, because they are critical for supporting the successful fulfillment of your SLPA responsibilities. They may vary specific to your employment setting or the state regulations under which you are hired but are closely aligned with the competencies previously described as those of an SLPA. Remember, you are responsible to your supervising SLP in all that you do. Your SLP has many years of education and is there to help you realize your goals. The relationship is intended to be one of reciprocal support in that you extend the services of the SLP and she supports and supervises your ability to do so. Specific guidelines for working with your SLP supervisor/mentor are addressed in Chapter 3 of this text. The relationship you establish will prove critical to your success as an SLPA. Your supervisor/mentor will be a rich resource for new and continued learning and will work with you in ensuring that your work is a source of satisfaction for you as you develop the competencies necessary to enhance the quality of care provided to the population you serve.

SCENARIOS AND STORIES THAT ADDRESS ROLES AND RESPONSIBILITIES

SCENARIO 1

A supervising SLP has taken ill and has asked her assigned SLPA to cover for her during an important discharge conference about one of the patients at a rehabilitation center program. She feels that her SLPA, Ted, is perfectly capable of sharing what has been going on in sessions and the progress that has been made with this patient because Ted has been involved in his care, has attended previous discharge conferences, and knows the team of professionals quite well. She also knows that the team is confident in Ted's abilities to share accurate information, and there will be another SLP from her department attending the conference.

Questions:
How would you handle this situation if you were Ted?
Do you think it is appropriate for him to attend the conference?
Should he sign the discharge note in the case record as the attending SLP?

SCENARIO 2

Joan, an SLPA at Braddock Elementary School, is carrying out a speech program developed by her supervisor/mentor with four children on a weekly basis. Each child in the group is working on velar sounds /k/ and /g/. The sessions are going well, but the data Joan has collected indicate that one of the children, Brian, is not making much progress. He is also getting frustrated because the other students notice his frequent mistakes. Joan is using phonetic placement cues and techniques as directed by her supervisor to improve target production, but this does not seem to be helping Brian. In her SLPA training program, Joan learned about the Hodson Approach and believes this approach might be better for Brian.

Questions:
Should Joan go ahead and try a different approach with Brian?
Should she try it with all the children in the group?
Discuss your response in light of the prescribed roles and responsibilities of the SLPA as outlined in this chapter.

SCENARIO 3

Kathy is working as an SLPA in a hospital under the supervision of an SLP who provides inpatient care to a number of patients who are recovering from strokes. Many of these patients have swallowing and feeding problems. One patient is being seen by the rehabilitation team, which includes a physical therapist (PT), occupational therapist (OT), and neuropsychologist as well as the supervising SLP. Kathy has been instructed to spend time with this patient practicing his speech output because he is severely dysarthric secondary to his stroke. The OT has requested that she also monitor and document his ability to drink fluids independently while she is with him during their practice sessions. Kathy is not sure what to do.

Questions:
How should Kathy handle this request?
Is this within Kathy's scope of responsibilities as an SLPA?
Discuss your response with your instructor.

SCENARIO 4

Clara, an SLPA in an early intervention program, is working with a bilingual Spanish-speaking child who was diagnosed with autism. Clara is a proficient bilingual Spanish speaker, having moved to California from Mexico as a young child. She is carrying out the treatment plan created by her supervisor by working on the child's initiation skills and expressive vocabulary development. When Clara works with this child, she often sees his mother who is also very involved in his program at the early intervention center. His mother frequently asks Clara about his progress and enjoys speaking with her in Spanish before and after preschool session. Clara has checked with her supervisor, who says it is okay for her to share information about what she does with Jose during the time she is working with him in his preschool classroom. Last week, Jose's mother asked Clara to be sure to work with Jose in his ability to put words together in both English and Spanish because she hopes to improve his ability to use both languages. Clara can relate to this mother's desire to preserve Jose's first language and culture even though he is enrolled in a predominantly English-speaking program. She is not sure how to respond.

Questions:
If you were Clara, how would you respond?
Is she working within her scope of responsibilities as an SLPA?

These are just a few examples of situations you may encounter as an SLPA. Take this opportunity to discuss issues regarding your scope of responsibility based on these examples. Use the information contained in this chapter about the scope of responsibilities of the SLPA and the supervising SLP as a guideline for your thinking. Refer back to the specifically outlined scope of responsibilities of each role as you encounter issues in your career. Chapter 7 also reviews issues in professionalism and potential "ethical dilemmas" in depth. Review this information carefully and refer back to it as you develop the necessary competencies for your role as an SLPA. You may be asked to complete activities or tasks that are outside your role and expertise. You need to be aware of potential conflicts that can occur in your position and the resources you have to resolve them. Reference to state regulations and licensure guidelines will also be helpful to you as you proceed with your training and competency development. Your supervising SLP should also be aware of the scope of responsibilities as outlined and will be a sounding board for your questions and concerns.

DIFFERENCES IN PRACTICE: MODELS AND SETTINGS

Models or types of service delivery vary, depending on the setting in which you choose to work as an SLPA. A school-based setting will look very different in practice patterns from that of a hospital, rehabilitation center, or agency. This will be influenced by the types of communication problems demonstrated by the individual patients, clients, or students as well as their ages and abilities. It will also be influenced by the basic model (medical versus educational) that characterizes the setting. For example, the hospital inpatient program interfaces with the medical team (physicians, neurologists, PT, OT service and other medically oriented professionals), to provide rehabilitative services, often using individual or sometimes group sessions within this context. As patients are discharged and become **outpatients**, services may continue as these individuals adjust to leaving the hospital or rehabilitation center routines and return home to families and communities. This may be in direct contrast to a school-based program in which you may be asked to provide practice sessions in the classroom or in small groups with children having very different types of challenges. You will be interacting with an educational team, including regular classroom teachers, principals, resource room teachers, and other special educators, as well as your supervising SLP to further the students learning and educational performance. In either setting, you will need to understand the "culture" and how it is influenced by applicable laws, policies, and practices. Chapter 13 provides additional information regarding models and settings.

CONCLUSION

This chapter has introduced you to the scope of responsibilities consistent with your future position as an SLPA. These are described with reference to the ASHA model that clearly delineates the specific tasks and activities that can be delegated to you in your role as an assistant to your supervising SLP. Remember, the basic educational requirements and practice responsibilities are also governed by the state in

which you choose to practice so they may vary considerably from this model. Take the time to consider these differences and how they might affect your future growth and development as an SLPA. The ASHA model also provides a vehicle for voluntary national registration as an SLPA if this is consistent with your state regulations and licensure laws.

There are many aspects of the scope of responsibilities associated with the SLPA position to consider. The ASHA do's and don'ts and the ASHA Code of Ethics (2001) set clear parameters for your practice if your state regulations are consistent with these policies. Roles and expectations of your supervising SLP in terms of knowledge and skills also provide support for your implementing your role within the prescribed boundaries of the SLPA position. However, there are always potential "gray" areas or situations and questions to consider when implementing your scope of responsibilities, as shown in the examples given and the discussion of variations across settings. This means that it is even more important to develop a "relationship that works" with your supervising SLP in whatever setting you choose to seek employment. The relationship with your SLP will ultimately "make or break" your satisfaction with your work as an SLPA regardless of setting, service delivery model, and specific policies and regulations that you will follow.

DISCUSSION QUESTIONS

1. Are your current program training requirements and state regulations for practice as an SLPA consistent with the ASHA model? How are they similar or different?

2. Describe the scope of responsibilities for the SLPA. How does the ASHA Code of Ethics apply? Will the guidelines and regulations ensure quality of care to the individuals you serve in your role as an SLPA?

3. There are many competencies to develop in your training and work as an SLPA. Reflect on these competencies and how your relationship with your supervising SLP can ensure that you develop the knowledge and skills you will need in this position. How will you continue your growth and development in this role?

4. Based on the information provided in this chapter, do you have a "feel" for the specific setting or population of individuals you want to work with as an SLPA? What do you think will bring you the most satisfaction as you enter this position and what supports will be critical to your success?

SUGGESTED ACTIVITIES

1. Discuss the specific scenarios provided in this chapter regarding the role of the SLPA in various settings. How would you respond to the specific questions following each scenario? What questions or concerns do you have about how to respond to each situation described? Take the time to discuss these situations with your peers and instructor. Use the information contained in this chapter regarding scope of responsibilities to further your thinking about these issues and questions.

2. You can find more information about the scope of responsibilities for the SLPA by observing across several potential work settings. Talk with SLPs, SLPAs, or both, about their specific practice. Be sure to investigate any nuances or variations in the settings based on applicable state licensure laws or regulations. Talk with them about how they see the role of the SLPA in their setting and how the specific "culture" and policies of the setting affect what the SLPA does or does not do.

3. Visit the ASHA Web site at http://www.professional.asha.org and search for all applicable documents that deal with the role and responsibilities of the SLPA and the supervising SLP. Are there recent changes that might make an impact on your training and scope of responsibilities as an SLPA?

4. Use the ASHA Web site to explore documents and descriptions of settings and populations served by the SLP. What new information is available that supple-

ments your knowledge about working with individuals with communication challenges? Do you have questions about how these recent developments might affect your role and responsibilities as an SLPA? For example, does the introduction of "telehealth" practice affect what you might be asked to do as an SLPA? What does the ASHA Code of Ethics say about this issue? How does this affect your need for continuing education as an SLPA practicing under the supervision of an appropriately credentialed SLP?

5. Learn more about individuals with communication challenges by participating in volunteer work in your community or service learning projects associated with your training program. These experiences can further your competency development as an SLPA.

REFERENCES

American Speech-Language-Hearing Association. (1996). Guidelines for the training, credentialing, use, and supervision of speech-language pathology assistants. *ASHA, 38,* 16, 21–34.

American Speech-Language-Hearing Association. (2000). *Background information and criteria for the registration of speech-language pathology assistants.* Retrieved March 2, 2002, from http://www.professional.asha.org/certification/

American Speech-Language-Hearing Association. (2001) *Code of Ethics.* Retrieved March 12, 2002, from http://www.professional.asha.org/resources/DeskRefVol1TOC.cfm

American Speech-Language-Hearing Association. (in press). Knowledge and skills for supervisors of speech-language pathology assistants. *ASHA Supplement.*

CHAPTER 3

Working With Your Speech-Language Pathologist Supervisor/Mentor

Key Concepts

■

Initiating and maintaining a respectful, collaborative relationship with your supervisor/mentor builds a foundation for success as an SLPA.

■

Mentorship and supervision are dual functions of your SLP supervisor/mentor.

■

Expectations need to be clarified to avoid conflicts and misunderstandings that can have a negative impact on your work as an SLPA.

■

Development of key interpersonal skills can facilitate your relationship with your supervisor/mentor.

■

Consistent use of strategies of self-reflection and self-assessment will ensure your continued growth and development as an SLPA and enhance your on-the-job productivity and success.

Overview

■

A Mentorship Model

■

Supervision and the Supervisory Process

■

Expectations and Expectation Discrepancies

■

Critical Interpersonal Skills for Maintaining Successful Relationships

■

Strategies for External Feedback

■

Reflective Practice: Strategies for Self-Assessment and Continued Growth

51

INTRODUCTION

The relationship you develop with your speech-language pathology (SLP) supervisor/mentor will be an important source of support and will contribute to your success as an SLPA. Your role as an assistant demands a close working relationship with your supervisor/mentor based on mutual respect and collaboration in order to ensure smooth delivery of quality service to individuals with communication challenges. The relationship has the potential to evolve from one that is strictly supervision to one that takes on the key characteristics of a true mentorship relationship.

Let us examine what we mean by mentorship and supervision. Application of these concepts to the relationship you will develop with your field-placement supervisors and your supervising SLPs will affect your future work as an SLPA.

SIDELIGHT: *Christine's Story*

As Christine searched for a position as an SLPA in her local neighborhood, she thought about what she wanted from a job. One critical piece for her was to be assigned to an SLP who was not only competent but also caring. Her experience with her first SLP supervisor after finishing her training was not a positive one. The supervisor was not really interested in having an SLPA but was directed to by her employer because of the severity of disorders of the children seen in that setting. Christine had tried to establish a communication system that worked for both of them but found herself either having a great deal of time on her hands because the supervisor had not thought through assigned tasks ahead of schedule, or being under a great deal of pressure to copy or prepare materials at the last minute. This was not a satisfactory relationship, and she was looking for something else in her next position. Christine's knowledge and training in collecting data and her effective interpersonal skills in working with children, especially those who use augmentative alternative communication (AAC) equipment, had been ignored. She rarely got to work with the children and considered the job to be one of a glorified and underused secretary. She wanted a different relationship with her new supervisor, one in which she felt respected for her abilities. She was willing to do the paperwork and materials preparation involved and actually enjoyed this part of the job. But she also wanted the opportunity to be a productive member of the team and work with children under the direction of her SLP. She hoped that her interests and skills in technology would be valued and used because she particularly enjoys working with nonverbal children who use AAC devices.

A MENTORSHIP MODEL

Mentorship is a term that implies more than supervisory management of an SLPA's assigned tasks and responsibilities. It is more than the process of directing or guiding you to accomplish the goals of the organization for which you work It is often described as a "caring and supportive relationship between an experienced, more knowledgeable practitioners (mentor) and less experienced, less knowledgeable (mentee) in which the mentee receives career-related and personal benefits" (Henry, Stockdale, Hall, & Deniston, 1994). The essence of the mentor relationship involves the more experienced individual taking a direct and sometimes personal interest in a less experienced individual; in this case that individual serves as an assistant. A successful mentor relationship calls for commitment on the part of the supervisor/mentor to support you as an SLPA by ensuring you successfully establish work habits that are effective for you; for the supervisor/mentor; for the individuals you serve; and for the agency, hospital, or public school district or organization in which you are employed.

Mentorship relationships are not entirely one-sided, with only the mentor providing time, advice, expertise, and support to the mentee. More recent descriptions of the relationship point out benefits for both the mentee and the mentor as depicted in Table 3-1. For example, the relationship may offer the mentor fresh ideas, an extra pair of hands, and a sense of satisfaction that comes from watching someone else develop skills. The relationship may offer the SLPA the opportunity for support, protection, and guidance (Henry et al., 1994). This may influence improved performance and productivity, development of new skills, increased likelihood of success on the job, increased social and emotional support, and increased awareness of the organization (Murray, 1991). Other authors, including Emily Fenichel (1992) in the Zero to Three *Learning Through Supervision and Mentorship: A Source Book,* add that a strong, positive mentorship relationship may also increase knowledge base, improve competency development in the assigned role, and enhance communication skills.

Table 3-1. A Comparison of Roles and Benefits for the SLPA and SLP

The supervisee/SLPA can benefit from opportunities to:

■ Broaden knowledge base about the profession

■ Self-reflect with a trusted person in a nonthreatening or "safe" environment

■ Determine and discuss personal goals and objectives for growth

■ Receive objective feedback about progress toward achieving personal goals

■ Learn how to self-reflect to increase understanding of self

■ Learn from a more experienced practitioner who provides clear direction, demonstrates techniques, and answers questions

■ Tap into a rich resource for ideas and strategies that work

The supervisor/mentor SLP can model and benefit from:

■ A mutually respectful, collaborative approach to monitoring performance while maintaining quality of care

■ Supporting a learning process parallel to the clinical process

■ Offering information and instruction that are relevant and helpful to the SLPA as well as the individuals served

■ Supporting the SLPA in dealing with stressful aspects of clinical work and reducing personal stress at the same time

■ Creating and maintaining an overall climate of inquiry, open communication

Characteristics of the Effective Mentor

The characteristics, qualities, and skills of effective mentors are consistently described in the literature (Gallacher, 1997; Hutto, Holden, & Haynes, 1991; Murray, 1991; Stott & Walker, 1992; Wildman, Niles, & Niles, 1992) and include the essential characteristic of "willingness to be a mentor"

(Gallacher, 1997). Think about someone you have worked with in your past or a special teacher or advisor who you felt cared about you and your success. What special qualities or characteristics did this person have? Was he encouraging and supportive? Was he helpful but not authoritative or inappropriately demanding? Do you remember him as being flexible, respectful of you and your abilities, enthusiastic about what he did for a living, patient, willing to share information, and willing to put himself out for you? Does this sound like someone you would like to work with on a daily basis? These are the typically listed characteristics of a mentor. As a mentor, your SLP will employ a variety of skills to support you in your role as an assistant. He may initially interview you, and then consistently observe you at work, communicate with you, provide demonstration and coaching sessions, be readily available to problem-solve challenging situations, be available for consultation, develop rapport with you, and gain your trust. You will find that your mentor/supervisor sometimes has challenges such as finding the time necessary to accomplish the mentoring activities described in addition to his many other responsibilities. It may be a good idea to build the time for one-on-one meetings into your work schedule from the beginning of the relationship. Take the initiative to set up these meetings, if it is not already in your work schedule.

The specific benefits of a successful mentor relationship may include increased job satisfaction, the opportunity to actualize your skills, demonstrate your abilities, expand your knowledge base, and the opportunity to grow and learn as you work with an experienced professional (French, 1997). As previously noted, you may gain in experience and skill, gain knowledge of your work environment, be provided social as well as emotional support, and enhance your communication abilities—all skills that will directly affect your success as an SLPA. Your assistance with work-related activities furnishes increased resources for your mentor/supervisor. He will quickly value and appreciate your abilities if this is the case. As you participate in this mentor relationship, think about what you can learn from this experienced professional that can contribute to your own growth and development and support any future career aspirations you may

have. The model provided, as well as the advising, feedback, and coaching can result in a positive relationship that is beneficial to you as you gain additional experience as an SLPA. Being a member of a productive team brings satisfaction and internal rewards in itself, but the ultimate satisfaction often stems from working effectively with individuals who need your help. A positive and productive relationship with your supervisor/mentor will ensure you have the opportunity to make the most of your work with individuals with communication challenges and disorders.

SUPERVISION AND THE SUPERVISORY PROCESS

It is clear that the amount and type of supervision your SLP supervisor provides will be based on your skills and experience, the service setting, the tasks assigned, and other factors (Gordon, 1992). While you are in training, the minimum amount of direct supervision required in the ASHA model is 50% of your time spent in direct service delivery (ASHA, 2001). Given the ongoing requirements for supervision and monitoring by your SLP, it makes sense that you need to build a working relationship in which you can listen and learn from feedback about your performance (Horton, Kavoler, Longhurst, & Paul-Bacon, 1997). This will only be to your benefit as you continue to refine your knowledge and skills as an SLPA. As a function of the relationship, your SLP supervisor/mentor is accountable for the work you do in extending services and support to individuals with communication challenges. Interest in and evaluation of the quality of your performance and ongoing competency development is thus part of his role as your supervisor. Performance evaluations should be timely and consistently scheduled as part of your ongoing routine and relationship. Consistent communication is an essential component of this process.

According to Sergiovanni (1991), effective supervision of performance accomplishes three broad purposes. When applied to your position as an SLPA, these include (1) quality control in which the supervisor is responsible for monitoring of your performance; (2) your development of competency as an SLPA in a particular setting; and (3) promoting your commitment to the position and the work in your setting, which in turn, can function to enhance your motivation. Individualizing methods of supervision to match your learning style and needs can be a challenge. This is why consistent communication regarding your performance and your development of specific competencies described in Chapter 2 is necessary and critical to the process of supervision.

KEY COMPONENTS OF SUPERVISION

Supervision can be described as involving key components such as:

- Defining and communicating the job activities and tasks that are within your scope of responsibilities as an SLPA
- Counseling and coaching for improved performance
- Providing job-related instruction including planning and organizing the work to be delegated to you
- Evaluating your performance
- Providing formative feedback
- Providing consequences for poor performance
- Arranging the environment to support a positive performance

What Can You Expect From Supervision?

In a chapter of her text on supervision, which addresses supervising SLPAs, Susan Dowling (2001) discusses the supervision of paraprofessionals as a relatively new component of clinical practice in speech-language pathology and references continuing confusions that exist between supervisors and assistants about supervisory requirements. She refers to the ASHA model and the specific scope of responsibilities described in Chapter 2 of this text as she describes what an SLPA might expect from the SLP supervisor. First, she discusses the need for "organizational acculturation" (p.195), stating it is certainly valuable for your supervisor to welcome you as a new employee and give you information that will help you get settled. Such orienting tasks as intro-

ducing you to others in the facility, outlining your responsibilities, and explaining your role to others are advised. You will most likely appreciate it if your supervisor also shows you where things are located. The "royal tour" will facilitate your adjustment and save time and need for interruptions. As Dowling suggests, providing you with a schedule and a place to work will also assist you in knowing what is expected and facilitate your timely adjustment to your new work setting.

Other aspects of supervision involve open discussions of your training and supervisory needs with your supervisor. This will help determine the specific tasks and activities you are initially able to do in a particular setting. Clarification of expectations will identify those tasks that you can competently perform while maintaining the quality of services provided. Discussion of the specific support functions you will initially be responsible for allows you the time you need to become familiar with the routines. As you demonstrate competency, with appropriate levels of supervision, you will most likely be asked to take on more complex tasks. This will result in increased intensity or frequency of services and support for those on your caseload.

Another key responsibility of your supervisor is to guide your development, including modeling of professional behavior, confidentiality, appearance, ethics, and appropriate interactions with patients, students, or other professionals in the particular work setting you have chosen. Because recipients of services and other professionals are often unclear about the role of a given service provider, it is the responsibility of your supervisor to introduce you and continually refer to you as an assistant.

Your supervisor may use several strategies in preparing you for your work as part of supervising your performance. These may include:

- Planning with you for step-by-step implementation of the procedures for you to use in sessions or planning your weekly schedule
- Role playing of procedures with you so that you practice
- Demonstrating therapy techniques and some of the more difficult aspects of therapy or demonstrating

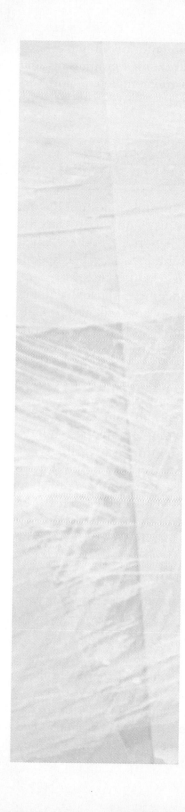

specific behavior management strategies used with a student or adult

- Co-therapy or working together with you during sessions until you are comfortable and confident about your role

- Explaining and demonstrating specific data collection techniques

- Asking you to observe other clinicians implementing specific aspects of a treatment plan

- Reviewing videotapes or audiotapes of your sessions so that he can keep informed about the individual as well as provide you feedback about your skills

- Providing you with verbal and written feedback and scheduling supervisory conferences during which you discuss your strengths and competency development as an SLPA

Documentation of your performance may take the form of a written log or journal, rating forms or other types of feedback instruments, copies of notes or communications regarding performance, drafts of written materials, and other records of interactions (Dowling, 2001). A **portfolio** of your work will provide a centralized place where feedback and progress can be kept and reviewed and highlight your development and success on the job. This is becoming a popular method to document personal growth and development and could be a way to collect data regarding key examples of your work and products you have created. The portfolio could then be helpful in job interviews at a later time or as part of the admissions process, if you chose to continue your education.

Feedback through checklists, written comments, and informal interactions are an expected part of the evaluation process (Dowling, 2001). However, a more formal written appraisal will most likely occur on a regular basis consistent with employment policies and procedures specific to your setting. Performance indicators most likely will be reflective of SLPA core competencies outlined in Chapter 1, but may also address more personal issues such as initiative, timeliness, reliability, appearance, and use of professional language and grammatically correct written language.

Conferencing with your supervisor/mentor on a regular basis is one way to prepare for your performance evaluations and ensure there are no surprises when you complete a more formal appraisal of your performance.

EXPECTATIONS AND EXPECTATION DISCREPANCIES

As the supervisory relationship begins, it is important for you and your supervisor/mentor to discuss and clarify specific expectations of each other. It is important to be explicit about general expectations for performance as well as specific activities and tasks to be undertaken. It is also very helpful to discuss the supervisor's specific philosophy about supervision and mentorship, tools to be used, and quality indicators so that there are no surprises when it comes time for a formal performance appraisal. Having more than one supervisor involved complicates the discussion, but it should take place, preferably with all involved, so there is a lower risk of miscommunication or expectation discrepancy. "Identifying discrepancies in perceptions and resolving differences are important for establishing an effective supervisory relationship and for opening up lines of communication" (Dowling, 2001, p. 195.) A simple format for setting the stage for this discussion is to prepare for it by completing a form, as the following story demonstrates. Think through what you would truly expect and hope for from your relationship with your supervisor/mentor. Are your thoughts similar to Charlene's?

SIDELIGHT: *Charlene's Story*

After a successful interview, Charlene was hired to be an SLPA in a large, private practice that saw a variety of clients with speech, language, and hearing disorders. She was excited about the position and looked forward to meeting with her SLP supervisor/mentor to learn more about what would be expected of her. Her supervisor was waiting for her when she arrived on her first day of work. She immediately liked her supervisor who was friendly and welcomed her to the office by showing her around and introducing her to the many SLPs who worked there. It was a busy place. Charlene then sat down in her supervisor's office and was given more information about the schedule, her supervisor's caseload, and the people she might be working with. They talked about the importance of starting out slowly and having the opportunity to get used to the setting and where everything was. It was a big office space, with several therapy and conference rooms, and each SLP had his own office. Charlene would also have a desk and share space with another SLPA in another room. She was shown the lunchroom, complete with microwave and refrigerator, the copy machine and supply closet, and the mailbox and phone systems. Charlene was beginning to feel comfortable when her supervisor suggested she get settled at her new desk, and take the time to complete an expectations worksheet (Figure 3-1). Her supervisor explained that it was something she often used to set the stage for a conversation about responsibilities and expectations. It would provide them with some specifics to talk about. She said she would be filling one out too and then they would compare their thoughts and frame how Charlene's position would be structured to meet both their needs. Charlene liked this idea but was a little nervous about what to say. She decided that her supervisor seemed nice enough and that honesty was the best policy. She might as well find out right away if this relationship could work. So she filled out her form as follows.

She wanted to be clear about her schedule, because she would have to leave no later than 5:00 P.M., on the dot, to pick up her child from childcare. The director of the practice who had hired her had said that would not be a problem, but she wanted to have this clear with her supervisor so she would know why Charlene could not stay longer, even if asked. Charlene also wanted to be sure she was not expected before 9:00 A.M., because she had to take her child to her sitter. It sounded like she would get to work with clients and not just do paperwork, but she wanted to be clear on what to do with each client because she did not want to waste anyone's time. Charlene and her supervisor shared the results of their respective worksheets. Charlene was pleased to see that her new supervisor's first expectation of herself was to respect Charlene's work schedule, and she had listed several other things that Charlene appreciated. They had a productive conversation and Charlene felt like they got off to a great start. Her supervisor provided Charlene with a suggested schedule of observation for the first few days on the job and a list of specific activities she would be expected to complete, with help. After her supervisor explained her philosophy of supervision, and that they would touch base daily and schedule a weekly conference to go over clients and update expectations, Charlene felt very comfortable. Charlene especially appreciated the opportunity to share what she felt she was good at and liked that the supervisor responded in a positive way. Her supervisor also outlined a strategy they could use to communicate assignments and decide which tasks Charlene felt competent in doing right away. She also asked what support or additional training Charlene might need in order to feel comfortable performing some of the activities she had planned. Charlene felt respected and supported. She thought she was going to really like this position.

Expectations of myself	Expectations of my supervisor
1. Be on time, all the time at 9:00 a.m.	1. Respect my ability
2. Listen to what is expected	2. Provide clear instructions
3. Follow schedule	3. Provide positive feedback
4. Follow my supervisor's lead	4. Let me know if I am making a mistake
5. Dress appropriately for work	5. Answer my questions
6. Be available (until 5:00 p.m.)	6. Observe my work
7. Ask for direction when needed	7. Show me approaches to use with clients, if I need help
8. Respect confidentiality of clients	8. Respect my schedule
9. Respect my supervisor's schedule	
10. Keep accurate data as requested	
11. Learn more about clients by reviewing records	
12. Be as helpful as I can	

Figure 3-1 Charlene's expectations

Charlene's story exemplifies the positive aspects of beginning a new relationship by clarifying expectations about roles and responsibilities. Knowing what to expect can save time and prevent misunderstandings from interfering with the development of a positive working environment. Charlene's new supervisor was prepared to be a mentor as well as a supervisor and was obviously interested in providing Charlene the support she needed to be successful on the job. If Charlene and her new supervisor had disagreed about certain aspects of the position, they would have had the opportunity to clarify their positions and reach resolution before the difference became a problem that interfered with the work they had to do together. They also began by establishing an open pattern of communication so that Charlene had a model to follow if she needed to address any questions or concerns at a later time. Again, establishing clear, open, and honest communication provides a foundation for a positive working relationship based on mutual respect and accountability.

SIDELIGHT: *Kim's Story*

Kim really wanted the position she was interviewing for as an SLPA. It was in a rehabilitation center that provides a variety of services to adults who were recovering from strokes, traumatic head injury, and other neurologic impairments. She knew she would be assigned to one of the master's level SLPs, but she hoped she would also be able to work with the PTs and OTs. She really was thinking about going back to school and becoming a PT, but she did not think she would tell this to her supervisor because it would not happen until her son was older and in school. She felt she interviewed well for the SLPA position. She had her AA degree and had done reasonably well in her field placement. She thought that she had better avoid the issue about her work schedule. They wanted her to be there by 7, but she was hoping she could change that because she has to take her son to childcare in the morning. She thought that if she just could get offered the position, she could work out the details with her supervisor later. Is Kim asking for trouble? Do you think she is heading in the right direction for establishing an open, honest basis for communication with her supervisor? What could she do differently?

CRITICAL INTERPERSONAL SKILLS FOR MAINTAINING SUCCESSFUL RELATIONSHIPS

Because supervisors and assistants typically work in a very close personal relationship, it is best if they respect each other. How can you build respect? What are the interpersonal skills that you have that others are drawn to in a working relationship? What can you do to develop your skills in these areas? Let us revisit the basic competencies listed in the interpersonal skill area for SLPAs, which was first addressed in Chapter 2. First and foremost, it is important to know the role you play as an assistant and the responsibilities you will have as an SLPA. This means you will need to be effective in developing clear channels of communication with your supervisor. You will need to be receptive to direction and constructive criticism and be willing to request assistance from your supervisor when necessary. You will be asked to actively participate in interactions with your supervisor and be honest about your limitations and abilities in your position. Clear and frequent communication that is open and nondefensive will enhance your ability to successfully complete delegated tasks and responsibilities. This will con-

tribute to the basic respect needed in your relationship with your supervisor/mentor.

Other interpersonal skills involve relationships with children and adults. Ask yourself how you can develop your skills in dealing effectively with attitudes and behaviors of the patient or students you work with. Sensitivity and understanding of frustrations related to difficulty in communication is key to establishing appropriate rapport with the patient, client, or students and their families. Being a good listener is a skill that will ensure your success. As you develop relationships with others, you will need to communicate your sensitivity, respond appropriately to their needs, and take into proper consideration cultural backgrounds and values. Respect for differences will be important as you learn to deal with a variety of challenging situations. Learning more about the type of disorders associated with communication challenges will also help you accept and understand variations in behaviors of those you work with. For example, learning about a recovering aphasic's frustration with remembering the correct words for a particular situation is critical to understanding how you can help cue the patient and reduce the characteristic frustration. This will help you develop the insight and patience needed to deal with challenging inappropriate behaviors. Seeing and understanding the frustration behind the struggle to "find the right word" helps you support the patient's ongoing attempts to communicate. Understanding that family members may be embarrassed by the individual's use of **perseveration** or use of inappropriate language when the patient is frustrated may be a key to a successful relationship with both the family and the patient. Your ability to handle such situations calmly makes a difference. Self-confidence in your skills will develop as you become familiar with characteristic communication behaviors of those with communication disabilities.

Think about how you can develop skills that reflect your intent to show respect to those you work with. Use of appropriate language that is consistent with the individual's age and educational level will be important in demonstrating your respect for him. Being courteous and respectful at all times is necessary. Using appropriate titles when addressing adult patients and their family members communicates your

respect for them. This is especially important when relating to those adults who may feel embarrassed at their inability to communicate their basic needs. Humor is an effective way to establish powerful connection. However, humor must be appropriate and must fit the situation. Inappropriate use of humor can be devastating to a relationship. You must understand and recognize that the inability to communicate even basic needs or complete an easy task is often frustrating and very embarrassing to those who have to seek your help. Children also demand your respect and patience. They can tell if you are "talking down to them" and will often continue their resistance to cooperate with your intended activities. Management of young children's behavior is both an art and a skill and demands your patience as well as your ability to redirect or change activities, pace, or sequence. You may find that children with communication challenges are often impulsive and distractible. This may be associated with their particular disability and not necessarily under their control. Appropriate preparation of materials and the ability to anticipate difficulty by "reading his or her cues" may prevent outbursts and disruptive episodes with any individual with frustration associated with the inability to communicate. Strategies and techniques for effective management of behavior are covered in Chapter 13 of this text and will help you develop competency in guiding behavior. This will be a much needed and appreciated skill in that it directly makes an impact on the productivity of your work as an SLPA.

Consider the personal qualities that will help you succeed as an SLPA. Your supervisor/mentor is looking for individuals who can manage their time effectively. This means being responsible and punctual in all assigned tasks. Arriving punctually for work-related meetings with your supervisor and others will be valued and appreciated. Maintaining your assigned schedule and completing all assigned tasks on time will go a long way in establishing respect from your supervisor/mentor and others you work with. Being prepared and organized is the critical piece that will maintain a credible working relationship with your supervisor/mentor. Prior organization and careful preparation of materials will be keys to your success. Preparation includes being prepared for last-minute changes in schedules, having materials ready when they are needed, and completing appropriate paper-work on time. Flexibility in being able to adjust to a new or challenging situation will be helpful to your supervisor.

SIDELIGHT: *Jim's Story*

Jim was working to help a small group of children practice target sounds introduced by their SLP. Their teacher had forgotten to tell Jim about a scheduled field trip to the zoo, and so the children were gone for the day when he went to collect them for their group session. Jim could have retreated to the staff lunchroom and taken the 45 minutes to relax. Instead, he used the time to catch up on the copying that his supervisor had requested be done for her meeting with a family the next day. He then took the time to organize his notes regarding the children's progress in generalizing their targeted sounds from the previous time he has spent observing them in the classroom. He reported these results to his supervisor so that he could get direction on "next steps" to be taken to further their progress. She expressed her appreciation for not only helping her prepare for the meeting ahead of time, but for using his unexpected 45 minutes in a productive way.

Other competencies to remember include understanding the need for and maintaining confidentiality. This is of the utmost importance. This means you need to develop skills in handling difficult questions about a person from those you are not able to discuss this information with. You will learn to defer these types of questions to your supervisor in a courteous and respectful way. You will be expected to direct patient/client or family and other professionals to your supervisor for information about testing results, treatment, or referral. It also means that you follow established guidelines regarding where and when you can discuss specific information about those you work with. Maintaining confidentiality regarding anyone you work with is a crucial component of quality care. Elevators and hallways can be tempting places to discuss an issue given time demands and schedules. However, avoidance of these situations is mandatory because unintended consequences can result from this misconduct. Breaches of confidentiality can be devastating to a patient, client, or family member. It is your responsibility to adhere to guidelines and respect the basic rights of privacy guaranteed to those individuals served. A thorough

understanding of this matter is essential to your success as an SLPA and is reviewed in depth in Chapter 7 of this text.

Appropriate conduct in the work setting also includes maintaining a personal appearance consistent with the norms of the workplace. This does not mean that you have to spend thousands of dollars to acquire a new wardrobe when you are hired. But it does mean that you have to observe any formal dress codes associated with your setting. This may mean that jeans and tee shirts remain in the closet, and you wear clean and comfortable clothing to work each day. This may also mean that obvious facial or body piercing and other elaborate personal jewelry items that will interfere or distract from your work may need to be removed during work hours. Because you may be working with children outside, at water tables, on the floor, and in sand boxes, slacks or what works in any particular setting may replace skirts and dresses for female SLPAs. Follow your supervisor's lead and request clarification of what is acceptable to prevent any concerns or misunderstandings about dress and appearance. Your setting may also require that you wear a lab coat, an identification name badge, or both, during work hours. It is best to observe both the formal and informal guidelines established. Your supervisor/mentor will expect and appreciate your adherence to these policies so that he does not have to waste valuable time in monitoring your dress and appearance.

Appropriate conduct in the workplace also means using appropriate language. It goes without saying that your use of appropriate speech and language will be a necessary and important aspect of your work with individuals with communication challenges. This does not mean that accents are unacceptable or that banter and humor cannot be used in informal conversations. However, it does mean that inordinate use of slang, swearing, or inappropriate terms will not be accepted in your conversations with professionals and patients/clients or family members. Use of language appropriate for the patient, client, or student as well as others you work with in terms of their age, educational level, or authority is necessary. Take the time to observe interactions in your work setting. What is the tone and level of language used? Can you adhere to these standards while maintaining your

own characteristic personality and manner or style of inter-action? Videotaping yourself in interactions with others is one clear way of seeing how others respond to your manner and style. Seek input from your supervisor/mentor if you have concerns about your performance in this area.

Evaluate your own performance in the interpersonal skill areas of competence. Use the opportunities in your training program to practice development of core competencies. Reflecting on your own strengths in this area will help you improve your competency and will make a difference in how you are perceived and valued for your work. Take time to assess your interactions with others, perhaps through role-playing exercises or videotape. Evaluate and assess:

- Others' responses to your patterns of speech and language
- Your ability to listen to others
- Your ability to ask appropriate questions
- Your interactions with different age groups
- Both your own and others' use of appropriate terminology
- Use of clear speech and appropriate language models

Potential employers will have expectations about your level of performance in these areas, so it is a good idea to make changes now that will increase your employability. Once you have been hired, you may be asked to use check-lists and review videotapes of your performance in sessions. These may be strategies your supervisor/mentor uses to document your performance for evaluation purposes. Use these opportunities as ways to obtain constructive feedback that can help you meet your goals of providing quality services to those you work with on a daily basis. Being able to evaluate your own performance is an indicator of your ability to improve and grow as an SLPA. Seek input regarding changes that may be necessary to improve your abilities in these areas.

In summary, you will be expected to demonstrate these basic interpersonal skills in your work with others. These skills are considered important and necessary attributes for successful performance in most work settings. Spend the time now to refine your communication abilities. Your future

supervising SLP will appreciate your effort to develop these basic interpersonal skills before you "hit the floor running" on your first job. They will appreciate your responsiveness to their requests and an overall pattern of behavior that reflects your commitment to the individuals with communication disorders who receive your services. An attitude that says, "How can I help? What can I do to make your job easier and more effective?" will be appreciated and valued in any setting in which you are employed. Care and commitment to doing a job well done will speak a thousand words and move you forward to developing a mutually satisfying relationship with your SLP supervisor/mentor.

STRATEGIES FOR EXTERNAL FEEDBACK

As discussed, your supervisor/mentor will most likely rely on several strategies to provide you with feedback about your performance and growth as an SLPA. These may include:

- Both formal and informal notes or verbal feedback
- Documented observations
- Periodic use of checklists
- Data regarding patient, client, or student progress
- Feedback from patient, client satisfaction instruments
- Feedback from other team members or staff
- Regularly scheduled or periodically scheduled conferences or meeting times
- Formal performance appraisal procedures

The discussion regarding expectations in the preceding section may be helpful in setting the stage for how your supervisor plans to share information and feedback with you. An honest and thoughtful look at expectations associated with your job description and responsibilities will support your knowing how to respond to requests and assignments. Knowing what to expect allows for communication about how you are to proceed in fulfilling delegated tasks and responsibilities.

Individual Growth Plans

Some supervisor/ mentors may also use the information from this candid discussion to develop an individual growth plan or similar instrument that puts in writing what is expected from each of you as you work together to meet the needs of those you serve. An individual growth plan can be revisited and updated periodically and serves as a tool to ensure ongoing communication and improve your performance through documentation and conversations with your supervising SLP. It might look something like Figure 3-2.

Individual Growth Plan

Name _____

Date _____

Supervisor _____

Strengths:

Areas for Growth:

Performance Goals and Strategies:

Supports Needed:

Supervisor Signature_____ Date _____

SLPA Signature _____ Date _____

Figure 3-2 Individual Growth Plan

Figure 3-2 provides a clear and simple way to help you define what is needed to improve your job performance, and it documents ongoing communication with your supervisor/mentor. It provides direction for you in personal goal setting based on your own strengths and areas for growth.

Your supervisor may periodically "check in" with you to determine how you are progressing and learn whether additional supports are needed for you to reach your performance. It becomes your responsibility to complete the activities or strategies delineated in your plan and to revisit and update the plan as needed with your supervisor. A completed plan may look something like Figure 3-3. Notice that an individual growth planning process always begins with strengths, then addresses areas for growth, and ends with a specific plan with strategies to continue development of targeted competencies.

SIDELIGHT: *Individual Growth Plan in Action*

Susan and Lynea have discussed Susan's work with several small groups after Lynea had observed several sessions. A growth plan is one way to structure feedback and document discussions about this type of session. Susan appreciated the small amount of time it took to organize what she needed to do to improve her work with small groups and was also appreciative of Lynea's recognition of her efforts to prepare and complete her assigned tasks on time. They discussed different strategies to increase productivity and practice during small group work, and Susan knew what she had to do to change what was happening in the sessions. She also valued the time provided to watch an experienced SLP in small group work and felt this was one way to support her growth and development in use of appropriate strategies and techniques. She often learns best by observing others, and this seemed to be what she needed at this point in time.

Conferences and Feedback Sessions

As noted, consistently scheduled conferences or periods of time set aside to discuss the individual plans for a client, patient, or student will help you improve your performance and abilities to assist your supervising SLP in her work. Conferences can be structured in such a way for you to gain

---

Individual Growth Plan

SLPA: Susan
Supervisor: Lynea
Date: 10/6/01

Strengths: Susan is

- Punctual and reliable
- Prepares for sessions ahead of time and sets up an attractive environment
- Consistently maintains schedule for small group work
- Interacts well with the children—they enjoy their time together
- Ensures children are returned safely to their classroom
- Documents practice and accurately takes data

Areas for Growth:

- Increased expectations for productivity
- Creativity in activities
- Management of distracting behaviors

Goals and Strategies:

- Increase number of responses during a session by restructuring activities so children can take more turns and repeat correct responses from baseline of 20 to about 50 or higher each
- Increase engagement by creating games and interactions that are fun and inviting and capitalize on interests of the children in the group
- Set clear limits and rules to play games and provide consistent verbal feedback about correct productions

Supports Needed:

- Observation of SLP with specific expertise in small group work

---

Figure 3-3 Susan's Individual Growth Plan

the information needed about the individual being served as well as to allow the time you need to ask questions or address concerns you have. It can also be a time to review progress of those you are serving so your supervising SLP can determine changes that need to be made with intervention protocols or activities.

You may want to work with your supervisor in structuring these meetings to include time set aside during each meeting to address your questions. Most work settings are

very busy, and it is easy to get sidetracked and to run out of time for important issues that need to be addressed so that you can function at your best. It is important that you use these meetings in a constructive way to get the direction you need to complete your responsibilities and also the feedback you need to improve your performance. It may work to begin each meeting with a rundown or review of your questions to be addressed and then proceed with the specifics of what is completed and what needs to be done regarding your assignments. Keeping on track is as much your responsibility as that of your supervisor. Organize your time so that you have clear feedback from your supervisor regarding your performance. Initiate these discussions with your SLP if he has not. Perhaps it is a new process for your SLP, and he would welcome the suggestion.

Formal Rating Forms

Many supervisors will periodically complete a more formal rating form much like Figure 3-4. This form could be used to assess and look at your overall competency development at any point in time. This type of a form may also be used to provide you with feedback during your field placements. It could also be used to assess your performance as part of a formal performance appraisal process that provides information to those responsible for maintaining the funding for your position or any merit raises you may be eligible for in a position. As you can see, this particular form closely follows the outlined competencies to be developed and maintained by the SLPA, consistent with the ASHA model explained in Chapter 2. You could also complete this same form about yourself and then use it to compare your own perceptions about your performance with those of your supervisor. This could lead to a productive discussion of your abilities and your areas for growth and development. If done periodically, it can provide a rich resource for an individual growth planning process. Figure 3-5 has also been included as a sample form that you might be asked to complete to provide feedback about your field placement. This form provides feedback to your direct supervisor and instructor about strengths and any areas of concern about the placement.

**SPEECH-LANGUAGE PATHOLOGY ASSISTANT
STUDENT PRACTICA EVALUATION FORM**

Student_____   Midterm grade_____

Semester_____   Final grade_____

Facility_____

Please rate each competency using the following scale:

– Needs improvement   O Meets expectations

+ Strengths   N/A Not applicable

A. INTERPERSONAL SKILLS (communicates honestly, clearly, accurately, coherently, and concisely)

1. Deals effectively with attitudes and behaviors of the patient/client
____ Maintains appropriate patient/client relationships
____ Communicates sensitivity to the needs of the patient/client and family
____ Takes into proper consideration patient/client needs and cultural values
____ Demonstrates an appropriate level of self-confidence when performing assigned tasks
____ Establishes rapport with patient/client and family
____ Demonstrates insight in patient/client attitudes and behaviors
____ Directs patient/client, family, and professionals to the supervisor for information regarding testing, treatment, and referral

2. Uses appropriate language (written and oral) in dealing with patient/client and others
____ Uses language appropriate for patient/client and others' age and education level
____ Is courteous and respectful at all times
____ Maintains appropriate pragmatic skills

3. Deals effectively with supervisor
____ Is receptive to constructive criticism
____ Requests assistance from supervisor as needed
____ Actively participates in interaction with supervisor

B. PERSONAL QUALITIES

1. Manages time effectively
____ Arrives punctually and prepared for patient/client appointments

Figure 3-4 Sample SLPA Practica Evaluation Form (continues)

____ Arrives punctually for work-related meetings (e.g., meetings with the supervisor, staff, etc.)

____ Turns in all documentation on time

2. Demonstrates appropriate conduct

____ Respects/maintains confidentiality of patient/clients

____ Maintains personal appearance appropriate for the work setting

____ Uses appropriate language for the work setting

____ Evaluates own performance

____ Recognizes own professional limitations and performs within boundaries of training and job responsibilities

C. TECHNICAL–ASSISTANT SKILLS

1. Maintains a facilitating environment for assigned tasks

____ Adjusts lighting and controls noise level

____ Organizes treatment space

2. Uses time effectively

____ Performs assigned tasks with no unnecessary distractions

____ Completes assigned tasks within designated treatment session

3. Selects, prepares, and presents materials effectively

____ Prepares and selects treatment materials ahead of time

____ Chooses appropriate materials based on treatment plan

____ Prepares clinical setting to meet the needs of the client of obtaining optimal performance

____ Selects materials that are age and culturally appropriate as well as motivating

4. Maintains documentation

____ Documents treatment plans and protocols accurately and concisely for the supervisor

____ Documents and reports patient/client performance to the supervisor

____ Signs documents reviewed and cosigned by the supervisor

____ Prepares and maintains patient/client charts, records, and graphs for displaying data

5. Provides assistance to speech-language pathologist

____ Assists during patient/client assessment

____ Assists with informal documentation

____ Schedules activities

Figure 3-4 (continued)

____ Participates with speech-language pathologist in research projects
____ Participates in in-service training
____ Participates in public relations programs

D. SCREENING

1. Demonstrates knowledge and use of a variety of screening tools and protocols
____ Completes training on screening procedures

2. Demonstrates appropriate administration and scoring of screening tools
____ Differentiates correct versus incorrect responses
____ Completes (fills out) screening protocols accurately
____ Scores screening instruments accurately

3. Manages screenings and documentation
____ Reports any difficulty encountered in screening
____ Schedules screenings
____ Organizes screening materials

4. Communicates screening results and all supplemental information to the supervisor
____ Seeks the supervisor's guidance should adaptation of screening tools and administration be in question
____ Provides descriptive behavioral observations that contribute to screening results

E. TREATMENT

1. Performs tasks as outlined and instructed by the supervisor
____ Accurately and efficiently implements activities using procedures planned by the supervisor
____ Uses constructive feedback from the supervisor for modifying interaction (interpersonal or otherwise) with the patient/client

2. Demonstrates skills in managing behavior and treatment programs
____ Maintains on-task behavior
____ Provides appropriate feedback as to the accuracy of patient/client response
____ Uses feedback and reinforcement that are consistent, discriminating, and meaningful to the patient/client
____ Gives directions and instructions that are clear, concise, and appropriate to the patient's/client's age level and level of understanding

Figure 3-4 (continued)

____ Applies knowledge of behavior modification during interaction with the patient/client

____ Implements designated treatment objectives/goals in specified sequence

3. Demonstrates knowledge of treatment objectives and plan

____ Demonstrates understanding of patient/client disorder and needs

____ Identifies correct versus incorrect responses

____ Describes behaviors demonstrating a knowledge of the patient's/client's overall level of progress

____ Verbally reports and provides appropriate documentation of assigned activities

Comments:

_____   _____
Supervisor   Date   Student Date

Figure 3-4 (continued)

PLACEMENT FEEDBACK FORM

Student_____   Semester_____

Supervisor_____   Site_____

Please rate the following items using the number corresponding to the appropriate rating.

N/A Not applicable

5   Outstanding

4   Above average

3   Satisfactory

2   Below average

1   Unsatisfactory

Supervisor

____ Established appropriate requirements for practica performance

____ Observed intervention for an appropriate amount of time

____ Exhibited skill in therapy and diagnostic evaluation and observation

____ Provided adequate direction and guidance

____ Demonstrated appropriate procedures for evaluating performance

____ Demonstrated appropriate professionalism

____ Demonstrated flexibility in response to feedback

____ Was responsive and encouraging in supervisory interactions

____ Demonstrated appropriate professional skills

____ Overall performance as a supervisor

Practica Placement

____ Contained adequate equipment, materials, and observational facilities

____ Offered appropriate interaction with other professionals

____ Offered adequate training in:

    ____ Screening and assessment of communication disorders

    ____ Intervention with communication disorders

    ____ Documentation and reporting procedures

    ____ Overall adequacy of placement site

Figure 3-5 Sample Feedback Placement Form (continues)

If the overall adequacy of the practica site was less than satisfactory, what changes or additions would you suggest?

Would you recommend this supervisor for future practica placement?

☐ Yes ☐ No

Would you recommend this practica for future placement? ☐ Yes ☐ No

How would you rate the value of your experience as an SLPA (in training) during the past semester?

Other comments:

_____

Signature   Date

Figure 3-5 (continued)

Notes and Checklists

When your supervisor observes your work, ask him to jot down what he sees that you are doing well and include those things that he would like to see you change. These notes can be another effective way to monitor your performance and help you receive both positive and constructive feedback about your abilities. Request that your supervising SLP share his observations with you, and use these notes in your regularly scheduled conferences or individual growth planning process. If he uses a checklist when he observes your performance, request a copy ahead of time so you can be aware of what he is looking for with regard to your execution of tasks and responsibilities. These can also be a helpful addition to your portfolio as time goes by and changes in your abilities are documented.

Other Sources of Feedback

Your supervising SLP may also collect data regarding your performance by looking at satisfaction surveys. There may be responses to specific questions that document your ability to establish and maintain rapport with those individuals you serve. This can prove to be a vehicle that affirms your interpersonal skill development as it affects those you work with. It can be a very positive source of feedback. Your supervising SLP may also seek input about your performance from others on the team of care providers in your setting or the teachers you come in contact with as you serve particular children in their classroom. Again, this feedback can be considered in your performance appraisal as it speaks to your abilities to fulfill the specific requirements of the position in your particular setting.

Formal Performance Appraisal or Evaluations

Many settings require a formal performance appraisal or evaluation process be documented on an annual or semiannual basis. It is important for you to be aware of the policy and procedures that dictate in your setting. Increases in pay

may be determined and continuation of your employment may be evaluated and it is critical that you are knowledgeable about these procedures. You may want to suggest sources that could be used to inform and document the quality of your performance or at the minimum at least be aware of what sources are being used in this process. You most likely will learn about these procedures from your supervising SLP or the human resources component of your place of work. It is important that you understand how and when you will be evaluated and that you are an active participant in this process. This will ensure a fair and valid appraisal of your work.

REFLECTIVE PRACTICE: STRATEGIES FOR SELF-ASSESSMENT AND CONTINUED GROWTH

Taking responsibility for evaluating and assessing your own abilities is an indicator of your professionalism and your willingness to learn, especially if you can be honest in your self-evaluation and be open-minded about constructive feedback. This is a sure way to build and maintain a positive relationship with your supervisor mentor and opens the door for you to benefit from his years of experience and practice. It is also a way to document your ongoing attention to improving your performance and produces data that track your growth, development, and ability to change as needed. Reflective practice is described as a process of "knowing thyself." This demands an honest and open-minded look at your abilities at several levels.

One strategy for self-assessment is to use a framework to evaluate your performance within the context of a single session or across time. Pick a context for your self-assessment and ask yourself this simple question: "On a scale from 1 to 10, how do I feel about my performance in a given situation or across time?" By the way, you cannot pick 5 because this is thought to reflect ambivalence about your performance. It becomes a forced choice. If you pick a number above 5, such as 6, then think of three reasons why you think

things went well during this period of time. List these reasons and then try to think of at least one more to write down. Then turn your attention to why you did not pick 8 or 9. There must have been something you felt was not going well. List three things you think you need to change that might improve the outcome you are looking for. Think of one more. If you chose a number below 5, first begin listing those things that you did not like and need to change. Be gentle with yourself and be sure to list at least three things that worked. Now you have data. Reflect on your lists and pick at least two things you will continue to do because you feel they worked to achieve the outcomes you are looking for. Then prioritize two from your lists that you will try to incorporate into your work plan to see if positive change results from your efforts. This is a short and simple way to self-assess your performance in any given situation and can lead to productive questions and discussions with your supervising SLP. Using self-assessment tools, checklists, or rating forms to gauge your self-perceptions of your abilities and performance can be a productive endeavor. Comparison with how your supervising SLP rates your abilities or performance can lead to insights about your abilities. These observations can provide you with the guidance you need to increase your competency level as an SLPA.

Another way to document your performance is to keep a log or journal of the work you are doing. Add this to your portfolio. Include positive feedback from your supervisor/mentor(s). Be sure to add any thank-you notes or letters of appreciation from patients, clients, or individuals you work with. You might also include samples of any written work or creative activities you have developed as part of your job responsibilities. Some individuals include pictures of products they have created or samples of videotapes of their work. Can you think of additional items that might be included that would speak of your abilities and growing confidence in your work as an SLPA? This may be a way for you to document your successes and learn from your mistakes. It can be a rewarding journey in self-reflection that leads to increased satisfaction with your growth and development as an SLPA and sparks your motivation for continued improvement.

CONCLUSION

There are many ways to succeed as an SLPA, but developing a productive working relationship based on mutual respect with your supervising SLP marks a clear path toward success. Establishing a relationship, in which your supervising SLP serves as a mentor or guide, will bring you closer to your goal of developing competency as an SLPA. Understanding how you can build on this relationship through development of your core interpersonal skills as a foundation for the technical skills and competencies you will need to be successful as an SLPA can lead to positive outcomes and increased job satisfaction. Such tasks as clarifying expectations, becoming knowledgeable about your responsibilities, and understanding how you will be supervised and evaluated, all contribute to positive working relationships and job success. Seeking and being open to feedback and support from your supervising SLP and engaging in self-reflective practice strategies described in this chapter will prove worthwhile in clearing your path and maintaining your direction for success as an SLPA. Setting the stage for your work with individuals presenting with communication challenges by establishing and maintaining a close working relationship with your supervisor will prove to be mutually beneficial to all concerned.

DISCUSSION QUESTIONS

1. Review the information about mentorship. Are the characteristics attributed to a mentor what you are seeking from a supervising SLP? If your supervisor fulfilled your expectations as a mentor, would you have increased job satisfaction and motivation in your work? What would make the difference?

2. Describe the dual functions of supervision and mentorship. How do these terms differ? Consider and discuss what specific attributes associated with these functions could help you in your work as an SLPA.

3. Discuss Kim's strategies for "getting the job" described in her story. Will they continue to work for her? What do you see as a potential "backfire" in her situation?

Compare her attitude with that of Charlene. Who do you think will last longer on the job provided that Kim is hired? Why?

4. Review the many strategies presented as tools for feedback regarding your performance. What might work for you? What do you think is most important in facilitating your development and performance? There is likely more than one strategy that can help you progress and succeed as an SLPA. Would some be more appropriate to use during training on the job? Does it have more to do with individual learning style?

SUGGESTED ACTIVITIES

1. Use the expectation discrepancy worksheet to outline what you expect from your instructor in this class and what you expect of yourself in completing the requirements associated with it. Ask that your instructor also complete the worksheet. Do the responses match? Does your instructor expect the same things of himself that you expect of the instructor? Do your expectations of yourself match those of your instructor? Discuss with others in your class. If there is a discrepancy, is there room for negotiation or resolution?

2. Select what you consider to be key factors or attributes that would speak to your abilities to interact with others in a helping situation. List these qualities and develop specific indicators that would demonstrate you had these skills. For example, if "active listening" was an attribute or a quality you should have in a helping situation, what might indicate you had this quality? Indicators might include: appropriate use of silence, use of nonverbal communication (head nods, etc.), and infrequent interruptions of other. Use this example and develop a self-assessment tool covering at least five other qualities with indicators you should possess that indicate your ability to interact with others in a positive way.

3. There are several sample forms included in this chapter. Figure 3-4 was developed to evaluate competency

development of an SLPA student in training in a field placement. Figure 3-5 was designed to be a placement feedback form that an SLPA student would complete about the field placement he experienced. Think about what you read regarding competency development of the SLPA and qualities of the supervisor/mentor. Do these forms address factors that are important to evaluate? What would you do with the feedback obtained? How would you like the results shared if you were the student or supervisor being evaluated?

4. Do you have a video camera? Videotape yourself in interactions with a young child, an adult, and a fellow student. Review the tape. What did you observe about your use of language and humor during these interactions? What did you like about your interaction skills? What, if anything, do you want to change? Are there things you might need to pay attention to or monitor when you interact with individuals with communication challenges?

REFERENCES

American Speech-Language-Hearing Association. (2001). *Scope of practice in speech-language pathology*. Rockville, MD: Author.

American Speech-Language-Hearing Association. (in press). Knowledge and skills for supervisors of speech-language pathology assistants. *ASHA Supplement*.

Dowling, S. (2001). *Supervision*. Needham Heights, MA: Allyn & Bacon.

Fenichel, E. (Ed). (1992). *Learning through supervision and mentorship: A source book*. Washington, DC: Zero to Three. National Center for Infants, Toddlers and Families.

French, N. (1997). A case study of a speech-language pathologist's supervision of assistants in a school setting: Tracy's story. *Journal of Children's Communication Development, 18*,103–110.

Gallacher, K. K. (1997). Supervising, mentoring and coaching. In P. Winton, J. McCollum, & C. Catlett, (Eds.), Transforming personnel preparation in early intervention (pp. 191–214). Baltimore: Paul H. Brookes Publishers.

Gordon, S. (1992). Perspectives and imperatives: Paradigms, transitions, and the new supervision. *Journal of Curriculum and Supervision, 8*, 62–76.

Henry, J. S., Stockdale, M. S., Hall, M., & Deniston, W. (1994). A formal mentoring program for collaborative culture, and the case of peer coaching. *Teaching & Teacher Education, 6*, 227–241.

Horton, A., Kander, M., Longhurst, T., & Paul-Brown, D. (1997). *Preparing and using speech-language pathology assistants.* Rockville, MD: American Speech-Language-Hearing Association.

Hutto, N., Holden, J., & Haynes, L. (Eds.). (1991). *Mentor training manual for Texas teachers.* Dallas: Texas Education Agency.

Murray, M. (1991). *Beyond the myths and magic of mentoring.* San Francisco: Jossey-Bass.

Sergiovanni, T. J. (1991). *The principalship: A reflective practice perspective* (2nd ed.). Needham, MA: Allyn & Bacon.

Stott, K. & Walker, A. (1992). Developing school leaders through mentoring. *School Organization, 12*(2), 153–164.

Wildman, T. M., Magliaro, S. C., Niles, R. A., & Niles, J. A. (1992). Teacher mentoring: An analysis of roles, responsibilities and conditions. *Journal of Teacher Education, 43,* 200–204.

Communicating With Families and Children

Key Concepts

The child or individual with a communication challenge must be considered in the context of their family.

◼

Family-centered practice is based on recognized values and principles that affect how service providers interact with families.

◼

Working with families implies a partnership that is focused on a "let's do with rather than let's do for" philosophy, recognizing and supporting family empowerment.

◼

Families most often know their child or other family member best. Service providers can learn a great deal about the individual they are serving by listening to family stories.

◼

Respecting and honoring differences in backgrounds, culture, priorities and lifeways means respecting the family as the key decision maker for the child or family member with communication challenges.

◼

Overview

◼

Your Role With Families

◼

Building Relationships Based on Family-Centered Practice

◼

Learning From Families

◼

Family Rights and Responsibilities

◼

Respecting and Responding to Individual and Cultural Differences

◼

Specific Strategies That Support Parent and Individual Participation and Involvement

◼

Focus on Talking With Young Children

Key Concepts continued

Most families want to be involved and participate in the program for their child or family member who has a disability. It is important to start from this perspective rather than assume otherwise, even though stereotypes of the uninvolved or noncaring parent are circulated. The provider's goal is to find ways to support family members' inclusion on the team.

■

Specific communication strategies used with young children parallel those used with adults. It is important to develop and use these strategies to enhance communication competence of individuals with disabilities.

INTRODUCTION

This chapter presents aspects of what is called family-centered care or family-centered practice and discusses how these concepts affect your role as an SLPA. It is important to realize that you may be providing services and support to many individuals, which means you will also be interacting with family members of those individuals. Building relationships that support the individual means building relationships with families

Research summarized in a text written by Guralnick (1997), as well as experience, demonstrates that family involvement is often the key component determining success in intervention programs. Families can also provide you with information that makes your job easier. A relationship based on respectful interactions is important in intervention and can bring you many rewards in your role as an SLPA.

This chapter also presents information to help you enhance your own communication skills because they make an impact on your work with families, adults, and young children. Focus on communicating with others involves specific suggestions regarding strategies that can improve language and learning. Reading about and practicing effective strategies for communicating with others builds the foundation for success regardless of the work setting you choose as an SLPA.

YOUR ROLE WITH FAMILIES

Building a relationship with family members is like building any relationship; it involves establishing trust and demonstrating respect for another's background and culture and listening to that individual's priorities, issues, and concerns. As an SLPA, you will engage with various family members in your role as a care provider. Effectively communicating empathy for their situation and focusing on listening to what they have to say is helpful to family members. It is important that you establish rapport with family members just as you do with the individual with a disability you are working with. It is important that you communicate your warmth and genuine caring about the individual being served and that your involvement is explained so that they are aware of your role with their child or family member.

Given your position as an assistant, it is critical that any information that centers on decision making, interpretation of test results, progress in intervention efforts, recommendations, referral sources, or discharge information be provided by your supervising SLP. You will not be in a position to offer advice or counseling to the family, but your opinion about progress or disposition may be sought given your involvement with the patient, client, or student receiving services. Remember, all information about what is happening in your work with these individuals must be filtered through your SLP supervisor. It is best to clarify with your supervisor how you will be introduced to the family so that your involvement as an assistant is clear and understood.

Family members typically want to be involved and participate in the programs that SLPs offer to their patients, clients, and students. They want to know who is working with their child, spouse, or family member. They appreciate knowing that you care, respect, and enjoy working with the individual who is receiving services. It is not only possible but necessary for you to interact positively with family members and establish a climate of interaction that is supportive and understanding of their concerns. This is critical to ensure that quality of care is maintained. It is also important to understand how interactions with family members can affect outcomes in intervention. You will read and discuss

key principles of family-centered care that build the foundation for partnerships with family members and guide interaction that support the quality of care for the individual receiving services and support from your supervising SLP.

Family-Centered Practice

Many authors have written about family-centered practice, especially in early intervention with young children (Bailey, 1991; Berman, 1994; Crais, 1991; Dunst & Bruder, 1999; McWilliam, 1992; Moore, Eiserman, & Ferguson, 1995). You will hear the term **family-centered care** or **family-centered practice** or one like it in every setting in which you work. These terms refer to an emerging focus that is currently taking place in both health care and education, which recognizes the rights and responsibilities of the family as the primary caretaker and key decision maker about family members. As a concept, family-centered care or practice is becoming more widely discussed across health-related and education professions. You will hear the term used in schools as it relates to procedural safeguards and the rights of family members to be on any team making educational decisions about their child. It is also used in the **Individuals with Disabilities Act (IDEA)**, which is federal legislation that all public schools must adhere to regarding special education programs. Family involvement in the child's **individual education plan (IEP)** or **individual family service plan (IFSP)** is mandated by law, but more than that, it is considered best practice. You will hear this term or one like it, *developmentally supportive family-centered care* (Als & Gilkerson, 1995), in reference to preferred practice patterns with young children born premature, with congenital issues, or genetic syndromes that need specialized care in **neonatal intensive care units (NICUs)**. You may hear it in rehabilitation centers and hospital programs, wherein SLPs serve adolescents or young adults who have suffered traumatic head injury.

Both children and adults with long-term developmental disabilities and elderly people who have been injured or are recovering from traumatic and life-threatening events such as stroke or progressive neurologic disease will benefit from interventions based on family-centered principles and practices. Whether it is about early identification and intervention, or newborn intensive care, or development of language and literacy or long-term care associated with recovery and maintenance of functional communication abilities, family participation and involvement stand out as primary factors influencing positive outcomes of intervention. This makes sense when one thinks about the steady support and long-term commitment of family members in their relationship to children, spouses, or other individuals in their family who are challenged by communication. It is thus critically important to understand the basic principles of family-centered practice and how you can assist your supervising SLP in establishing positive interactions with and supporting the involvement of parents and other family members in the care of individuals with disabilities. Having the family members as active participants in their child's program provides opportunities for extended support of communication attempts in everyday routines, activities, and places. This is also true of the adult recovering from a stroke or attempting to maintain functional communication following diagnosis of a debilitating, progressive or neurologic disease.

Principles of Family-Centered Practice

Family-centered practice is a multifaceted approach that looks different for each individual receiving services and for

SIDELIGHT: *A Parent's Perspective*

Linda is the mother of three children. Her oldest daughter was born with Down syndrome. Linda was involved in several early intervention programs that provided assessments and services to her child. In sharing her experiences she talks about how difficult it was to work with certain providers, because she did not feel respected by them. She says this interfered with her acceptance of services. She remembers the first evaluation of her daughter as a very negative experience. She remembers that the therapists did not listen to the information she shared and actually ignored her reports of what her daughter was doing at home. Linda says, "to make progress and have a family go in a positive direction, the family has to feel valued; that the information they are sharing is just as important as the information the professionals are sharing. For the family to feel this way is critical to success." —Linda Ryan Yager, parent

each family, setting, and situation, but it is refocusing providers on evaluating how they relate to families.

A demonstration model project (Moore et al. 1995) at the University of Colorado in Boulder actually worked with families to formulate several belief statements as underlying basic principles of family-centered practice. Examples of principles or values generated by this group of families are consistent with other conceptualization of what is meant by family-centered practice and include key belief statements such as:

1. Recognize the family as the constant in the life of the individual with a disability. Care providers or services may change over time.

2. The family should be considered as the key decision maker about the child or family member's services or educational plan. Teams need to support family members' priorities.

3. Recognition of family strengths, resources, resilience, and individuality involves respect for different ways of coping with disability.

4. Family members' perspectives and the information they share should be believed and valued.

5. Sharing of unbiased and complete information with parents or family members about their child's care or therapeutic program is essential on an ongoing basis in an appropriate and supportive manner.

6. The individual, ethnic, racial, and socioeconomic diversity of families should be acknowledged and honored.

7. The health care and educational systems serving individuals need to be flexible, accessible, and responsive to family needs.

Can you think of other examples of basic principles or belief statements that could guide your interactions with family members?

Although it is important to discuss these principles of family-centered practice and how they are implemented in a health care setting or an elementary school, it is equally

important to consider all the principles as a whole. Family-centered practice is not just implementing one of these principles in interactions with families. Each type of belief statement reinforces and facilitates the implementation of the others. Together these beliefs convey a shift in philosophy of practice, moving from a traditional medical model, where an expert or doctor solves the problem at hand, to a model that is both collaborative and cooperative and includes the knowledge and expertise of all the people involved with an individual with a disability. The family is obviously central to the concept of family-centered practice and is surrounded by a team of experts and service providers who support the care or education of the individual with a disability. The team may involve physicians, teachers, and related service personnel such as SLPs, occupational therapists (OTs), physical therapists (PTs), and support personnel, like the SLPA, who extend the services provided to the individual with disabilities. The team may change in its makeup depending on the services and support needed, but its purpose remains clear.

Principles of family-centered practice are, in part, based on an ecological theory of human development (Bronfenbrenner, 1977, 1979) that looks at the infant, child, or individual as the center of a series of expanding concentric circles or "nested environments," each contained within the next. The individual is surrounded first by family and then by others living in their home, childcare, school, or community daily life. Each person's circles of influence may be different, depending on the circumstances. People around each individual child will change with experience of differing life events and age. However, as a concept, this model speaks of the involvement of the family, extended family, or caregiver system as typically the first, and often greatest, system of influence and interaction. It is interesting to make comparisons between circles of support that surround each one of us. What people are in your circles of support? Do the people in your circles of support look different than those of an individual with a disability? Should they?

SIDELIGHT: *Kevin's Story*

When my son Kevin was born with Down syndrome, life changed. At first, I said, "Why me? Why us?" I stayed at home for days after we got out of the hospital and just cried. I Isolated myself from friends and family. Eventually, former friends stopped calling. My life revolved around doctor appointments and early intervention therapies. I took Kevin to the program 3 days a week. He then began individual therapy in OT, PT, and, eventually, speech and language. It seemed I was always in a waiting room at the hospital, doctor's office, or in the car. I felt surrounded by well-meaning people but they were professionals. They were not necessarily supporting me as a parent. They were working with Kevin. After about 2 years, I realized I had not seen a number of my friends and family for months and was spending all my time taking care of Kevin and simply trying to survive. It was a very difficult time. One of the therapists noticed how I spent most of my time with Kevin. She talked with me about the need to take care of myself as well as Kevin. She suggested I contact another parent who had an older child with Down syndrome. We met for coffee and talked. I began to see that even though my life had changed with Kevin, I needed to surround myself with circles of support beyond the professionals in his life. I began to talk with family and friends again. I began to do other things besides therapy. I actually came to feel more competent as a parent and felt able to deal with the many challenges in my life with a disabled child.

—Rochelle Williams, parent

BUILDING RELATIONSHIPS BASED ON FAMILY-CENTERED PRACTICE

Many parents and family members agree that once they have a child or other family member identified with a disability, their life changes dramatically. They may have once spent time at work and at home with family or socializing with friends, going to church, and engaging in other recreational activities or hobbies, but suddenly find themselves spending time at numerous weekly therapy appointments, doctor's appointments, on the phone with insurance companies, or meeting with professionals who care for their child or family member with a disability. They find themselves interacting with a whole constellation of people and "systems" that take up a great deal of time and energy (Crais, 1992). The people and activities in their daily life may change on a weekly, monthly, or yearly basis as well. Regaining balance is often

very difficult and in some cases may be impossible to achieve, especially by the family involved with adjusting to having a family member with a disability. The family may find they have less time for family and friends or activities they used to like to do. Families often speak of the need for support in adjusting to new and different experiences and needs. They often report a lack of empathy, understanding, and respect from those who work with their child or family member with a disability.

Principles of family-centered care recognize that our systems of health care and education need to address these issues. Families need support, understanding, and respect, and we need to understand that they may cope with their life changes in many different ways. Many families speak of the cyclical nature of adjusting to traumatic events in their lives, such as identification of a disability in a family member. Many providers use a grief model to explain what is happening to the family system and discuss stages of grieving that may be involved. Stages that encompass emotions such as anger, denial, bargaining, and acceptance are described in the literature by authors such as Kenneth Moses (1983). The parallel is made to a family who is trying to adjust to and "grieve the loss of their dreams," what they thought their child would be like, or the way life was going to be as a couple growing old together when they retired.

Families may recycle through these stages or phases as they deal with transitions or new events in their lives. Transitions that involve leaving the security of the hospital and going home, or transitions that mean one's child is entering the public school or leaving school to live an adult independent life may be especially difficult for families. It is important to understand that this may be what is happening within a family system as they cope and adjust to life changes. Professionals should not take it upon themselves to take over the decision-making process or make assumptions or judgments about a family. Families often report feeling disempowered or angry because service providers tell them how they should act or feel in these situations. Professionals, although often with good intentions, may see the need to "protect the family," withhold information because a family is "not ready," or make a judgment that a family is in "denial"

simply because they disagree with the recommendations that have been made.

These principles and key components can be applied easily to individuals receiving services from an SLP in any setting, and thus apply to your extension of those services. Another definition from a parent (Browne & Smith-Sharp, 1995) involved in developing a family-centered practice in NICUs in Colorado is as follows:

> Family centered care is the compassionate, open, total inclusion of family in the care and decision making process for their baby. In order to accomplish this, a great deal of information must be provided and education must occur, not only regarding medical facts, but also about rights, values, priorities, expectations, and needs of the family. The goal is to leave the power with the family, that is never take it away in the first place, necessitating "empowering" the family at a later date. (p. 13)

Family involvement is also considered essential to improving educational results for children with disabilities. As IDEA legislation emphasizes, family involvement is a strong factor affecting learning and school performance. The several levels of parental rights articulated by IDEA include consent, notification, participation in educational decision for their child, and participation in policy making. These are fully explained in Chapter 8 of this text. But the concept of family-centered practice must extend beyond legislative compliance or the opportunity for true collaboration inherent in the concept may be lost. The research of Carl Dunst and Mary Beth Bruder (1999) extends this concept to include what family members do by engaging their children in a rich array of everyday learning activities. They note that "parents can be partners in reinforcing school learning at home, especially if good communication has been established between the school and home and if the goals on the individual education plan (IEP) or individual family service plan (IFSP), have been written to promote collaboration" (Dunst & Bruder, 1999, p. 2). In their work, Dunst and Bruder have integrated this research into a model for early intervention, which can be summarized as based on chil-

dren's learning opportunities across a variety of situations, parental support that strengthens existing parental knowledge and skills, and family and community supports provided in a family-centered manner. This makes sense for working with all individuals, whether in early intervention, in life skill programs, or in nursing home settings.

A key component that takes place across any setting is the need for communication with those around you. Opportunities to regain functional communication skills may be best practiced in the meaningful context of daily routines and real-life situations with family members or other caregivers in the individual's environment. You will find that effective interactions with families can extend what you are trying to accomplish with individuals you serve. Not only are family members a rich source of information about their family member, their support and understanding can only serve to support the communication abilities of those in need of your services. Encouragement and authentic support of family involvement will further the goals you and your supervising SLP are working toward. Family-centered practice is key to establishing effective working relationships and achieving the goals established in any intervention program you may be involved in.

The concept that families are central to your work is one that you may not have thought of when you decided to become an SLPA. You may have thought, "I just want to work with patients, clients, or students. I don't want to have to deal with the family." Although you may not be directly responsible for sharing information or counseling family members, your relationship with them is important. An attitude of respect, support, and understanding in a nonjudgmental manner may significantly make an impact on your work with a particular individual and must be taken into consideration as you interact with family members and fulfill your responsibilities as an SLPA.

LEARNING FROM FAMILIES

Listening to family stories is not only an effective way to gather information about the patient, client, or student you are working with, it also can solidify your relationship with

family members. Being a good listener may be an integral part of your work. You might ask if this is really necessary. According to Stonestreet, Johnson, and Acton (1991), establishing relationships with families is critical to resolving expectation discrepancies and misinterpretations of behavior that can interfere with the intervention a patient, student, or client is receiving. When asked about their interactions with providers, parents often commented that a communication gap prevented them from understanding what the therapist was doing for their child. Comments included "interventionists or professionals don't listen to us" and "they don't take time with us" (p. 40). According to Stonestreet et al. (p. 40), parents also commented that they were frequently overwhelmed by the vocabulary used to describe their children and that they felt "besieged by acronyms" such as IEP, IFSP, LRE. They also voiced concerns about interventionists and professionals who do not answer their questions. School personnel were reported to sometimes respond to questions with comments like "that is not my area" or "I will refer you to the psychologist." Parents also voiced concern about physicians who say, "he'll out grow it" or "let's wait and see." They also questioned why professionals hedged and often could not just say, "I don't know, but I'll help you find out." Parents also spoke of the professionals who tried to make decisions without their input. The authors (p. 43) also describe the companion concerns expressed by interventionists regarding their interactions with family members. Such comments as "parent's just don't listen to us" or "parents keep information from us and want us to make a decision for them" also point to the gaps in communication that can occur. It is easy to see how these misunderstandings or misperceptions could interfere with any type of intervention program and certainly speaks to the need for open, honest, and respectful channels of communication with family members.

What can you do as an SLPA to improve family member participation in the process? How can you recognize and assist your supervising SLP in responding to the specific needs of particular parents? Here are some helpful ideas adapted from Stonestreet et al. (1991, p. 43), which may facilitate interactions with family members:

- Support an atmosphere of exchange with your SLP and family members.

- Recognize the individual needs of particular parents or family members.

- Refrain from use of professional jargon or terms they may not be familiar with.

- Provide helpful information and resources, which are always filtered through your supervising SLP.

- Be sensitive to the many challenges families face when dealing with emotionally charged situations.

- Recognize the strengths and resilience of families in dealing with difficult situations.

- Invite family members to participate in activities or sessions planned with your SLP.

All of these suggestions are based on your development of active listening skills. It is very important to listen completely before formulating any type of response. Your body language will be important as you listen and acknowledge what you are hearing. Sometimes family members just need a nonjudgmental ear to listen to how their day is going. It may be difficult to suspend judgment about a particular family member's course of action or decision. Perceptions, decisions, and priorities of the family may change from day to day with new circumstances that affect their actions. Sometimes, it is through talking and "trying on" different opinions that family members discover what the best course of action may be for their family or family member with communication challenges. A nonjudgmental and supportive attitude will help you establish relationships with families that can make a difference.

Communication skills that are important to refine when you are working with adults and family members include:

- Active listening skills that let a family member know of your interest and acceptance of the situation

- The ability to wait and listen and not interrupt

- Use of open-ended questions that allows families to share what they choose to share

TOURO COLLEGE LIBRARY

- Development of nonverbal behaviors that communicate your interest and attention to what families are sharing
- Adoption of a nonjudgmental attitude
- Use of silence to allow family members the time they need to share
- Use of nonverbal affirmations to show that you are interested and listening to what is being shared
- Providing respectful affirmations of a family's feelings, including head nods and verbal comments such as "yes, that is an issue" that reflect your listening without judgment about what they are saying

These are active listening skills that you will also use in interactions with patients, clients, or students you work with. It is important to not only develop your listening and communication skills but also to share what you learn from families with your supervising SLP, because the information relates to planning and implementation of successful intervention programs.

Learning from families also involves observing them with the individual you are working with to find out what supports and elicits behaviors that relate to successful communication. Information that comes from family members is often key in determining what works with a particular individual. It is often the parent or family member who can share strategies that have elicited communication attempts or successful communication exchanges. This information can help you learn more about the patient, client, or student's interests, likes, and dislikes, and key strategies for increasing communicative competence in a variety of situations. It is important that you discuss this information with your supervising SLP so that sessions planned and techniques used can be as facilitative as possible for the individual concerned.

FAMILY RIGHTS AND RESPONSIBILITIES

As noted, the family has certain rights and responsibilities that affect your work with patients, clients, or students. It is

important for an SLPA to learn about specific family rights and responsibilities because implementation of related policies and procedures may differ from state to state or across settings. The procedural safeguards afforded patients and family members under the applicable legislation of IDEA and various other federal laws are discussed fully in Chapter 8 of this text. It is important to note that implementation of the intent of the law may vary in terms of the procedure used within a specific setting. However, the rights remain the same. For example, under IDEA, a family has the right to due process, which includes the right to be notified if their child or student is being considered for special education placement before any testing takes place. Multidisciplinary assessment cannot take place until the family has received appropriate notification or has signed a document allowing the assessment to happen. Records and results can only be shared with others outside of the setting, given informed consent of the legal guardian or parent. It is important to realize that there are both legal mandates and ethical considerations involved when working with family members. Although your supervising SLP will take the lead in ensuring that family rights and procedural safeguards are met, you will need to be aware of what is involved so that quality of care is ensured. It would certainly seem that all individuals have the "right" to consent, notification, and participation in the decision-making processes about their child, student, or family member. (See Figure 4-1.)

RESPECTING AND RESPONDING TO INDIVIDUAL AND CULTURAL DIFFERENCES

"The implementation of family centered practice often seems like an elusive goal, even when working with families, matching our own backgrounds, but is further complicated when working with culturally and linguistically diverse populations whose views and language are different from our own" (Sanchez, 1999, p. 351). This is especially complicated when the family speaks a language other than English. Appropriate use of cultural mediators, translators, and inter-

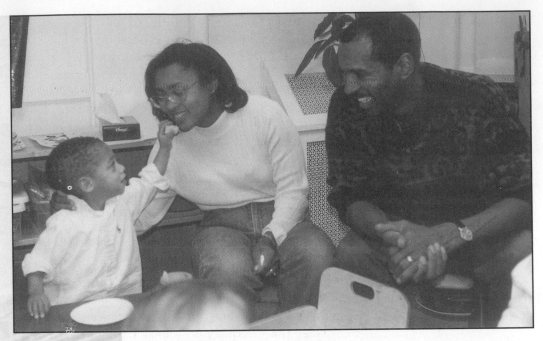

Figure 4-1 A family visiting school

preters, may prove essential with families whose culture or language is different from your own. It is important to read Chapter 6 of this text, which further details cultural and linguistic considerations, when working with individuals from diverse backgrounds. It is also important to understand that we must move beyond stereotypes and overgeneralizations such as "they don't care about their children's education" or "they never show up at meetings" to better understand why a family is making the decisions they are in a given context. Being sensitive and empathic to family concerns, priorities, and resources also reach beyond those families that come from a background different from your own. It includes families that may have chosen a different lifestyle, such as "two-mother families" or adherence to strict religious beliefs and practices that demand different lifeways. Legislative mandates certainly speak of prohibitions against discrimination of any kind, based on racial, ethnic, gender, religious preference, or sexual preferences, but will you be able to move beyond stereotypes or beliefs you have as you work with a variety of parents and family members? Will your skills hold even in situations where you do not agree with the decisions or lifestyle choices of those you work with? Are there situations or people you have worked with in which this has been an issue? How will you deal with these situations if they come up in your work with your supervising SLP?

SIDELIGHT: *Fawzi's Mother*

Fawzi's mother came to this country with her husband to escape religious persecution in her country of origin. She and her husband are practicing Muslims. When they had their second child, who was born with a disability, this family sought support and special education services through their local school district. Fawzi's father was the person who talked at the IEP meeting, although Fawzi's mother attended. She always deferred to her husband if asked questions about her daughter. This proved to be a somewhat uncomfortable situation for the team members, who wanted more information about Fawzi's behavior at home. The SLP could not understand why Fawzi's mother would not respond to her questions or talk with her about things to do at home to improve Fawzi's language abilities. Both she and Fawzi's mother appeared uncomfortable and frustrated with the situation. Fawzi's parents seemed upset when they left the meeting. Fawzi's mother did not return to the next meeting held about her daughter's program. What questions do you have about this scenario? What preparations could the team have made to make this an easier meeting for the family and still obtain the information they needed for program planning?

SPECIFIC STRATEGIES THAT SUPPORT PARENT AND INDIVIDUAL PARTICIPATION AND INVOLVEMENT

What kinds of situations will allow you to make a difference for a child or adult? Situations may include everyday routines at school such as getting ready for an activity; putting materials away before recess; transitions between activities or places that the student is asked to go; literacy activities like book reading, storytelling, physical play, or other play activities inside or out on the playground; classroom or school celebrations; or socialization activities such as talking with friends. Similar activities may apply for the adults with whom you work. Everyday activities and interactions within a meaningful context are key to a successful intervention.

This also means that the SLP and SLPA consider the need for continuity between home and school or home and work. In the case of a child, it is important to inquire what a child likes to do. Is it any different for an adult you may be working with? What makes a person smile may be the piece of information that can guide your interactions and improve success. Family members may be your primary source for this type of information. This means that ongoing communication is a critical tool in helping your supervising SLP and you to relate to families and, most importantly, to the individuals you work with. What can you do to enhance your communication skills in order to improve interactions with all concerned? Review the list of ideas presented in the previous section on learning from families. How do they apply?

QUOTE

Communication does not begin with being understood, but with understanding others.

—W. Stephen Brown

FOCUS ON TALKING WITH YOUNG CHILDREN

Because we are talking about communication skills that you need to use with individuals and families you work with as an SLPA, we have included a section that focuses on parallel skills you can adopt when working with young children. It is important to recognize that you will be working with children who demonstrate challenges in learning language and developing their communicative competence. Thus how you talk with children will, in itself, provide an opportunity for them to develop improved language and speech skills. As an SLPA you can use strategies to enhance the communication skills of young children and model for family members (Figure 4-2) how they can adapt their own speech and language use to be supportive of their child's language learning opportunities.

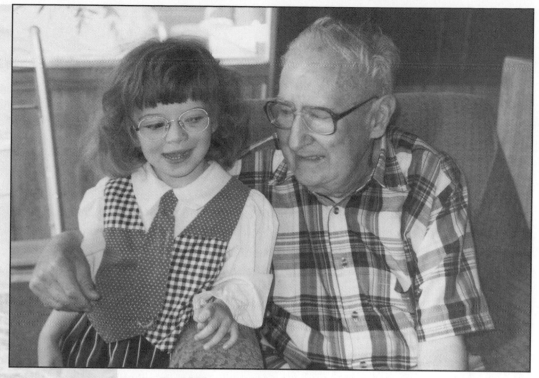

Figure 4-2 A little girl and her grandfather engaging in "family talk"

Interactive Communication Strategies

Children's learning of language is based on responsive relationships. Children learn language(s) through interaction with family members, caregivers, teachers, and peers in the context of their world of everyday routines, activities, and places. Ideally, these interactions are engaging, fun, and frequent. The child is not a passive learner of language and does not have to be directly taught language. In fact, the child is an active participant in the learning of language. It is important to recognize this fact because that is the only way the child can become a competent communicator. However, as teachers, caregivers, and parents, we can facilitate the child's optimal development of language in many ways. Experience certainly supports development of oral proficiency through use of interactive communication strategies in the classroom and home setting.

TALKING POINTS AND FAMILY TALK: INTERACTION IS KEY!

What are the interactive strategies that foster a child's acquisition of language?

■ Following the children's lead during interactions helps them use language with their conversational partners. Partners need to respond to children with interest and provide them with information that relates to what they are talking about. The information must be relevant and appropriate to the children's language level so they can use it to build on what they already know.

■ Wait time is a strategy that provides children an opportunity to talk or initiate conversations. Adults often need to WAIT to allow children to initiate a conversation. Wait for 3 to 5 seconds and see if a child will initiate, and then take your turn.

■ Turn taking provides the foundation for conversation. Babies learn the foundations of conversational turn taking in the back and forth "dance" of cooing and babbling they do with their caregivers. Turn taking is a part of conversation that becomes second nature to most children. Some children with disabilities need help learning turn taking. Once established, children can then adapt their turn-taking knowledge to the situation at hand.

■ Mirroring what the child has said (repeating) or done (nonverbal match) is sometimes helpful. It allows you to first clarify (check in) what the child is trying to say and then provides a basis for you to continue your turn with a model or expansion. This simply involves doing or repeating what the child says. Others may describe it as matching the child's level of language use.

■ Self-talk is sometimes helpful when children are reticent to interact verbally. This can be for many reasons, including when they are exposed to learning a second language, they are shy, or maybe they have been identified as a child with specific language challenges. When a parent or teacher talks about what she is doing while she does it, it is providing the child with a model to help her learn the words being used and to understand communication expectations. However, it is always important to balance the use of self-talk with wait time so that the child has a chance to initiate. Sometimes more talk is not necessarily better.

■ Modeling provides children with information about how we put words together to make complete sentences in our language. For example, a child at a certain level of language development may say, " I gots lots of those at home" or "I runned so fast, he didn't catch me." The teacher or parent will provide a model, such as "You have lots of those at home" or "Oh, you ran so fast, he couldn't catch you." It is important to use descriptive speech and clear articulation, because children will often imitate the model provided. Again, the teacher or parent does not need to correct the child

("You said that wrong...say it this way"), but simply supply a positive model (sentence or clear articulation) for the child to imitate. Children will learn from positive models and be successful in future attempts to put words together in longer and more complex sentences consistent with their language system.

■ Expansion is a way to build on what a child says. As children become more proficient in the verbal communication, as they talk more and use longer and more complex utterances, it helps to " bump up" or "up the ante" and provide an expansion, or an addition, to the sentence structure they have used or the concept they are talking about.

Example: Child says: " Right now! I want to go now!"
Parent says: " You want to go right this very minute! You are ready to go to the park!"

Example: Child says: " They ran across the bridge.
SLPA says: " You're right! The three billy goats all ran across the bridges to get away from that big, mean, ugly troll."

Expansions in themselves, provide models, fulfill your turn, and are responsive to the children's level of language development. They provide a scaffold or framework for the child to add to as they develop improved competence as a communicator.

In summary, use of less directive talk with children is effective in eliciting responses from them (McDonald & Carroll, 1992). Supportive interactions by adults through use of the strategies outlined above will provide the facilitation needed with children who are developing their language(s). For many years, such authors as Weiss (1981), McLean (1989), Snow (1977), and Weitzman (1992), among others, have suggested that less directive talk facilitates the language learning of all children and especially those with identified disabilities. Directive demands for language such as "Tell me..." "Say..." "Tell me the name of this..." "Give me the..." often are less successful in eliciting verbal language with children and often restrict their eagerness to talk.

Sample items from the *Talking Points* (Moore, 2001) self-reflection tool can help you look at your use of the strategies explained above and can be integrated into your work with your SLP supervisor. The *Talking Points* tool (Figure 4-3) is intended for your use as you explore and refine your techniques about how you talk with young chil-

Talking Points: A Self Reflection Tool

Things to Consider

Did I

☐ Watch, observe, and listen before initiating or responding
☐ Allow the children to initiate by using appropriate "wait time"
☐ Ask too many questions
☐ Give too many directions at once
☐ Talk too fast
☐ Interrupt the child
☐ Match the child's level of language and check for comprehension
☐ Encourage questions from the children
☐ Use open-ended questions to scaffold responses
☐ Reduce test questions
☐ Provide choices for answers when needed to scaffold successful responses and participation

Did I

☐ Provide a strong language model—use appropriate grammar and use words appropriately in terms of their meaning
☐ Mirror or repeat what the child is trying to say
☐ Use self-talk by talking about what I am doing
☐ Match the child's level of language
☐ "Bump up" or "up the ante" and expand to the next level
☐ Stay with the child's topic and expand if appropriate
☐ Take advantage of the teachable moment for language and literacy enhancement

Did I

☐ Introduce "new words"
☐ Explain the meaning of words with "word alikes" (really big—large—huge) and negotiate the meaning of new words
☐ "Prime the pump": prepare the child by ensuring he/she knows key words in an activity
☐ "Frame" and incorporate basic concepts ("beginning—middle and end") into conversations
☐ Provide a variety of activities and books to solidify new learning

I'm really good at ...

I need to think about how I ...

Figure 4-3 Talking Points: A Self-Reflection Tool

dren to facilitate their language learning in a developmentally appropriate sequence.

Did you know that research in classrooms regarding talking behaviors indicates that engaging children in conversations and use of a wide vocabulary by teachers is correlated with the children's success in developing language and literacy (Dickinson & Smith, 1994)? Another study by Philips (1987) shows the quality of conversation in the classroom and the amount of one-on-one or small group conversational interactions are highly related to language learning. As noted in the 1998 report on *Preventing Reading Difficulties in Young Children* by the National Research Council, the quality of adult-child talk is important, as is the overall amount or frequency of such interactions. Dickinson and Smith report that the amount of talk that children experience is correlated with the amount of time they talk with adults. An extensive study by Hart and Risley (1995) also indicates that the amount of talk and the kinds of vocabulary words used in conversation at home make a difference in how well children develop their language. Studies have shown that the quality of verbal interactions and exposure to interactive storybook reading experiences with teachers and caregivers make a difference in language and literacy learning (Kontos & Wilcox-Hertzog, 1997; Layzer, 1993; Neuman, 1995). Our observations of behaviors in classrooms are consistent with the conclusions in the studies listed above. Observed behaviors of teachers suggest that they ask questions more often than they comment on what a child has said or done. Many teachers ask a very high proportion of "test" questions when they already know the answer. Observations indicate that teachers and therapists initiate more often than they allow children to initiate, and that teachers often choose a topic for conversation rather than responding to a child's initiation. It is important to note that when a caregiver's or a teacher's talk dominates, the child's language is restricted.

Janet Stone (1993) discusses the concepts of responsive talk versus restrictive talk. She explains responsive language as talk that conveys a positive attitude and respect for and acceptance of a child's individual ideas. She provides examples of teacher requests or commands expressed in nur-

turing ways that help the child to understand as responsive talk. Restrictive talk is described as language that involves teacher control, reflected in threats, punishments, and criticisms or disrespectful commands such as "Get that out of here" or "Sit down now" (p. 150). Restrictive language involves lectures versus explanations. Use of restrictive language can discourage independence and verbal give and take. Use of nurturant language such as "I need each of you to put your books back on the shelf so we can go outside" instead of "No one is going outside until this is all picked up!" It is important to think about how you talk with children because how you talk and what you say can influence how the child feels about herself or whether or not she becomes a competent communicator. It is also helpful to remember these ideas when you are talking with adults. A positive attitude, respect, and patience are necessary with any individual who is having difficulty with communication.

Other Helpful Strategies

As an SLPA, how can you balance the use of questions and comments to scaffold a child's learning? How do you use the right type of questions, at the right time and in the right way? Following are some thoughts to consider about four types of questions:

- Do you ask test questions, which is a question that requires an answer you already know the answer to or that the child knows the answer to?

    Examples: "What color is that?"

    "What is your name?"

    "How old are you?"

- Are you asking authentic questions that require information that you might not know about?

    Examples: "Did you have fun yesterday when you went to the park?"

    "What did you do?"

    "Who went with you?"

- Are you asking a closed question that may only require a nod of the head or a one-word answer?

Will this work to encourage the child to talk more or just give a one-word answer?

Examples: "Did your daddy bring you to school today?"

"Do you want a turn?"

■ Are you asking an open-ended question that would allow the child to use language at the level she is capable of and provide you with a sample of how she uses language to express herself?

Examples: "I wonder what will happen next?"

"My, that's a interesting picture...tell me about it?"

In summary, asking questions is a balancing act. Some children may benefit from your use of different types of questions at different stages in their development and at different times, depending on why you are asking the question. However, it is critical to know about and use the types of questions that can facilitate and expand on what children know and can tell you about their world (McDonald & Carroll, 1992). Watch your SLP in sessions. How does she use questions effectively to elicit responses?

SUGGESTIONS FOR SUCCESSFUL COMMUNICATION

When talking with young children or adults with communication challenges, it is sometimes helpful to keep the following summary of suggestions in mind:

■ Reduce conversational overload. "Talk, talk, and more talk" is not necessarily better.

■ Slow down the pace. "Rapid fire" speech or too many questions at once may overwhelm children or any individual, especially if their receptive language skills are limited or not fully developed.

■ Change or adapt the language you use to help the child or adult understand what you are trying to say

■ Use comments and questions to continue the conversation, not control the conversation

■ Avoid questions that STOP the conversation.

Elaine Weitzman (1992, p. 79) talks about three strategies for talking with young children. She uses the terms *observe, wait, and listen*. This helpful hint comes from the HANEN program as described in *Learning Language and Loving It: A Guide for Promoting Children's Social and Language Development in Early Childhood Settings* (1992). This text is a rich compilation of information that you can also use with family members to explain how young children develop and acquire their language. Weitzman (1992, pp. 48–65) presents a summary review of the stages of communication and language development. In general, the language you hear from young children increases in length and complexity from about 12 months of age through the early childhood years. It is commonly believed that babies are born with the ability to acquire language and learn the language(s) they are exposed to from their family and culture. You need to be aware of and review information about when and how young children develop language.

According to Weitzman (1992, p. 150), *observing* means paying close attention to the child so you can see exactly what she's interested in or what she's trying to tell you. This is a critical skill so that you can match the child's language level as you respond and take your turn. Weitzman (p. 151) also discusses the importance of waiting as a powerful tool because it allows the child the opportunity to initiate. This supports the child in becoming an active learner versus a passive learner of her language. It provides the message "you're in control and I know you can communicate and I'll give you the time you need." Listening (p. 150) means paying close attention to what the child is saying so that you can respond on the topic, following the child's lead, and in doing so you convey the message that what the child is saying is important. Active listening involves not interrupting the child or assuming that you understand what she is trying to say before she has finished speaking.

Another way to remember these strategies is SOUL, as described by Weiss (1981, p. 41). SOUL stands for Silence, Observation, Understanding and Learning. If you are silent and take the time to observe and understand the level at which the child is functioning and listen to what she is trying to say, you can match the level that is needed to facilitate the child's language learning. According to Weiss, this provides a basis for knowing which responsive talking strategy to use next with a child. It allows the child time to initiate, and it allows you time to know how you can support the child's communication through mirroring or matching what the child says, modeling through conversational interactions, self-talk or talking about what you are doing as you do it, parallel talk about what the child is doing during play, or expansion and elaboration of what the child has said.

Your supervising SLP might suggest using the *Talking Points* self-reflection tool as a quick and easy way for you to explore your own "talking" style the with children you are seeing. Take a moment to look at this tool. What is your first reaction? Could it help you to really know more about how you talk with young children? Many teachers, therapists, and family members benefit from videotaping a segment of conversation with an individual child or a small group of children. Try it and explore ways to optimally refine your conversational interactions with young children.

CONNECTIONS TO HOME

Preparing materials with children that they can take home to share with their parents, brothers, sisters, and grandparents is another way to help children practice what they are learning. Parents also benefit from learning about "helpful hints" or ways of talking with their children. As an SLPA, you might help develop the following:

- A newsletter article that could go in the school publication about "helpful hints for talking to your child"

- A bulletin board for the hallway in your school that illustrates "helpful hints"

- A handout to be sent home that explains different strategies for talking with young children

Other Ways to Support Young Children's Language and Literacy Development

It is also critically important that we move beyond the how's of talking and explore what we say to young children that can

enhance their language and literacy learning. Some techniques to consider as you work with young children in the context of learning new information may be helpful to review.

Priming the Pump

Priming or priming the pump is a technique used by many early childhood teachers, SLPs, and other interventionists to target specific concepts or new vocabulary before introducing a new book or activity. You introduce and review targeted concepts in a meaningful context through play or other activities so that children have the information they need to participate in a new activity or comprehend a story you are reading to them. This is especially important to second language learners who may not have specific experience with a word or concept.

Example: Introduce and integrate basic concepts such as "butterfly," "cocoon," "caterpillar," and "change" as well as days of the week when reading *The Very Hungry Caterpillar* by Eric Carle, by using a calendar repeatedly to plan what will happen on Monday, Tuesday, or Wednesday. Have a butterfly in the room, visit the butterfly pavilion on a field trip with parents, post pictures of butterflies on the walls, and place related books on the bookshelf. Talk about the words and concepts with children during different times of the day and at snack time. Ask questions such as "I wonder what butterflies eat?" and wave your arms like a butterfly during music and movement activities. This is a way to integrate new learning and expand on what the child already knows.

Predicate the Topic

Predicate the topic means introducing topics with the relevant predicate so the appropriate context for the topic is provided. Young children need high context, lots of clues, and cues to ensure comprehension of new words and concepts. We might assume they know a word or concept through experience, but they may need the repetitive and various

contextual examples to expand their knowledge. This again is especially important for second-language learners who may not have the links needed to make sense of how a new word is used. Children learn through experience and then map their world knowledge with words. Use visual cues, props, and actual experiences to highlight connections and ensure understanding.

Example: When talking about food, talk about it in context of "buying food, eating food, and shopping for food at the grocery store."

Story Extension or Elaborating Schema

Story extension activities or elaborating the schema means systematic use of play and sensory-motor experiences (cooking, art, science, toys you can handle, music, and movement) to extend and elaborate existing schemas (or what the child knows about a specific topic) through use of "scripts" and "routines" to help the child, especially preschool age children, learn new vocabulary and language.

Example: Use the Happy Birthday song as a "script" for having a birthday party for a child and integrate and expand through activities such as making party invitations, pretend baking of a cake, etc. This a wonderful opportunity to read *Arthur's Birthday* by Marc Brown and talk about how all the children celebrate birthdays in different ways at home.

Here to Then Connections

Here to Then Connections are made by extending conversations beyond the "here and now" to provide opportunity for children to talk about past or future events and practice the higher level language structures that denote this in their grammar. Children with language challenges sometimes have difficulty using high-level syntactical constructions that denote their intended meaning.

Example: "Today is Monday and we are getting ready for a trip. Where will we go on Friday? What will you need to bring for the trip?"

Making Explicit What Is Implicit

Making explicit what is implicit is about making inferences. This is often difficult for young children learning language. It is difficult to teach inferencing but you can build a foundation for this developing ability by offering a model of how we connect thoughts by filling in missing links with more information and through use of redundancy. Say it again in another way to help the children understand the connections.

Example: "How did that caterpillar become a butterfly? How did he change? First he built his cocoon and stayed inside for several days. It took time for him to change just like it takes time for you to grow up. You need time to grow and get ready to be big. As you grow up, you will change too. You might grow taller and stronger. When the butterfly was ready, he came out of that cocoon. He was ready to be a butterfly and fly away. You will get ready and when you are older, you will go to another school."

Return to the Story

Children enjoy activities that relate to a story that retells tasks and acting out the story. Using flannel board pictures for story reenactment and making puppets and props available for play are all ways to help children return to the story and replay it in a multitude of ways. Some children use this as an opportunity to practice new words learned and solidify their understanding of new concepts. Through repetition and practice, children become less dependent on high context and props and increase their ability to abstract information and use it in new situations.

Example: Jason's SLPA made a troll character and found three goats that Jason could use during play after he read the book. At first Jason wanted to be the "mean ugly troll" so he could try and catch the three billy goats crossing the bridge out on the playground. All he did was growl fiercely, and then with more practice he started using the script, saying, "Who is that crossing over my bridge?" He loved to use the three billy goats in the sand table and reenact the drama with the bridge that he had built with blocks in the

sand. He practiced so many times, he could say the parts of the billy goats as well as his own as the troll.

Negotiating the Meaning

Negotiating the meaning means using questions to clarify and expand on the meaning of words. Sometimes children do not understand how to use a new vocabulary word and need help learning its meaning in a particular context.

Example: "It says he's exhausted. Hmm, I thought that meant he was very tired. What do you think it means? How do you think he feels after running so far?"

Scaffolding With Questions

Scaffolding with questions involves the skill of prediction. Prediction and knowledge of sequence are important for building the foundations for later success in reading comprehension. Use of leading questions to facilitate a child's ability to organize story events or activities is helpful in building this foundation.

Example: "Oh, it is scary. What do you think will happen next?" or "You're right, we are going to put the cookies in the oven, but what do we need to do first?"

Create Stories

Once children are knowledgeable about a basic storyline or the sequence of an activity is established, they enjoy changing the events, involving new or "made-up" characters and elaborating on the events. Supplying graphics, pictures, and materials for children to use to create their own story is a way for them to bring something home and share their new learning. "Stories" that go home and are read, illustrated, or retold and discussed with parents or siblings are wonderful ways to extend new learning and involve family members in their child's program.

Example: After reading the story of the three bears so many times, Alex made up a story about the three dogs based on the theme of the three bears. He dictated the story to his

SLPA while he was practicing his speech. He then illustrated the story and took it home to read to his parents. He also was practicing correct productions of his target sounds /d/ and /g/ each time he read the story.

Framing

Framing means providing a framework that helps children comprehend basic vocabulary concepts they need in school. Expectations are high for young children entering kindergarten to know and be able to use basic concepts. Basic concepts such as *first*, *second*, *last*, *before and after*, *in front of*, *behind*, and *through* are used in helping children negotiate the meaning of everyday activities and routines. Use of basic story-grammar frames helps children organize and sequence such concepts as *beginning*, *middle*, and *end*. Help children frame their world by introducing and using these basic concepts in their everyday routines. Recognize that some are learned earlier and those that are more abstract are learned later as children develop competency in the nuances of their language. Use these concepts in your everyday conversations with children, explaining them if needed. Find out what kindergarten teachers expect and help children prepare for transition by incorporating these concepts into their everyday routine activities and places.

Example: Although John seemed to understand the concepts of first, second, and last, his SLP suggested that these concepts be reviewed and integrated into a number of activities he was doing in therapy. She knew his kindergarten teacher would expect him to know what came first, what was second, and what came last. The SLP wanted him to have practice using these concepts in a number of different situations so he would be ready for kindergarten-level work.

In summary, there are many developmentally appropriate ways to support young children's learning of their language so that they become competent communicators and are "ready for school." The preceding suggestions are examples of successful ways you can enhance and build foundations for language and literacy learning with young children receiving service from your supervising SLP. These strategies can also be adapted and shared with family members

through newsletter articles on "Helpful Hints" for talking with their child at home, attractively displayed on parent bulletin boards, during parent conferences, or in other parent education program efforts.

It is important to note that every child is respected as an individual learner and has her own timetable for acquiring language. However, we know language learning is predictable and occurs in stages (Weitzman, 1992). As SLPAs, it is helpful for us to know where a child is functioning at any given point in time as well as what would be the "next steps" in her development. Knowing next steps helps you choose effective strategies and techniques to facilitate children's growth and development in language. Your supervising SLP will help you understand what is next so that you understand what you need to do to support and improve children's and adults' speech and language abilities.

CONCLUSION

This chapter contains a great deal of information regarding how you can improve your skills when interacting with family members, individuals with communication challenges, and young children. The information presented revolves around the central theme of interactive and responsive communication. Your development and improvement of your own communication abilities can affect the relationships you develop with those adults you work with and their families. It is also critically important to understand and refine your abilities to interact with young children if you are going to work with this population, because what you say and how you say it can make an impact on their language learning and help build the foundations for later development of literacy. Communication is key on several levels, and attention to refining your skills in this area will serve you well in any context in which you choose to work. Communication skills will lay the groundwork for building relationships with other personnel and teams you work with, which can make your chosen career rewarding and enjoyable.

DISCUSSION QUESTIONS

1. What are the key components of family-centered practice? How do they apply to your work as an SLPA across settings and with different populations?

2. What is your role with families? What attitudes and skills will be helpful to you in enhancing your relationships with families? Do these vary across settings?

3. Review what you know about how young children learn language. Based on principles of language acquisition, do the talking points make sense? What about different styles of interaction and how they can make a difference in your interactions with young children?

SUGGESTED ACTIVITIES

1. Take the time to have a conversation with the family members of an individual who has a disability. Listen to their stories. What can you learn from these stories about how family members might react to the identification of a disability in a member of their family? What are their priorities, concerns, and resources that come into play when discussing the situation? Ask them to share with you what they consider to be important skills a care provider must have when working with their family.

2. Role play an interaction with a peer and have a third party observe the ways you communicate both nonverbally and verbally. Notice who says what to whom and how it is said. Discuss how nonverbal communication can change the intent of the words you use if misinterpreted by another.

3. Brainstorm situations wherein listening to families may prove critical to the success of an intervention program for an individual with communication challenges. Discuss how you can work with your supervising SLP to gather and use this information in a productive way.

4. Videotape yourself in interaction with a young child or adult. Review the videotape. Refer to the *Talking Points* self-assessment tool (Moore, 2001). Reflect on your use of the specific strategies and techniques outlined in this chapter and listed on the tool. How did you do? Are there specific strategies or skills you need to develop to enhance your interactions with others?

REFERENCES

Als, H., & Gilkerson, L. (1995). Developmentally supportive care in the neonatal intensive care unit. *Zero to three, 15,* 2–10.

Bailey, D. (1991). Building positive relationships with families. In M. McGonical, R. Kaufmann, & B. Johnson (Eds.), *Guidelines and recommended practices for the IFSP* (2nd ed.), (pp. 29–38) Bethesda, MD: Association for the Care of Children's Health.

Berman, C. (1994). Family-directed evaluation and assessment under the Individuals with Disabilities Education Act (IDEA): Lessons learned from experiences of programs and parents. *Zero to Three, 14,* 16–22.

Bronfenbrenner, U. (1977). Toward an experimental ecology of human development. *American Psychologist, 32,* 513–531.

Bronfenbrenner, U. (1979). *The ecology of human development: Experiment by nature and design.* Cambridge, MA: Harvard University Press.

Brown, M. (1996). Arthur's Birthday. New York: Random House Media Products.

Browne, J., & Smith-Sharp, S. (1995). The Colorado consortium of intensive care nurseries: Spinning a web of support for Colorado infants and children. *Zero to Three, 15,* 12–15.

Carle, E. (1989). *The very hungry caterpillar.* New York: Putnam.

Crais, E. R. (1991). *A practical guide to embedding family-centered content into existing speech-language pathology coursework.* Chapel Hill: North Carolina. Carolina Institute for Research on Infant Personnel Preparation, FPG Child Development Center, University of North Carolina at Chapel Hill.

Crais, E. R. (1992). Moving from parent involvement to family-centered services. *American Journal of Speech-Language Pathology, 1,* 5–8.

Dickinson, D. K., & Smith, M. W. (1994). Long-term effects of preschool teachers' book reading on low-income children's vocabulary and story comprehension. *Reading Research Quarterly, 19,* 104–122.

Dunst, C., Trivette, C., & Deal, A. (1988). *Enabling and empowering families.* Cambridge, MA: Brookline Books.

Dunst, C., & Bruder, M. (1999). Family and community activity settings, natural learning environments, and children's learning opportunities. *Children's Learning Opportunities Report, 1,* 1.

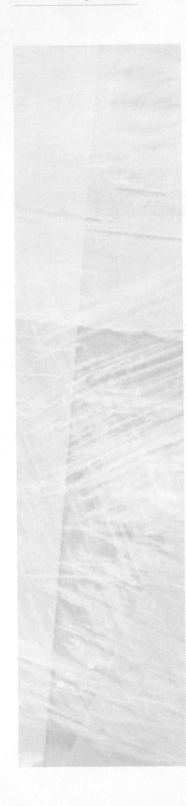

Guralnick, M. J. (1997). *The effectiveness of early intervention.* Baltimore: Paul H. Brookes.

Hart, B., & Risley, T. R. (1995). *Meaningful differences in the everyday experiences of young American children.* Baltimore: Paul H. Brookes.

Kontos, S., & Wilcox-Hertzog, S. (1997). Teacher's interaction with children: Why are they so important? *Young Children, 52,* 4–12.

Layzer, J. J. (1993). *Observational study of early childhood programs* (Final Report, Vol: 1). Life in preschool. Cambridge, MA: Abt Associates.

McDonald J., & Carroll, J. (1992). A social partnership model for assessing early communication development: An intervention model for pre-conversational children. *Language Speech and Hearing Services in Schools, 23,* 113–124.

McLean, J. (1989). A language-communication intervention model. In D. Bernstein & E. Tigerman (Eds.), *Language and communication disorders in children* (pp. 203–228). Columbus, OH: Merrill.

McWilliam, R. A. (1992). *Family-centered intervention planning: A routines–based approach.* Tuscon, AZ: Communication Skill Builders.

Moore, S. (2001). Talking points: A self-reflection tool. In S. Adams, S. M. Moore, & D. Wittmer (Eds.), *Ready to read, write & relate handbook* (pp. 24–28). Denver: Great Kids Head Start.

Moore, S. M., Eiserman, W., & Ferguson, A. (1995). *The Spectrum Project.* U.S. Department of Education, Office of Special Education Programs (No. H024D60007). University of Colorado at Boulder.

Moore, S. M., Eiserman, W., & Ferguson, A. (1996). *Information sharing and program planning processes: A self-reflection tool* (Project ACT). Colorado Department of Education, University of Colorado at Boulder.

Moses, K. (1983). The impact of initial diagnosis: Mobilizing family resources. In J. A. Mulick & S. M. Pueschel (Eds.), *Parent professional partnerships in developmental disability services* (pp. 11–34). Cambridge, MA: Academic Guide.

Philips, (1987). Child-care quality and children's social development. *Developmental Psychology, 23,* 537–543.

Sanchez, S. (1999). Learning from the stories of culturally and linguistically diverse families and communities. *Remedial and Special Education, 20,* 351–359.

Snow, C. (1977). Development of conversations between mothers and babies. *Journal of Child Language, 4,* 1–22.

Snow, C., Burns, S., & Griffin, P. (Eds.). (1998). *Preventing reading difficulties in young children.* Washington, DC: National Academy Press.

Stone, J. (1993) Caregiver and teacher language: Responsive or restrictive. *Young Children, 48,* 149–155.

Stonestreet R. H., Johnson, R. G., & Acton, S. (1991). Guidelines for real partnerships with parents. *Infant Toddler Intervention: The Transdiciplinary Journal, 1,* 37–46.

Weiss, R. S. (1981). INREAL: Intervention for language handicapped and bilingual children. *Journal of the Division of Early Childhood, 4*, 40–51.

Weitzman, E. (1992). *Learning language and loving it.* Toronto, Ontario, Canada: A Hanen Center Publication.

CHAPTER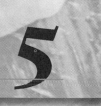

Working With Personnel in Your Setting

Key Concepts

■

Teams of professional work together in a collaborative manner to ensure quality of care and education for all individuals served regardless of the setting or disciplines involved.

■

Teams may look different depending on the model of interaction used, such as multidisciplinary, interdisciplinary, or transdisciplinary. The model used is often influenced by the setting and function to be performed.

■

Teams that function well require leadership, expertise, time to develop, and collaborative strategies that demand open, respectful communication.

■

Roles and boundaries between disciplines must be respected to promote positive interactions among all concerned.

■

It is important to understand the "culture" of your work setting, be it a hospital, school, rehabilitation center, agency, or private practice.

■

Strategies that promote positive interactions between team members focus on open and honest communication and collaboration.

Overview

■

Knowing the Team

■

Team Models and Teaming

■

Understanding Your Setting

■

Boundaries and Interactions Associated With a Specific Setting

■

Strategies to Promote Positive Interactions and Experiences

125

INTRODUCTION

This chapter focuses on the roles of the team members you may interact with in a particular setting and the "culture" of different settings you may choose to work in with a supervising speech-language pathologist (SLP). As a speech-language pathology assistant (SLPA), you might choose to work in a school district, hospital or agency setting, private practice, or another setting that serves individuals with communication challenges. It is important that you choose a setting that serves the population you are interested in working with. If you know you want to work with children, you might choose to work in a public school, a community-based setting, or a children's hospital that serves the pediatric population. If you want to work with adults who have communication problems such as aphasia after a stroke or motor speech problems associated with head injury, or communication challenges associated with progressive neurologic disease processes, then you may choose to work in a hospital or rehabilitation setting. However, you will find some overlap in the ages of individuals served and types of disorders identified across settings. For example, an SLP or group of SLPs in a private practice setting may see many different individuals with a variety of challenges, including stuttering problems, vocal abuse or other voice problems, and learning disabilities. It is important to start thinking now about the population you want to work with and the setting you would like to work in.

FOR YOUR CONSIDERATION

To be ready for your setting, you will need to do the following:

- Review the types of disorders, medical conditions, or developmental challenges associated with communication, speech, or language problems.
- Learn about the roles of various professionals, representing several disciplines, who may function on a team in a given setting and provide services to a particular individual.
- Understand the different types of service delivery models that may vary across settings.

This chapter also addresses issues associated with maintaining positive relationships with the individuals you

may work with in a variety of settings. It is important to understand how a particular team may function given the setting and services provided. Each setting will present an individual "culture" or environment that has many unspoken rules or norms for interactions with team members and the individuals served. A hierarchy may exist that dictates policy and procedures that affect how services are delivered and how people interact in a given setting. Knowing the background, the history, and context of a given setting will help you establish and maintain positive relationships not only with your supervising SLP, but also with others you may work with in that setting.

KNOWING THE TEAM

You will be working directly with your supervising SLP as an extender of services to individuals with communication challenges. As noted in previous chapters, you are directly responsible to your supervising SLP and need to work closely with him to clarify your role and expectations in any given setting. As you work with your SLP, you may find that you are also interacting with a larger team of professionals that are all providing services to individuals who may have concomitant motor problems, social emotional challenges, or other intervention needs in addition to their speech, language, or hearing challenge. You may come in contact with occupational therapists, physical therapists, nutritionists, psychologists, various medical professionals, nurses or physicians, classroom teachers, special education teachers, principals and other administrators, depending on your setting.

Physical therapists (PTs) are trained to assess and provide intervention in relation to physical movement abilities or disabilities. They are interested in motor development or motor performance and functional movement patterns that have to do with mobility and stability. They help individuals develop strength, mobility, and range of motion in joints and muscles to facilitate activities of daily living. They often have a bachelor's degree but many have a master's degree or area of specialization. You will hear PTs talk about **range of motion** and **neuromuscular** impairments. They may discuss muscle tone and **neurodevelopmental** status. They can be

very helpful as a member of a team in determining if a motor problem is interfering with functional abilities and are a rich resource for strategies to work with individuals in terms of their seating and mobility. They can provide stabilization techniques and other very functional considerations that affect how an individual will be able to benefit from a session that focuses on listening and communicating. For example, if a young child with cerebral palsy is not seated appropriately in a supportive and stable position, they will find it very difficult to concentrate on the specific speech and language tasks you may be presenting to them. It would be difficult for you to concentrate on reading this book if you were off balance and worried about falling out of your chair. Physical therapists are often seen in hospital settings or rehabilitation settings with both children and adults and provide important information to the team about managing motor impairments.

Occupational therapists (OTs) are also concerned with motor function and may be on the team in a school-based program as well as in a more medically related setting, such as a hospital or rehabilitation center. They often work with students to also improve skills in activities of daily living such as walking, writing, access to keyboarding, and self-feeding skills. They are skilled at using the muscle strength and range of joint movement developed by the PT to adapt and teach activities of daily living. Some school employees question the need for an OT in the schools because they assume that OTs are trained to focus on adults who are undergoing occupational or vocational rehabilitation, to reenter the workforce after an accident or other physical trauma. However, OTs are often a rich resource for helping to determine home or classroom adaptations or adaptive equipment that facilitates access, especially if fine motor tasks are involved. Access is about being able to effectively reach, point, or use equipment or materials in the environment of the individual. OTs often have a bachelor's degree and designate their credential by adding OTR after their name. This stands for registered occupational therapist. They are employed in various settings to provide services to both adults and children. You will hear terms such as *motor planning (praxis)*, defined as smooth execution of fine motor movements during learned tasks like writing. You may also hear OTs talk about sensory processing and sensorimotor

integration (SI), which involves how a student or child receives and perceives information through a variety of sensory systems. They may talk about a child being underresponsive or hypersensitive to various stimulations. For example, an OT may be very concerned about a young child's hypersensitivity or **tactile defensiveness** to various materials or sensations. OTs and SLPs often work in tandem or collaboratively in a pediatric or early childhood setting to improve the sensory motor as well as related language challenges and behavioral issues associated with sensory defensiveness and difficulty or inability to use communication.

As described by Longhurst (1997), the therapists from the three disciplines (OT, PT, and SLP) often collaborate and integrate services on related service teams to support teachers and improve classroom learning for students or in hospital and rehabilitative settings with both children and adults. Their intervention skills are often seen as complementary and closely interrelated, and more often therapists from these disciplines are trained together to work in an interdisciplinary or transdisciplinary fashion. Each of these disciplines now uses a multiskilled, multilevel workforce that incorporates the use of assistants. All three therapy professions, represented by their respective national associations, the American Physical Therapy Association (APTA), the American Occupational Therapy Association (AOTA), and the American Speech-Language-Hearing Association (ASHA), have established formal scope of responsibility statements and personnel preparation standards for support personnel. The AOTA and APTA, and individual states recognize support personnel through formal credentials. The AOTA and APTA also accredit training programs. As noted, ASHA registers SLPAs and approves training programs as well. You may find more information about how support personnel are credentialed and used in your state's practice acts, licensure statutes, or certification regulations.

There are many similarities across the three disciplines in their training and use of assistants or support personnel. Although the amount, level, or type of training may vary, each assistant works as an extender of services of intervention programs, designed and supervised by their supervising professional. The amount of supervision and degrees of independence based on training and experience as well as dele-

SUPPORT PERSONNEL

The support personnel for each discipline—occupational therapy, physical therapy, and speech-language pathology are described as follows:

■ The physical therapist assistant (PTA), typically completes a two-year associate degree in an APTA accredited program and delivers services in the practice of physical therapy as delegated by and under the supervision of the practicing physical therapist. PTs and PTAs work in a variety of clinical settings. This team is concerned with increasing quality of movement through range of motion exercises and uses all types of supportive equipment as well as therapeutic techniques to improve seating and mobility of individuals with motor impairments.

■ The certified occupational therapy assistant (COTA) also completes a two-year education in an AOTA accredited program that includes coursework and field work. The COTA is a qualified assistant who provides services under the supervision of the OTR and carries out the treatment for an individual that has been designed by the OTR after the OTR's evaluation. OTRs and COTAs help individuals attain or regain more independence in their individual activities of daily living. As noted, with young children, the OT team may focus on sensory processing, sensory perception (awareness of sensations from joints, muscles, and skin receptors) and praxis (motor planning, including how to get from here to there and smoothly and effortlessly executing motor behaviors). The OT team may work with those children who are hypersensitive (too much) or hyposensitive (too little) to touch; children with concentration, attention, or hyperactivity behaviors; children with balance issues and who may appear clumsy or have difficulty organizing and planning what they do. OT and SLP practices sometimes overlap with regard to feeding activities because OTs are concerned with the daily living activity of independence of feeding and thus often are concerned with oral motor and swallowing function, and SLPs are concerned with oral motor development and function as it relates to communication as well as swallowing disorders (dysphasia).

■ As an SLPA you will also complete specified training in an accredited SLPA program at the two-year level consistent with the current ASHA model, or you will complete another training program, perhaps at the BA level consistent with the practices or licensure regulations in your state. You will complete tasks that have been designed or developed by your SLP and under the direct supervision of your supervising SLP, as described in Chapter 2 of this text.

gation of specific responsibilities may vary for each, depending on the state or setting. Specific guidelines and scope of assigned responsibilities can be found in organizational documents or state licensure laws. It is important to note that in some states, other levels of support personnel may be recog-

nized and have a different level of training such as therapy aides across the disciplines who have a much lower level of responsibility (e.g., transporting patients, preparing materials, restocking supplies, etc). They often receive on-the-job training after high school and are not trained to deliver intervention service under supervision.

The three disciplines—occupational therapy, physical therapy, and speech-language pathology—are often part of an interdisciplinary or transdiciplinary team model of intervention in a hospital or rehabilitation setting. The three disciplines thus have a number of things in common despite differences in typical level of education and scope of practice. Because of these commonalities, the three professional organizations at the national level have formed a tri-alliance, and work together to promote improvements in health care and education practices for consumers through collaborative activities.

There are many other professionals from various disciplines whom you may come in contact with as you work with your supervising SLP. In health care settings, you will be interacting with a number of medical personnel, which may include physicians with the following specialties:

- Pediatrics or children (developmental pediatricians)
- Neurology or brain function (neurologists)
- Specialized care of premature infants (neonatologists)
- Ears, nose, and throat doctors (otolaryngologists)
- X-rays and other radiographic ways of determining disorders such as swallowing dysfunctions (radiologists)
- Rehabilitation of individuals after injury or those born with medical conditions (physiatrists)

You will most likely learn a great deal about the specialties within the medical profession if you choose to work in this setting. You may work with the nursing staff that has also chosen to specialize in a specific area such as neonatal intensive care or oncology (cancer), and you may also interact with respiratory therapists, social workers, psychologists, neurodevelopmental specialists, and, of course, audiologists,

who may be in your same department and are in charge of assessment and management of hearing disorders.

In school settings you may be interacting with professionals in an educational context, including what are considered to be related service personnel. These may include professionals who deal with:

- Emotional or social-emotional challenges and behavioral challenges (educational psychologists or school psychologists)
- Reading disorders (reading specialists)
- Fine motor, sensorimotor or sensory-integration issues (OTs)
- Gross motor challenges (PTs)
- Achievement problems related to learning issues (special education teachers)
- Regular classroom teachers
- Paraprofessional support staff that may be assigned to a specific child or classroom
- Bilingual specialists or English language learning (ESL) teachers
- Administrators such as special education coordinators or directors
- Assistant principals or principals of the school
- Audiologists

The SLP and audiologist often work very closely together given the overlap in expertise and interests regarding those individuals who are deaf or hard of hearing. In community-based settings you may interact with some of the professionals mentioned above as well as mental health professionals, community health nurses, family advocates, as well as family resource consultants, depending on the age served and the function of the agency. In private practice you may be interacting with the referring physician, social workers, neuropsychologists, and others, depending on the focus area of the practice. It is important for you to learn about the roles and responsibilities of all the professionals you may interact with in a particular setting.

In any school, department, or agency, you will most likely learn about the hierarchy of the organization and who is responsible for what in terms of scope of practice, administrative responsibility, and the sometimes overlapping matrix of professionals who work on teams to improve health care and supports. You may be exposed to differences in territorial functioning or turf battles among team members given their training, interests, perceived scope of responsibility, or the stringency of application of the traditional medical model as well as history of the organization.

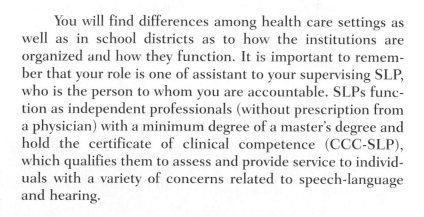

SIDELIGHT: *OTs or SLPs?*

Tracy worked as an SLPA in a children's hospital setting. She was amazed at the turf war that was taking place between the OTs and SLPs. Members from both departments were constantly talking about who was better qualified to handle patients with swallowing and feeding problems. It was a major topic in cafeteria discussions. It seemed that both disciplines thought swallowing and oral motor work were in the scope of practice. They disagreed about who would handle the patients needing swallowing evaluations and therapy. OTs said they had been working on feeding for years and thus swallowing was within their scope of practice. Tracy was feeling compromised because she had several friends who worked in the OT department. They were constantly badmouthing her supervisor. She hated being in this situation because she respected her supervisor and knew she had recently come to this hospital with many years of experience and specialized training in **dysphagia** and feeding. She felt the need to defend her mentor and supervisor. She was so happy when the administrators in both programs got together and decided to develop a team approach wherein both disciplines were involved in the evaluation and assessment process. This seemed to alleviate a great deal of the tension surrounding this issue. It was a beginning. The therapists from both departments began to work together to increase the quality of care for these patients.

You will find differences among health care settings as well as in school districts as to how the institutions are organized and how they function. It is important to remember that your role is one of assistant to your supervising SLP, who is the person to whom you are accountable. SLPs function as independent professionals (without prescription from a physician) with a minimum degree of a master's degree and hold the certificate of clinical competence (CCC-SLP), which qualifies them to assess and provide service to individuals with a variety of concerns related to speech-language and hearing.

TEAM MODELS AND TEAMING

In her book, *Building Early Intervention Teams*, Margaret Briggs (1997) defines team as "a group of individuals who are committed to a shared purpose, to each other, and to working together to achieve common goals" (p. 12). At one level, you will be working with your supervising SLP as a "team," to improve practices and achieve intervention outcomes for individuals who have communication challenges. As noted in Chapter 4, many in the profession of speech-language pathology consider the individual as well as family members to be integral "team members" in achieving this purpose. As described, the " team concept" expands as you work with your SLP and other professionals to achieve a common purpose or goal for those individuals who have communication challenges as well as other developmental or acquired impairments associated with medical conditions or that interfere with educational outcomes. When learning about the concept of team in a variety of settings, you need to be aware of and understand the structure of the team. Teams are typically configured in a variety of ways that influence the interaction between members. They also frequently develop in stage-like sequence that also affects their productivity and effectiveness. Specific patterns of communication, collaboration, and commitment significantly influence how team members interact and function. Characteristics of well-functioning teams include the type of support available to the team in terms of administration and management.

Let us first examine team models or specific structures that may have an impact on how and when team members work together toward common goals. Child Development Resources in Lightfoot Virginia distinguishes between three models for team interaction as adapted from Woodruff and McGonigel (1988).

Multidisciplinary Teams

Multidisciplinary teams are often described as teams that recognize that other disciplines have important contributions to make to the work with individuals with disabilities.

However, team members may conduct separate assessments by discipline and develop and implement separate plans for intervention within their own area or discipline. Generally, they may meet with families separately and lines of communication are typically informal. However, it is recognized that all involved are working toward a common goal. The goal involves improvement of the functioning level of the individual with a disability. There is an acknowledgment that many perspectives are needed to provide a complete picture of what needs to be done in terms of assessment and intervention regarding an individual who presents with a disability. As Briggs (1997) notes, in the schools and in early intervention, under the provisions of IDEA, multidisciplinary teams of professionals are required. Although the law requires that assessment and intervention from the necessary professionals be provided, it does not necessarily stipulate how the arrangements and interactions of the professional will be structured. In some settings, because the structure and resulting communication between professionals is so loose, families are left with dealing with conflicting opinions and fragmented information that can be confusing and overwhelming. (See Hannah's Story.) They may appreciate the information and multiple perspectives from the professionals involved, but often would benefit from assistance in placing the information provided into a meaningful context so that they can make informed decisions about intervention paths and recommendations.

SIDELIGHT: *Hannah's Story*

Hannah was born with a cleft lip and palate. She had a lip repair when she was 3 months of age and a repair of her palate at about 9 months of age. She also received speech therapy to help her develop intelligible or clear speech patterns and language abilities. At around 4 years of age, her family was referred to a craniofacial team by her developmental pediatrician and her current SLP. Although her speech was somewhat developed, she was frequently unintelligible to those who did not know her. Her voice was very hypernasal. You could tell the sounds were coming through her nose. Her family brought her to a series of appointments at a local children's hospital and she was seen first by the audiologist, then the SLP, had x-rays taken in radiology, and after lunch, she and her parents were seen by a genetic counselor. Her family then took Hannah to dentistry, which was followed by an appointment with the cleft palate surgeon, who after examination, said that Hannah needed another surgery. Her parents were confused because they thought the need for surgery would be discussed at a follow-up meeting with all the professionals involved. They were led to believe this would happen after they received the results of all the evaluations that had taken place. They wanted to know about all the options available before they made a decision, although they knew surgery was a possibility. Then they thought they would make a decision after discussing the results with their pediatrician and their SLP. They were confused when the cleft palate surgeon suggested they make a preliminary appointment with his office manager to discuss the surgery and how it would be done. They left the hospital confused and overwhelmed and angry with the cleft palate surgeon who did not seem to have time to explain his results or answer their questions.

Interdisciplinary Teams

Interdisciplinary teams are often described as a group of helping professionals who are willing and able to share responsibility for intervention across several disciplines, and families may meet with the team as a whole or its representatives. According to Foley (1990), this is done in appreciation for the multifaceted nature of disabling conditions and the need for expertise from several disciplines. The team meets regularly for conferencing or consultation with each other and although they may assess the individual separately, they typically share results and goals to form one service plan. Results may be shared in an integrated report. The team member may implement parts of the plan for which the team's discipline is responsible. Although, as Briggs (1997) noted, there is collaboration and, in some instances, there may be a crossing of "discipline boundaries." For example, two professionals who provide cotreatment will still practice within their defined roles and areas of expertise. Yet there could still be a lack of cohesion for the family, and the individual may be receiving services or several separate services scheduled at different times and in different places.

Transdisciplinary Teams

Transdisciplinary teams are characterized as including family members as full team partners (McGonigel, Woodruff, & Rozmann-Millican, 1994) with primary decision-making authority. Team members typically commit to teach, learn, and work across disciplinary boundaries to plan and provide integrated services. Thus staff development becomes a critical factor in team development and team building. The team would meet regularly to share information and to implement intervention plans. Typically, staff and family participate together in an arena assessment focused on the individual looking across disciplines rather than from a specific discipline perspective. So the team would not focus on communication alone to the exclusion of social-emotional and sensorimotor abilities. Transdisciplinary teams are most commonly found in early intervention programs wherein there is a focus on sharing responsibility and all aspects of intervention with the family based on family needs, resources, and priorities. Some professionals would also characterize the developmentally supportive care model in neonatal intensive care units (NICUs) as approaching the transdiciplinary structure, or teams committed to a specific focus area, such as augmentative alternative communication (AAC) may attempt to structure their services around the transdisciplinary model.

SIDELIGHT: *An IEP Team Staffing*

After meeting with their son's individual education plan (IEP) team, the Setterlands felt like they understood their son's learning problems and why he was having difficulty in school. The services that he would be receiving from the SLP, OT, psychologist, and a reading specialist seemed to fit, but they were concerned that their son would be pulled out from the regular classroom for a minimum of 45 minutes to 1.5 hours on any given day. This seemed fragmenting and they were afraid the program would be so separate that he would not get what he needed to achieve in the regular curriculum. They wondered whether all these different sessions with different people were really necessary and if their son would be able to learn.

The transdisciplinary model is probably the one to achieve because it demands highly collaborative work and because it is based on an evolving team concept, which demands that disciplines "step outside" their comfort zone. Most professionals continue to be trained within their discipline so that they are most comfortable doing what they have learned to do in their personnel preparation programs. However, there is a trend for teams, especially in early intervention, to commit to transcending traditional roles and

boundaries to focus on the individual needing services as a whole. This demands implementation of a family-centered, culturally responsive perspective versus a discipline-focused perspective.

Regardless of the structure of the team, there are several characteristics of a team that apply to any setting or purpose. Larson and La Fasto (1989), Parker (1990), and many other more contemporary authors such as Senge (1994) have described key characteristics of well-functioning teams. In any setting, a team must understand its mission. Many intervention teams spend time reaching consensus on what their mission is so that there is a clear understanding of why they exist and their purpose. Many teams also write down their mission statement and periodically revisit it, especially as new members come onto the team. Teams need leadership and resources, including human resources or members, time, and other forms of support from team leaders and administrators. Team members need to be affirmed and rewarded for doing an effective job. Time often proves to be a critical factor in how effectively team members adhere to a specific structure, especially given current pressures in health care regarding productivity and accountability. It is all well and good to say communication between team members is important, but unless the system has built-in time for members to meet and communicate, it will not happen effectively. Communication is probably the one most important variable teams need to establish to function effectively. Teams must also have the necessary expertise and knowledge base to fulfill their responsibilities. If one specific team member does not come onto the team with the requisite knowledge and experience needed, then the whole team process and product is affected. The process and procedures the team is going to use are important to establish and also revisit through feedback and evaluation to maintain the quality of team functioning. Processes used must be understood and agreed upon by team members so that all members know what is required and expected. This leads to trust and respect among team members, which are also essential for a successful team to develop and function.

Many teams report that they fluctuate a great deal in their effectiveness in functioning together. This may be influenced by where they are in their evolution as a team.

For example, a cyclical process of team development that moves through stages of forming, norming, storming, performing, and transforming has been extensively described in the literature (Blanchard, Carew, & Parisi-Carew, 1990; Montebello, 1994; Parker, 1990) about teams and the teaming process (Briggs, 1997). As with any relationship, there may be a period of excitement and orienting at the very beginning. Then members of a relationship often establish the "rules" or norms that they will live by. Often, with time, as we become more comfortable in a relationship, conflicts occur because of differences in opinion or perspective. How these conflicts are resolved will often determine the success of the relationship and whether it lasts over time. Teams are curious creatures and may take on a life of their own. They certainly are an effective way of meeting the multiple needs of individuals with disabilities and if they comprise competent team members who are committed to collaborate and communicate in a family-centered, culturally competent manner, they can effect improved quality of service as well as improved systems for meeting the needs of individuals with disabilities in our society.

UNDERSTANDING YOUR SETTING

The "Culture" of the Schools

Speech-language pathologists have a long history of service in the schools. In this setting, they are often the therapists with whom teachers, administrators, and students and their families are most likely to be familiar. They are sometimes referred to as the SLP, the communication specialist, or the speech-language pathologist. The greatest proportion of SLPs work in the schools (American Speech-Language-Hearing Association [ASHA] Omnibus Survey, 2001). As you know, they most often have a master's degree as the entry level for the profession and designate their credentials with MA, CCC-SLP following their name to note they have the certificate of clinical competence. Their practice has

changed as changes in educational service delivery systems have changed. Increasing number of students who need services for communication disorders and technological advances have also affected their scope of practice. SLPs are the professionals most often involved in developing communication systems through AAC.

In public school systems, you will encounter every type of disability seen in childhood associated with communication challenges. Given federal mandates, such as IDEA, and the move toward full **inclusion** of children with disabilities in their neighborhood school, you will see children who have been identified with congenital anomalies such as cleft lip and palate that may or not be associated with specific syndromes such as Down syndrome, or other medical related conditions. Parents of children who formally went to special residential programs, such as children who are deaf or hard of hearing, blind, or who may be described as autistic or severely developmentally delayed, now often choose to have their children educated through the public school system. Your supervising SLP may have students on her caseload who are identified as functioning in the spectrum of pervasive developmental delay (PDD), or children with neurologic impairments related to cerebral palsy or head injury who need AAC. You will most likely see a number of children identified with language learning disabilities (LLD). In 1991, the U.S. Department of Education estimated that nearly half of all children receiving special education services had LLD. Sometimes these children are described as demonstrating a "perceptual communicative handicap" (PC) or simply as learning disabled (LD). Then there are children who are seen by the SLP because of specific speech or language problems related to phonological impairments or articulation issues that interfere with intelligibility, voice problems, or stuttering problems.

The caseload refers to the number or types of communication problems seen by an SLP working in a school. As noted, this can be varied or be very similar, depending on the program. For example, some SLPs are "itinerant" in that they move from school to school seeing children identified as needed for their services. They may use a **pullout** model of service delivery. That is, the student is excused from his regular class to attend an individual or small group session with

the SLP. There is an identified trend in many states for SLPs to use a collaborative consultation model and actually work with the student in the context of his regular classroom, which many consider to be the least restrictive environment (LRE). Other SLPs may work in a **center-based program** with an intervention team that provides intensive services to children with severe needs such as autism or pervasive developmental delay or who are deaf or hard of hearing. Districts will use different disorder categories to determine the priority for types of services needed on the IEP. Students you see in a school-based setting may fall into one or more of the categories used to determine eligibility for services under IDEA, as explained in Chapter 11. There is great variety in the types and the severity level of children seen in a public school setting, yet all must meet eligibility requirements used by the school district to determine need for services in special education. In the schools, the systems of service delivery will also vary, depending on the philosophy of the SLP you work with, the number of students on caseload, and the needs of the students. Remember, the IEP will be developed by the team of professionals who work in special education in the schools, not just by the SLP alone. The team may consist of an SLP, psychologist, special education teacher, learning disabilities specialist or resource room teacher, and an audiologist, PT or OT, social worker, or other team specialists as needed (Figure 5-1). The classroom teacher and of course the parents and sometimes the principal or director of special education will also be key members of any school-based assessment or staffing team working with a student.

You will hear the term **Child Find** team. This is most often a team of related service personnel in a school district or county. The team often includes the SLP as well as other related service personnel, including an OT, a PT, social worker, psychologist, special education teachers, regular classroom teacher, and family members. Some districts will also have bilingual teams, depending on the geographic representation of the population they serve. This staffing team works together to screen and access those students who have been referred to special education from a variety of sources. Concerns about a student's achievement, ability to benefit from education in a regular classroom setting, speech or language abilities, or other identifiable disabilities would poten-

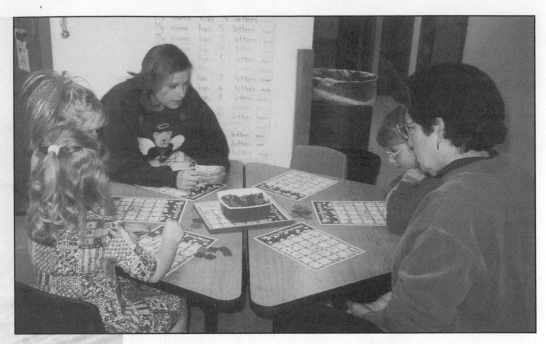

Figure 5-1 Co-therapy: An SLP and SLPA working together

tially qualify the student for services under part B of IDEA. The law stipulates that a multidisciplinary evaluation or assessment is needed to determine current functioning level of the student and to specify the needs and service that should be made available based on the child's disability and needs. Child Find teams often provide assessment evaluations to children from birth to 21 years of age as stipulated in IDEA. They work with professionals serving children within the school-based site to design programs that meet the individual needs of the children or students identified. There may be other specialty teams in a given district that focus on service delivery for a specific population such as deaf or hard-of-hearing students, students in need of AAC evaluations and program design, early intervention teams serving children at the preschool level, and behavior intervention teams that design and problem-solve challenging behavioral problems facing some children with disabilities. Again, the exact makeup of each of these teams may vary and the supervising SLP you work with may work with several teams as part of his responsibility in the district.

The "Culture" of the Hospital Setting or Rehabilitation Center

Your supervising SLP in this setting may also work with different types of teams, depending on the age level of the population served and the focus of services. For example, if you work in a children's hospital, you might be exposed to interactions with the cleft palate team or craniofacial team that provides specialized assessment for infants born with congenital anomalies or syndromes such as **Pierre Robin sequence** or **Down syndrome**. On this team, you may be assisting your SLP in screening or assessment of speech and language problems associated with cleft lip and cleft palate. You may interact with genetic counselors, plastic surgeons, orthodontists, and others concerned with the multiple challenge often faced with young children and families with such medically related issues. You may also assist your supervising SLP in the inpatient work she does in various hospital settings. He may be involved in a head injury or brain injury team or a newborn follow-up clinic that periodically sees and reevaluates graduates of the NICU or an orthopedic clinic that follows children with cerebral palsy and needs the combined expertise of several specialists to determine the access, communication, seating, and mobility needs of a particular individual.

SIDELIGHT: *Newborn Follow-Up Clinic*

Marsha, an SLP, works with the newborn follow-up clinic team to monitor the growth and developmental progress of babies born in the NICU. Frequently, babies return to the hospital at 6, 18, 24, and 36 months of age because parents have been told to keep in touch about the infants' growth and development. Sometimes parent have questions about their babies' development. They want to know whether their baby is developing at the rate expected. Marsha works with a PT, OT, social worker, and developmental pediatrician on this team. Assessment with the multiple professionals on the follow-up team helps parents identify issues early or prevent challenges from developing.

Your supervising SLP may, again, provide services in this setting in a variety of ways. Service delivery models in a medical setting will change, depending on the age, level of care, and targets of intervention. Your supervising SLP may have you supplement his direct therapy with a patient with several practice sessions to increase intensity of services and generalization of targeted outcomes. You will be following the treatment plan the SLP has developed. You may be working with him in a small group situation to support the intended goals and objectives for several patients. You may be working with your SLP to implement an educational program for family members, to help them learn specific techniques and strategies that work for the patient after discharge from the facility. You may be working with a patient individually to practice targeted behaviors using a piece of equipment or a computer program you have received training on and understand what is needed. There are many interesting and varied ways you will assist your supervising SLP and interact with others in this setting.

SIDELIGHT: *Computer-Based Practice*

When Tom began his job as an SLPA in the hospital setting, he received training about how to use the visipitch program with patients who needed feedback regarding the loudness of their voice. He also learned how to use other software programs to motivate patients to practice their speech in therapy. He found he enjoyed working with patients at the computer because they were motivated to practice given the immediate feedback provided by the software programs. Tom could also easily track the patient's individual progress on targeted speech objectives given the special features of the computer programs.

The hierarchy in a medically related setting may seem more explicit than that of an educational setting and is often seated in the historical or traditional model of the medical profession. It will also be significantly influenced by health care reform and the reimbursement procedures available, as explained in Chapter 9 of this text. With changes in health care and the advent of increased federal and state regulations through Medicaid and Medicare reimbursement procedures, productivity and accountability has become more and more central to the practice of the SLP. It is important to work closely with your supervising SLP to learn the particu-

lar protocol and procedures in the medical setting so that you are savvy and knowledgeable about boundaries and specific areas of responsibility in any given situation you encounter.

The different types of teams are varied and interesting, depending on the site of employment. Your supervising SLP will guide your interactions with these other professionals. Do not be overwhelmed with the numerous acronyms and specialty designations at this point. You will learn more about the culture of your setting and the particular models of service delivery and team makeup when you become employed in a particular setting.

BOUNDARIES AND INTERACTIONS ASSOCIATED WITH A SPECIFIC SETTING

Paying attention to hierarchy provides some cues as to how decisions are made in various settings. The boundaries between professional disciplines also determine who may lead in making one type of decision over another. For example, in a medical setting the physician may characteristically have the last word about any services the patient may have access to receiving. Unfortunately, third-party reimbursement procedures or insurance coverage have a negative impact on how long and how much therapy a patient may receive. But many settings operate according to a team structure that also dictates how professionals interact in any given situation. As described, in the school setting, the IEP process demands that the students' needs are determined through a multidisciplinary assessment process. Team members are supposed to work with families and share results so that an individualized plan based on the students' strengths and needs can be developed. Procedural safeguards should be in place, and the team, including family, is directed by mandates and best practice to collaborate in goal setting and program planning. Teams may operate differently, depending on the individual served, the types of setting, and the types of decisions that need to be made. Unfortunately, sometimes the process is not as collaborative as intended. Clarification

of leadership roles and team structure and function is thus key in determining how professionals interact as a team in any given setting. Your role on any given team will be determined by the role you fulfill as an SLPA with your supervising SLP. Sometimes boundaries become fuzzy and you might be asked to complete tasks that are outside your scope of responsibility. It is important to discuss these issues with your supervising SLP, become familiar with the team structure of your setting, and adhere to the guidelines set forth regarding your position as an SLPA.

STRATEGIES TO PROMOTE POSITIVE INTERACTIONS AND EXPERIENCES

Developing respect for your supervising SLP and acknowledgment of your own strengths and competency as well as limitations on your scope of responsibility can lead to a positive relationship with your SLP. As you clarify roles and expectations, you will hopefully develop the trust and maintain the ongoing communication characteristic of a well-functioning team. Again, the support and mentorship provided by your supervising SLP can also lead to positive interactions and productive work.

Knowledge and respect for others you work with in whatever setting you choose will also lead to positive relationships and new learning of respective roles of professionals practicing from several different disciplines. An open mind to how you can learn more about what others contribute to the welfare of patients, students, or clients will lead to improved practice and understanding of the needs of the individual with a communication challenge. Positive interactions with those you work with on a daily basis can be a satisfying aspect of your position as an SLPA.

As you work together with your SLP and interact with other team members, there are bound to be problems that arise. When trying to meet the needs of individuals with communication challenges, much perspective must be taken into account. Sometimes problems can occur as teams try to reconcile these perspectives and agree on a course of action.

Sometimes the problems can occur closer to home and reflect unresolved issues between you and your supervising SLP. Regardless of the source of conflict, there are strategies that can help you work together to resolve problems and de-escalate conflicts or issues of concern.

Collaborative Problem Solving

Steps to collaborative problem solving provide a framework from which you and your supervisor/mentor can approach an issue to be resolved. First of all, it is important to define the problem accurately. This first step is critical because you want to be able to clarify exactly what each of you thinks about the issue. Misunderstandings and misperceptions can be resolved more easily if the problems are clarified. Then you need to determine the needs or desired outcomes for the situation.

SIDELIGHT: *Caught in the Middle*

Your supervisor, Beth, is concerned that you be punctual and keep to the scheduled times for sessions. You have tried to be consistently on time in picking up a group of students you have scheduled for small group work twice a week as a supplement to your supervisor's session with them on Mondays. The classroom teacher is inconsistent about letting them go with you at the designated time, especially if it is interfering with completion of a class activity that is "running over time." The teacher wants the children to be able to finish the activity before they leave for their session with you. You have been as flexible as you think you can be under the circumstances. If it means a few minutes delay, you have adjusted to her wishes. But you now see a pattern developing, and the students have missed as much as 10 minutes of their scheduled session. Beth is concerned about your ability to adhere to the schedule, and she is also concerned about the implications of this situation in terms of the students receiving the services that they have been determined to need based on their IEPs. The students are also reacting to the uncertainty of their schedule and you feel this is interfering with the progress they can make on their designated goals and objectives. You have not been able to implement all of the activities on the intervention plan as outlined by Beth. This is becoming an issue with Beth, and you feel somewhat caught in the middle, because you do not want to jeopardize your relationship with either the teacher or your supervisor. So you explain the situation as best as you can to Beth and suggest a quick meeting be scheduled with you, Beth and the classroom teacher to resolve the problem. You all attend the scheduled meeting and clarify the problem from each of your perspectives. The teacher does not want interruptions that interfere with the students' ability to finish their work or participate meaningfully in an activity. You do not want to be put in the situation of interfering with the teacher's schedule nor be considered inconsistent in your ability to fulfill your responsibilities. Beth is concerned that the students are not receiving the designated services as stipulated on their IEP. Once all perspectives have been clarified and the outcome of providing the students the services they need consistent with their IEP has been articulated, the brainstorming of possible solutions can occur. Maybe the teacher can adjust her schedule so that the activities that she wants these students to participate in can happen at another time. Maybe the students' scheduled time with you can be changed. Maybe you could integrate the work you are doing into the classroom activities. After brainstorming other ways to deal with this issue, Beth and the teacher choose the solution that best meets their needs and develop a plan of action that hopefully will resolve the problem for you and the children.

It will be up to all of the players to cooperate in implementing the plan and check back to determine or evaluate whether the solution worked to eliminate or resolve the problem. If a problem like this is left unattended, it can escalate into a problem that can affect your relationships with your supervising SLP and others as well as how they perceive your work.

Apply these eight steps to problem solving to other situations in which you think a systematic approach to developing a solution could work (Fisher, Ury, & Patton, 1992). These steps are representative of commonly used strategies to help organize the process and move forward to solutions.

1. Define the problem.
2. Clarify the perceptions and perspectives of those involved.
3. Determine the needs or outcomes.
4. Brainstorm possible solutions.
5. Select the solution that will best meet the needs of all concerned and achieve the desired outcome.
6. Develop a plan of action.
7. Implement the plan.
8. Evaluate whether the solution is working and provide feedback.

It is critical to monitor whether the solution or proposed plan of action is working to solve a problem. For example, the SLPA working with Beth needs to monitor if the new plan for picking up children from the classroom is working. This affirms the process and helps you figure out if you need to step back and brainstorm other possible solutions and reengage in the process. If you incorporate this model for problem solving into how you typically address issues of concern, you will find it useful in de-escalating misunderstandings or misperceptions that can interfere with your work and your relationships with people you interact with in a daily basis. The use of mutual problem-solving processes can facilitate cooperative working relationships that result in improved services for those individuals involved.

Other issues may arise based on conflicts that are more difficult to resolve. Conflict is considered to be a naturally occurring process, though sometimes unwelcome, that occurs in any working relationship (Gerlach & Lee, 1997). Sometimes use of other strategies that help you address conflicts may be appropriate to consider. Thomas and Kilmann (1974) identify specific types or approaches to conflict as a way to decrease conflict and resolve challenging situations. Gerlach and Lee also address these ideas. First, they suggest pausing and taking a breath or stepping back to put the conflict into perspective. They suggest focusing your energy in a productive way. This often involves separating the people from the problem so that you step away from blaming someone and work to see the problem as an issue that can be resolved.

Move away from the temptation to see the conflict as a personality issue between you and someone else, or move away from judging their actions. "That mother never comes to meetings. She just doesn't care about education or the program for her child." This step can be very effective in defusing the intensity of emotions that arise with a challenging situation.

Second, name the conflict. Put the issues on the table and clarify the factors that contribute to the problem. Gerlach and Lee (1997) suggest you ask yourself the following questions to clarify your thinking: What is the exact source of conflict? Do all involved have the same informa-

tion? Is the information complete? Are the goals of each person involved compatible? Are the methods used to address the issues effective? Is it comfortable or "allowable" to disagree? Asking yourself questions in a given situation often helps you clarify and identify exactly what the piece or pieces are that are bothering you. Now, you can move on to doing something about it.

Third, examine how you are contributing to sustaining the conflict. What role, if any, are you playing in fueling the fire or preventing resolution. Thomas and Kilmann (1974) identify five typical responses to conflict, including avoidance, compromise, accommodation, competition, and collaboration. They suggest we all have a typical style or preferred way to deal with difficult situations. Each style or response can be useful in its own way in a given situation. For example, it may be appropriate to use avoidance in a highly emotional situation when a cooling off period after a confrontation is needed. The solutions to the problem might then be reached in a more thoughtful or rational manner. Avoidance is also appropriate if your safety is being threatened in a given situation. However, nobody really enjoys confrontations, and avoidance of a problem over time can lead to escalation of the conflict. Therefore, use of this strategy must be examined in terms of its long-term effectiveness.

Accommodation may mean "giving up the battle to win the war." This sometimes means that you go along with someone else's solution to a problem, even if you believe your solution is better. You would do this in the interest of preserving harmony and maintaining a good relationship. You might employ accommodation and tell yourself that it is not your place to escalate the issues by digging in and presenting a view that disagrees with others' thoughts. Keep in mind though that inappropriate use of this conflict resolution strategy may not always be in your best interest or the best method for team effectiveness (Thomas & Kilmann, 1974). Burying your ideas may not help in the long run, even if it eliminates the immediate conflict. But remember, each situation must be examined in terms of using this strategy.

Another strategy discussed by Thomas and Kilmann (1974) is compromise. Compromise is often suggested as an effective strategy for dealing with a conflict. This means giving up some of your own demands or ideas and making concession for the "good of the order" or to achieve a common goal. Are you willing to compromise and put aside some of your own needs and ideas if it means a better working relationship and improved services for those you work with? Oftentimes, a mutually acceptable solution can be reached so that a course of action is agreeable to all. However, inappropriate compromise must be avoided if it means "giving up" what is best for the patient, client, or student concerned.

RESPONSES TO CONFLICT

Thomas and Kilmann's (1974) five typical responses to conflict are:

Avoidance
Compromise
Accommodation
Competition
Collaboration

Competition is another strategy discussed by Thomas and Kilmann (1974). It is a strategy that may involve one person deciding what is right for all and thus may not incorporate the thinking of others. If a decision needs to be made quickly, it may be that the person with the authority makes this decision for all. Again, it may prove to be an effective and necessary strategy in a given situation but can also prove contrary to a fair and thoughtful approach and in time escalate other conflicts or contribute to the development of ineffective work of team relationships.

Thomas and Kilmann (1974) also describe a process of collaboration. Collaboration is a concept that is thought to describe a cooperative and creative form of conflict resolution. It means that members of a team or those involved in the conflict are open to each other's ideas and each contributes his ideas in a spirit of mutual satisfaction and agreement. It is described as a strategy that promotes all members of a team feeling involved in the resolution process. It means a resolution is reached, which could not have been reached but for the involvement of all concerned. All feel valued and a positive relationship is maintained. This is a preferred

strategy for conflict resolution, especially when there are numerous players such as in the IEP process. Collaboration takes time and energy, but if used appropriately the time spent will result in improved services for the individual involved. The time involved in collaboration, sometimes precludes its use, and those in authority must determine some decisions. For example, using a collaborative process to decide where and when to hold a certain event can be very time consuming as people check their calendars and discuss the pros and cons of certain locations. Sometimes, it is more important for someone in authority to make a decision based on the best available information because the teams' time could be better spent in other ways.

What is your preferred style for conflict resolution? Thomas and Kilmann (1974) have developed a tool to help individuals self-reflect on their use of these strategies. Your instructor may suggest you complete this instrument to examine your preferred or characteristic ways of dealing with conflict. However, it is more important to realize that you will most likely use all of these strategies based on the situation at hand and that development of your skills in negotiating conflict and examining how you interact with others will help you to know when to use one strategy over another.

Another strategy to create and maintain positive relationships when conflicts occur is to examine your options. Gerlach and Lee (1997) and Pickett and Gerlach (1997) suggest some questions to ask yourself that may help you determine your course of action. Do I want things to continue as they are? Can I address the issue with my supervising SLP or other key people involved in the conflict or situation? Can I develop a new way of thinking about the conflict? They suggest you then choose your best option and go with it, after having considered the potential consequences and impact of your actions. Your supervising SLP may prove to be an excellent sounding board to discuss your use of specific strategies in any given situation. If you have established an honest, open communication channel with your SLP and he fulfills your idea of what a mentor should be, then you have a rich resource to help you determine the effectiveness of any given strategy in a particular situation. Using your supervisor/mentor in this way can promote your relationship of trust and build the concept of teaming that can characterize your interactions.

CONCLUSION

This chapter has introduced and discussed several concepts that affect how you will interact and work with professionals in various employment settings. It is important not only to know the players involved and understand their roles, but also to gain insight about the culture of the particular setting in which you choose to work. It may be critical to be aware of the norms established for interaction in any given setting. These are often based on tradition, history, or "this is the way it's always done," accepted medical or educational models that influence conduct, and team structures that may be used. Boundaries, lines of authority, and opportunities to learn in any given situation must be understood to promote positive interactions, regardless of the setting you work in. It is important to be able to address various issues, which may include communication breakdowns; parental or family concerns; behaviors of your individual patients, students, or clients; scheduling conflicts; interpersonal relationships; or district, hospital, or agency policies. Adoption of specific strategies that promote collaborative problem solving and conflict resolution can enhance your relationships with your supervising SLP and the many other professionals you interact with as you all work together to reach the common goal of quality services for individuals you serve as an SLPA.

DISCUSSION QUESTIONS

1. Think back over your site observations in a hospital or school setting. What professionals did you see as involved in service delivery in a hospital setting versus a school setting? Is there overlap in roles and responsibilities among these professionals? Describe the characteristics of the "culture" of the school or hospital in which you observed an SLP at work.

2. What types of team structures have you observed in action? What were the pros and cons of each? What role will you play on a team given your scope of responsibilities as an SLPA?

3. Imagine a potential conflict that might occur between an SLP and OT as team members trying to see the same patient in a rehabilitation setting. What strategies might come into play as you work with your supervising SLP to solve problems or de-escalate conflicts that arise between team members.

4. Imagine you are involved in an IEP staffing and your supervising SLP has recommended that the student in question receive therapy three times per week to work on vocabulary development and basic language concepts that are needed to improve expressive language and reading comprehension. She is suggesting this service be provided as part of a comprehensive program to address the student's delays in academic functioning. Assessment results indicate the student is demonstrating word retrieval problems and is performing significantly below age level on various tests of vocabulary comprehension and use. The psychologist on the team expressed the opinion that speech and language therapy will be a waste of time because the student first needs to address his significant behavioral outbursts and distractible behaviors that interfere with his engaging in classroom work. He feels that until these behaviors are under control and modified, the student will not be able to benefit from a therapy. The classroom teacher agrees that the behaviors interfere with the student's ability to benefit fully from classroom activities but also sees these behaviors as stemming from the student's frustration with comprehension and making sense of his world and his frustration of not being able to adequately express what he wants to say. The parents of this student also see a number of the behavioral issues as related to their child's difficulty in expressing himself and knowing the words he wants to use at a given time. They want the IEP to address this need. Describe what you hope you observe in this IEP session in terms of resolving the differences in opinion between the psychologist and other members of the team. What specific strategies might be helpful in resolving this conflict?

SUGGESTED ACTIVITIES

1. If you have not observed in a potential employment setting that is of interest to you, arrange an observation as soon as possible. Observe who and when the SLP interacts with other professionals in this setting. What types of team structures are used? What strategies does the SLP use in resolving potential problems or conflicts?

2. Research the Conflict Mode Instrument (Thomas & Kilmann, 1974) or the Parker Team Player Survey (Parker, 1991) listed in the reference section of this text. Use them to explore your own preferred strategies for interaction and conflict resolution. Do the results fit with your perception of yourself? Do you feel competent in handling conflicts that might arise in your work setting? Will you need to develop your abilities to implement several of these strategies to improve your working relationships with others?

3. Pick a problem you consider to be interfering with your optimal learning or performance in your training program. Sit down with a trusted friend or mentor and apply the eight-step collaborative problem resolution strategies described in this chapter. First identify and clarify the problem. Proceed through the eight steps and use your trusted confidant as a sounding board for your ideas and reflections. Develop an action plan and implement it over time. How will you evaluate the effectiveness of your plan?

REFERENCES

Blanchard, S., Carew, & Parisi-Carew (1990). *The one minute manager builds high performing teams.* New York: Williams Morrow.

Briggs, M. (1997). *Building early intervention teams.* Gaithersburg, MD: Aspen Publishers.

Child Development Resources. (1991). The team approach in early intervention. In *Transdisciplinary training material.* Lightfoot, VA: Author.

Foley, G. M. (1990). Portrait of the arena evaluation: Assessment in the transdisciplinary approach. In E. D. Gibbs & D. M. Teti (Eds.),

Interdisciplinary assessment of infants (pp. 271–286). Baltimore: Paul H. Brookes.

Fisher, R., Ury, W., & Patton, B. (1992). *Getting to yes.* New York: Houghton Mifflin.

Gerlach, K., & Lee, P. (1997). Team building: Communication and problem solving. In A. L. Pickett & K. Gerlach (Eds.), *Supervising paraeducators in school settings: A team approach* (pp. 171–205). Austin, TX. Pro-Ed.

Larson, C. E., & La Fasto, F. (1989). *Teamwork.* Newbury Park, CA: Sage.

Longhurst, T. (1997). Team roles in therapy services. In A. L. Pickett & K. Gerlach (Eds.), *Supervising paraeducators in school settings: A team approach* (pp. 55–89). Austin, TX: Pro-Ed.

McGonigel, M. J.,Woodruff, G., & Rozmann-Millican, M. (1994). The transdisciplinary team: A model for family centered early intervention. In J. B. Jordan (Ed.), *Meeting early intervention challenges: Issues from birth to three* (2nd ed., pp. 95–131). Baltimore: Pail H. Brookes.

Montbello, A. R. (1994). *Work teams that work.* Erlanger, KY: Pfeiffer.

Moore, S. M., & Kovach, T. (1993). Reflections on leadership: The mentoring process. *ASHA, 35,* 47–48.

Parker, G. M. (1990). *Team players and teamwork.* San Francisco: Jossey-Bass.

Parker, G. M. (1991). *Parker team player survey.* Tuxedo, NY: Xicom.

Pickett, A. L., & Gerlach, K. (1997). *Supervising paraeducators in school settings.* Austin: Pro-Ed.

Senge, P. M. (1990). *The fifth discipline: The art and practice of the learning organization.* New York: Doubleday.

Senge, P. M. (1994). *The fifth discipline fieldbook.* New York: Doubleday.

Senge, P. M. (1999). *The dance of change.* New York: Doubleday.

Thomas, K., & Kilmann, R. (1974). *Thomas-Kilmann conflict mode instrument.* Tuxedo, NY: Xicom.

Woodruff, G., & McGonigel, M. J. (1988). Early intervention team approaches: The transdisciplinary model. In J. B. Jordan (Ed.), *Early childhood special education: Birth to three* (pp. 164–181). Reston, VA: The Council for Exceptional Children.

6

Working With Diverse Populations

Key Concepts

■

When working with individuals from cultural or language backgrounds different from your own, you must apply knowledge of second-language acquisition processes and acknowledge differences in values and lifeways that can affect your work.

■

Knowledge of first- and second-language acquisition and bilingual behaviors can help distinguish between a language difference and a language disorder.

■

Although it is important to learn about the cultural backgrounds of individuals you work with, it is equally important to consider each person and family as unique and not assume they adhere to a cultural belief or practice just because they are from a certain background or culture.

■

Being individually responsive to a person and family you are working with includes acknowledging and respecting differences in culture that need to be considered when providing services to that individual.

Overview

■

Cultural and Linguistic Considerations

■

Moving Beyond Stereotypes

■

Language Acquisition, Language Difference, and Language Disorders

■

Implications for Practice

INTRODUCTION

As you begin your work as a speech-language pathology assistant (SLPA), you will be expected to work with many individuals who come from backgrounds different from your own. You may be providing services and support to these individuals and their families, or you may be working side by side with others who represent a variety of backgrounds or speak languages other than English. The United States is a nation of great cultural and linguistic diversity. This presents an opportunity to learn and share both similar and different experiences. There will most likely be opportunities to learn about people from different backgrounds and cultures. You will also have the opportunity to share your own cherished heritage and traditions with others. You may have the opportunity to support bilingual or multilingual abilities that can serve to preserve an individual's native language and culture and that can enhance their abilities in meeting challenges from a global perspective. You bring much strength to your work as an SLPA. Cultural competence, based on positive considerations of difference and elimination of prejudice, can enhance your work with many different individuals regardless of the setting.

CULTURAL AND LINGUISTIC CONSIDERATIONS

The United States continues to experience dramatic shifts in population growth (U.S. Census Bureau, 2000). Demographics are changing throughout the country. There is a significant influx of people who speak other languages and come from backgrounds that may or may not be similar to your own. As the population becomes increasingly diverse, it is expected that school districts, urban as well as rural regions, and populations identified with a variety of communication challenges will also become increasingly diverse.

It might be expected that increased diversity is most evident in urban areas rather than suburban and rural areas. However, changes in the population may also be related to agriculture, industry or recreation, and other socioeconomic

DIVERSITY STATISTICS

What has previously been considered a minority population is expected to comprise more than 40% of the U.S. population by 2035 and 47% of the U.S. population by 2047 (U.S. Census Bureau, 1996). More recent statistics (U.S. Census Bureau, 2000) indicate a significant growth since 1990 in the Hispanic population (58%), Asian population (72%), and African American population (22%) in our country.

factors that reflect a changing population in many regions of the country. Where do you live now? Do you hear different languages being spoken in the supermarket or in elevators in your community? When visiting a hospital or school, do you encounter patients or students from a wide variety of ethnic, religious, and cultural backgrounds? When walking across the street, do you see individuals dressed in clothing that indicates they are from a different country or practice a religion different from your own? How do you react to these differences?

DIVERSITY IN COLORADO SCHOOLS

In 2001 the Colorado Department of Education released figures indicating that over 114 different languages were spoken by children and families enrolled in Colorado public schools. Of those who speak a language other than English, 80% reportedly speak Spanish. Many school districts now report a majority of what was previously termed a minority population represented in their student enrollment. For example, one urban school district in Colorado reports that over 86 different languages are represented in the student body currently enrolled in the district. Over 50% of the population comes from Hispanic backgrounds, which, when considered with other racial and ethnic backgrounds, make up close to 68% of the student population of this district (Colorado Department of Education, 2001). One school district in a mountain region of Colorado reports a significant increase in preschool children coming from families who speak Spanish. In fact, one preschool reported that 98% of the children enrolled were from families who speak Spanish as their first language. The Colorado Department of Education reported a 118% increase between 1993 and 1997 in students who speak Spanish. The 2000 census indicates that 17% of the population in Colorado is of Hispanic or Latino origin (http://www.quickfacts.census.gov/gfl).

For many, these changing demographics provide a rich opportunity for cross-cultural learning and sharing. All too often, however, this increasing diversity is seen as a problem to be addressed. "Perceptions about the various ethnic com-

munities we work with are formed early in life, often without having any meaningful experiences or personal connection with members of those communities" (Sanchez, 1999, p. 351). In the fields of health care and education, this lack of knowledge of cultural and linguistic factors that may affect an individual's response to intervention or disability may stem from a lack of direct contact with diverse families and often raises concerns, barriers, and even fear among providers. Many providers voice concerns about being expected to meet the diverse needs of a population they do not understand. They may ask, "How do we provide services to an individual and family who hold values that are different from those held by the professional providing services?" Many families may hold beliefs about health care and education that are different from the mainstream. They may also speak a language other than English. They may present role differences and child-rearing practices that are different or unfamiliar and stem from their cultural backgrounds, traditions, religious beliefs, and lifeways. How, as service providers, do we work together to build systems in health care and education that afford all the opportunity to access health care services and educational support, especially for those individuals in need of services and support because of an identified disability?

Cultural Competence

In order to develop skills of cultural competence as a provider, one must consider the concept of **culture** itself. What do we mean when someone comes from a cultural background different from our own? This is somewhat of an ethnocentric perspective because we are using our own culture as the standard by which we measure others. If we all come from a particular culture, how do we describe or define this concept? According to Anderson and Fenichel (1989, p. 8) "culture can be conceptualized as the specific framework of meanings within which a population, individually or as a group, shapes its lifeways. It is an ongoing process within which individuals are constantly reworking or trying out new ideas and behaviors." Do you agree with these conceptualizations of culture? If so, then it seems appropriate to think of culture as a dynamic concept. Everyone has a culture and it may change over time. How then do we develop cultural competence as we work with others who hold values and practice lifeways that are different from our own? It is important to consider that competence implies more than beliefs, attitudes, and tolerance, although it also includes them. Roberts (1990) explains *competence* as having the skills to take on another person's perspective and consider her beliefs, attitudes, and orientation when deciding on a course of action. Moving beyond tolerance of differences is important so that recognition, acceptance, and, ultimately, sharing, appreciation, and celebration of differences can occur. This can begin early in life as depicted in Figure 6-1. It is maybe more meaningful to move toward the ultimate outcome of recognizing individualization within a culture as the true standard for cultural competence.

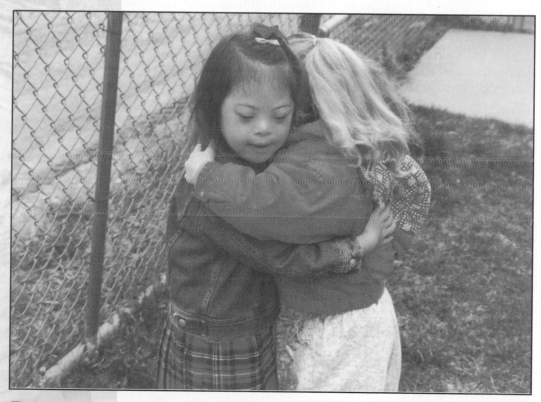

Figure 6-1 Good friends embracing and celebrating diversity

MOVING BEYOND STEREOTYPES

In a book that speaks to the richness of differences across cultures and the concern of nonacceptance of others, Mary Catherine Bateson (2000, p. 13) writes, "Prejudice and stereotyping are ways of making intellectual and emotional sense of a puzzling world; easy solutions to the challenge of difference. They offer the assumptions of commonality within one group, denying the differences that are there." How we perceive and consider differences points out the negative consequences or the negative influence of stereotyping. It is important to realize that cultures are not generic. Similarities across families may exist within cultural backgrounds. However, this does not mean that every family who may describe themselves as Southeast Asian, Native American, or African American holds the same beliefs or values. Actually, each of these categories may encompass numerous cultures, and even though their individual members may share tendencies in some areas, they may not in others. Individuals and families will be found to lie along different points of their cultural continuum (from traditional, for example, to fully bicultural) (Anderson & Fenichel, 1989). In an article written about increasing opportunities for partnership with culturally and linguistically diverse families, Eva Thorp (1997, p. 2) states, "all families in fact, vary greatly in the degree in which their beliefs and practices are representative of a particular culture, language group, religious group, or country of origin." This implies that we need to move beyond assumptions about a particular individual or family based on their background or culture. In fact, few cultures lend themselves to simple description. It is true that it may be helpful to learn about differences in cultures to develop a knowledge base and appreciation of different traditions, child-rearing practices, or lifeways of a particular culture, but this information must be used with caution (Lynch & Hanson, 1998). Such information can lead to faulty expectations that may be based on stereotypes and thus may not hold true for an individual or family you are interacting with in your work. Walls between you and others can be built when reliance on faulty assumptions interferes with your understanding of a situation. This can contribute

to misunderstandings and misperceptions about why an individual or family makes a particular decision or behaves in a way that seems contrary to a desired outcome.

In the book, *The Spirit Catches You and You Fall Down*, Fadiman (1997) tells the story of a young child and her family and their interactions with the health care system. This is a Hmong family who had immigrated to this country from Southeast Asia and was referred for medical intervention for their child because of a seizure disorder. After many misunderstandings, miscommunications, and concerns about the use of prescribed medications, the health care providers discover that they had acted on assumptions that were not true for this family. The family believed "qaug dab peg," which means "the spirit catches you and you fall down," was the source of Lia's epilepsy (p. 20). The family's culture explained this behavior as "soul loss" because Lia's sister slammed the door and "the noise had been so profoundly frightening that Lia's soul had fled her body and become lost" (p. 20). As the story progresses, the providers come to understand that the family may not be all that invested in stopping the seizures because, although serious, the Hmong consider "quaug dab peg" to be an illness of some distinction (p. 21). This is a dramatic story that illustrates how miscommunications and a lack of understanding of culturally based beliefs can interfere with what are assumed to be desired outcomes. In order to meet the needs of individuals and families, it is important to understand and appreciate our basic assumptions and those of others. Lia's story is even more meaningful when one considers the frequent assumptions that are made about second-language learners who are attempting to learn English and are often perceived as lower in intelligence or abilities because they are not proficient yet in their second language. It is important to understand the issues and challenges presented when learning a second language and what factors influence this process.

LANGUAGE ACQUISITION, LANGUAGE DIFFERENCE, AND LANGUAGE DISORDERS

It has been documented that a current critical concern in special education is the overidentification of second-language learners as having a language disorder. The incidence of overidentification of minority populations, including second-language learners within special education, means that there are far too many students identified as disabled when compared to the expected number predicted by the population figures available. For example, it has been documented that up to 12% of the school-age population demonstrates a language or learning disability or communication disorder of some type. Based on these predictive statistics, you would expect no more than this incidence figure within a particular population. However, incidence figures of disability are often higher than expected in traditionally underrepresented groups such as African American and Hispanic students. This begs the question of whether we are confusing a language difference for a language disorder and suggests careful examination of why individuals from what has been termed minority populations are over represented in special education. There is also the paradoxical concern that because we know so little about second-language processes and the development of English as a second language, or because we are unaware of the specific types of language disorders common to a given population, we may underestimate the needs of a group of individuals. It is thus important to review what we know about how language is acquired, how second languages are acquired, and the specific bilingual behaviors that characterize this process.

Defining Language

Language has been defined as a complex combination of several component rule systems (Bernstein & Tiegerman-Farber, 1997). It is a multidimensional concept that requires the interaction of linguistic structures, communication skills, domains of language, and knowledge of a language.

Linguistic structure refers to the subsystems or rule systems of a language, which include the following:

- Phonological system or sounds and rules for putting sounds together into words (phones and phonemes) of the language

- Semantic system or word "meaning," sometimes referred to as the lexicon or vocabulary bank of the language

- Morphological, syntactical, or grammatical rule system of the language that governs how words are put together to make meaning and formulate utterances or sentences

- Pragmatic system of how language is used in a social context

Oftentimes these conceptual rule systems are described or separated as form, content, and use (Bloom & Lahey, 1978). It is important to recognize that current theories of language acquisition view these subsystems as interrelated and interdependent. However, they are useful in helping to describe an individual's proficiency with a language. It is possible, for example, to describe an individual's pronunciation of English as difficult to understand and the order of words may not be grammatically correct; however, the verbal delivery of a complex concept may still be achieved given the vocabulary knowledge of the individual. Thus the individual's language proficiency may be "high" with respect to vocabulary knowledge and meaning, but "low" with respect to the use of sounds and grammar or syntax.

Communication skills encompass comprehension or understanding (receptive) of both oral and written language (listening and reading), and expressive (speaking and writing) of oral and written language. An individual may have developed strengths in one modality or process over another. For example, the individual may understand the language when spoken but have minimal ability to formulate verbally or decode the written symbols of the language in question. It is important to note that there is also a developmental timetable to consider when discussing acquisition of language processes. For example, the 12-month old understands a great deal more that she can express. Domains of a language are used to describe the context of language use. For example, the language spoken in the home may differ from that spoken with peers or from that used in the classroom or in the community. The pronunciation of words, the words used, and the level of complexity may vary from setting to setting, depending on the norms and use of language in that context.

PRINCIPLES OF LANGUAGE ACQUISITION

Knowledge of how language is acquired is helpful when trying to understand the principles of second-language acquisition. Principles to consider include:

■ Any language is learned by using language in a social context.

■ The focus in language learning is meaning and function (not form). Language learning initially requires "high context" or concrete referents as individuals develop comprehension of meaning.

■ Language learning is self-directed, not imposed by others. Motivation to learn is a contributing factor to success.

■ Language learning is personally important so that ideas, needs, and thoughts can be expressed. It is functional in nature.

■ The conditions for language learning are essentially the same for all. Exposure to a language is key.

Language Difference

Concepts about how a second language is acquired are reviewed by Moore, Beatty, and Perez-Mendez (1995) and include several points for your consideration:

■ Second-language acquisition is similar to, although not identical to, first-language acquisition (Ortiz, 1986).

■ Language is acquired, not learned. The implication of this is to focus on facilitation of acquisition by integrating language use into all aspects of daily activities, rather than only teaching language as a subject through drill and practice.

■ Cummins (1992c) and other authors document second-language acquisition as a developmental process that requires time and adequate exposure to

achieve proficiency: 1 to 2 years for conversational skill (basic vocabulary, grammar, pronunciation), and 5 to 7 years to develop the academic linguistic proficiency (literacy, problem-solving, and critical thinking skills) needed for academic success.

■ The development of competence in English as a second language is a function of the level of competence previously developed in a first language (Cummins, 1992; Kayser, 1995; Krashen & Terrell, 1983; Ortiz, 1994).

When second-language learning is considered for individuals coming from diverse cultural backgrounds and languages, it is important to ask, "What is known about bilingualism and biculturalism?" Considerations include the following points:

■ Children who are bilingual are a heterogeneous group, with a wide variety of exposure to languages and culture. For this reason, specific information from the family regarding cultural and linguistic background is essential in assessment of language proficiency or presence of a language disorder. For example, there is literally a world of difference between what one might expect in terms of language proficiency from a child being adopted from an orphanage in Bosnia at age 18 months into an English-speaking home versus a child of the same age who has immigrated to this country from Mexico and has been exposed to both English and Spanish since birth.

■ It is possible to be bilingual without being bicultural. (One may study Japanese without ever acquiring an understanding of the Japanese culture.)

■ Bilingualism is a fact in many countries in the world. It is considered an asset rather than a problem and is rarely confused with a "disability." Selected studies reported by Roseberry-McKibbon (1995) suggest individuals who are bilingual have a cognitive advantage; that is, individuals who are proficient bilinguals are thought to be cognitively and meta-linguistically more advantaged than those who are monolingual.

- Many consider those who are bicultural to have the advantage of the ability to view the world from more than one cultural perspective.
- It is recognized that individual and societal factors influence the process of second-language acquisition as well as adaptation to another culture.

Factors That Influence Second-Language Acquisition

There are multiple factors that influence the learning of a second language. According to a review of the literature completed by Moore, Beatty and Perez-Mendez (1995), the age of acquisition is a very important factor. For example, children who have been exposed to both languages since birth are described as simultaneous bilinguals. They come to learn both languages simultaneously. Preschool successive bilingualism are children who learn a second language after 3 years of age and school-age successive bilingualism are children who learn a second language after 5 years of age. Given your knowledge of first-language acquisition, how can the age of exposure to a second language make a difference in the acquisition of that language?

Other factors that influence second-language learning may be environmental in nature. For example, a child who grows up in a situation in which the family language is valued and both languages are fully supported is considered to be in an additive environment. Additive bilingualism is defined by Roseberry-McKibbon (1995, p. 137) as achievement of high levels of proficiency in the first and second languages. Subtractive bilingualism occurs when there is pressure to learn only English, because the home language is considered nonfunctional in the child's world or educational setting. Children or individuals in these circumstances may certainly experience a partial loss or gradual decline in their first language, particularly if they are forced to learn a second language to the exclusion of the first. This may be happenstance for some children who are adopted from other countries where a different language is spoken. They will certainly learn their second language of English and most likely completely lose their first language because there is no continued exposure to it in their environment.

SIDELIGHT: *Mimi's Story*

Mimi Valdez grew up in the San Louis Valley in a large family with an extensive history stemming from their Hispanic heritage and traditions. As the second oldest in a family of eight, she was told to only speak English when she left her home to go to school every morning. As she grew up, Mimi began to realize that those in her school and her community did not accept the language of her family. She quickly learned that she needed to speak English when outside her home. Her parents did not support her maintaining her Spanish and she found herself speaking more and more English with her brother and sisters and other family members. Now that she is in college, Mimi regrets not spending more time with her grandmother speaking Spanish because she feels she can still understand quite a bit, but cannot speak fluently, read, or write in Spanish. She is angry that she was not encouraged to preserve her first language but understands why her family did what they did. She regrets their decision and wishes that her family, school, and community had valued bilingualism when she was growing up. She especially resents the fact that she cannot communicate easily with her grandmother and has thus missed learning about her family's long history and the source of their family traditions.

The negative aspects of a subtractive environment can also influence the child's self-concept as well as her feelings about her family and background (Valdez, 1996). There are many stories of children who give up speaking their first language at home because they receive the message that society does not value it. Thus they lose vital connections to grandparents or others who can pass on family history and traditions. We certainly can see how this happened with many children from tribal reservations when they were sent away to government schools. There is a current effort in many tribes to revive the native languages and the cultural traditions of their heritage through reconnections and learning with elders.

Other terms used to describe bilingualism include *incipient, passive, active,* and *balanced.* Incipient bilinguals are individuals who are just beginning to learn a second language, whereas passive bilinguals understand a great deal of the second language yet cannot speak it. For example, many

bilingual children and adults understand but do not speak the language of their parents. Active bilingualism refers to individuals who use two languages for communication, and a balanced bilingual has a mastery of two languages comparable to monolinguals of each language. It is difficult to achieve balanced bilingualism because it infers a continued and consistent exposure and active use of both languages in daily situations.

Other factors that influence acquisition of a second language involve internal influences such as basic motivation, perceptions of value, style of language learning and use, cognitive abilities, and personality type. External factors that influence acquisition of a second language include age of exposure and other environmental factors such as amount of language support, opportunities for consistent exposure and use, positive consequences versus negative consequences for use, and quality of models or formal instruction. It is important to note that multiple factors will influence the rate of acquisition, yet research (Cummins, 1992c) indicates that time is needed to develop proficiency in a second language.

Stages of Second-Language Acquisition

Because you are involved in working with an increased number of individuals who may be in the process of learning English as a second language, either in school or in the community as an adult, it is important to learn more about the stages of second-language acquisition. This knowledge is very important when trying to understand a language difference versus a language disorder. When you are asked to collect spontaneous language samples or observe behaviors, it is important to document the situation as accurately as possible and record all that you hear. This will help your supervising SLP understand the stage of acquisition that the individual is in and shed light on the bilingual behaviors that are present. This will also enable your supervising SLP to interpret the information and use it appropriately in determining if a language difference or a disorder exists. The stages of second-language acquisition referred to by several authors (Hamayan & Damico, 1991; Krashen & Terrell,

1983; Kushner & Ortiz, 2000; Roseberry-McKibbon, 1995) are explained in the following sections.

Silent Receptive/Comprehension Stage

This stage is sometimes called the "silent period," because second-language learners are often quiet. They appear to be focusing on observing all that is going on around them so they can make sense of the new language and what it means without worrying about speaking or attempting to speak. Behaviors such as listening, pointing, matching, gesturing, drawing, miming choosing, or acting out characterize this stage. These are behaviors that you might observe the second-language learner doing. Think of these behaviors as guidelines for what you might expect of the individual in terms of her participation in a communicative interaction or learning environment.

Early Production

During this stage, speech may emerge naturally. Primary focus is still on development of listening comprehension, and early speech may contain many errors. Typical stages of progression include understanding and answering yes/no questions, providing one-word answers, listing answers, using two-word strings, and demonstrating an ability to categorize and use appropriate labels. The preschool-age child may use some commonly used vocabulary such as greetings, "don't," "no," or "my turn." At this stage the child is taking risks with use of the language and needs support to continue the process. The child will also benefit from good models and expansions in communicative interaction using the new language.

Speech Emergence

Given sufficient exposure to the second language and sufficient input, speech production will improve. Sentences will become longer and more complex and a more extensive vocabulary will emerge. Numbers of errors will likely decrease. Progression of behaviors observed may include:

increase in the number of three-word utterances and short phrases; ability to summarize; increasingly longer, more complete sentences; extended discourse or conversations; and an ability to recall the exact words or information, thus increasing dialogues. Narration skills to tell a story or describe an event and an ability to accurately define words or explain word meanings improve. The individual's ability to engage in longer conversations, use words appropriately to denote the intended meaning, and an increase in length and complexity of utterances emerge as she develops proficiency in the second language.

Intermediate Fluency

With continued exposure to adequate models and opportunities to interact with fluent speakers of the second-language, second-language learners will develop excellent comprehension, and their speech will reflect fewer grammatical errors. Opportunities to use the second language for varied purposes will broaden the individual's ability to use it in a variety of situations. You may observe the individual giving opinions, analyzing situations, defending arguments, creating new meanings, debating, evaluating, justifying, and examining using language.

Bilingual Behaviors

As you can see there are obvious parallels between the stages of first-language acquisition and second-language acquisition. It is important to review the stages of first-language acquisition, because it will help you understand that second-language acquisition, although very similar to first, presents patterns that are typical only for those learning a second language. Yet, even though there are different patterns or behaviors that characterize this process, they do not reflect disordered language comparable to an individual who needs clinical intervention. Some typical bilingual behaviors or processes described in the literature (Damico & Hamayan, 1991; Kayser, 1993; Roseberry-McKibbon, 1995) that can affect an individual's performance in communicative interactions or language tasks are outlined in the following sections.

Silent Period

This describes the language acquisition phase in which the individual focuses on comprehension of the second language, often referred to as L2, versus use of the first language, or L1. This period has been described as lasting up to a year in young children after their initial exposure to L2 (such as the first year in preschool). Again this period is marked by responses that are nonverbal or limited to one or two words. Progress can be interrupted or slowed down if the individual is forced to perform too early in the second-language acquisition process.

Language Loss

This often occurs when individuals spend more time in all-English-speaking situations. Their first language (L1) skills diminish from lack of use and reinforcement. Family members may remark that the individual uses her first language less and less at home. This can also happen to gains or proficiency developed in the second language if exposure and use are not maintained.

SIDELIGHT: *What Do You Think?*

After moving to the United States from Mexico, Clara made frequent trips back to Mexico with her children to visit her family. She found that when they went back for an extended visit and spoke nothing but Spanish for 2 or 3 months, it took her awhile to readjust and regain her proficiency in English when she returned to the United States. She was concerned that this may also be making an impact on her children who were developing English as a second language. Is this a problem?

Reduced Exposure

Reduced exposure to both the first and second languages may result in underdeveloped conceptual development. In what situations might reduced exposure to both languages occur? Consider that poor performance in either language may result from limited exposure to a rich vocabulary.

SIDELIGHT: *What Do You Think?*

Almir's mother learned Spanish from her grandmother and mother when she was growing up in this country. She also learned English as her second language, and she graduated from high school. She married a man from Russia who spoke Russian as his first language and with his friends when they came to visit, although he was acquiring English as his second language. Almir was born premature and was slow to develop in language. He was diagnosed with cerebral palsy and presented with oral motor problems that affected his ability to speak. Almir's pediatrician advised his mother to only speak to him in English. She said she would try to do this and told her mother to do the same. Almir spent most of the day being cared for by his grandmother, who spoke to him in Spanish, because her ability to speak in English was limited. Almir's mother was concerned that he was not being consistently exposed to proper English models at home and she felt guilty for having to work. Do you think the limited English models provided by the grandmother and father affected Almir's learning of English? His mother also found it difficult to only speak English at home because other members of her family spoke mostly Spanish or Russian. Was the pediatrician's recommendation appropriate given the home situation?

Code Switching

Code switching is changing from one language to another in the same sentence or paragraph (e.g., "Mi abuelita is picking me up after school today). Code switching is commonly used by fluent bilingual speakers and is modeled for many children in their home and community. Code switching is a typical bilingual behavior and in itself does not signal a communication disorder. However, it is often suggested that code switching within an utterance or a sentence not be used when modeling or teaching a child a second language. Having one family member speak to the child in one language the majority of the time (L1) and the other family member use the other language (L2) is suggested to reduce confusions. This approach of keeping the languages separate to a certain extent is emulated in dual language programs.

Interlanguage

This has been described as a temporary language system that fluctuates as the individual learning a second language

tests out or tries to apply different rules systems about the languages being used. The individual modifies the rules as a result of these trials based on models of appropriate use provided.

Interference

Interference is very similar to interlanguage and results when the individual applies rules from the first language to attempt to formulate or construct sentences in the second language. For example, a child who is dominant in Spanish who says, "the boy tall" instead of "the tall boy" is applying the rules of Spanish grammar or syntax. In Spanish the former sequence would be correct. This may happen as a child is learning two languages and thus means that the person assessing proficiency must be familiar with the rule systems used in each in order to determine if the error in sequence can be attributed to interference as a typical bilingual behavior.

Fossilization

Fossilization occurs when a person who has achieved proficiency or fluency in the second language continues to use certain patterns in structure or vocabulary that let you know she is a second-language learner. It is often associated with the charming characteristics of the first language persisting as the individual speaks the second language.

All of the bilingual behaviors described have been written about by Schiff-Meyers (1992), Kayser (1993), and Roseberry-McKibbon (1995). Please refer to these references for a more complete description of these behaviors and how they may apply to your work with English-language learners.

Second-Language Acquisition Versus Language Disorder

Key concepts of second-language acquisition and the implications for English-language learners must be understood in order to differentiate between a language difference and a

language disorder. Alba Ortiz (1986) from the University of Texas in Austin has written and presented extensively on this topic. She presents a key concept and then speaks to its implication for learning a second language as well as the implications for determining if a student or individual needs special education. For example, she notes that there is a common underlying pattern for developing proficiency for first- and second-language acquisition. Second-language acquisition is similar to, although not identical to, first-language acquisition. This implies that speaking a language other than English does not interfere with the acquisition of English, nor is it evidence of a disability. Conversational skills may take 1 to 2 years to acquire, but academic language proficiency may not be acquired for 5 to 7 years. Unfortunately, many students may be exited out of special services (English as a second language [ESL]) when they have acquired conversational skills in English. If they experience academic problems, they may be related to lack of academic language proficiency versus cognitive deficits or learning disabilities. It is important to distinguish these factors to prevent overidentification of English-language learners in special education. What if you were able to study abroad in a non-English-speaking country? If you spent 2 years in that country and spoke only the language used, you would most likely be able to communicate your needs, have lengthy conversations with others, and order from a restaurant menu. But would you be able to complete a college degree in that amount of time, given your lack of academic language proficiency in your second language?

Ortiz (1986) presents another concept. Because acquisition of language is developmental, you cannot hasten it. This implies that individuals must be given adequate time to acquire English-language skills. As students are in the process of acquiring English, they may make many errors related to typical bilingual behaviors. These are considered to be developmental and thus do not necessarily indicate a language disorder. Rather than which language a child speaks, the more critical variable is the quality of interaction she experiences with adults. This implies parents should be encouraged to speak to their children in their dominant language so that young children are exposed to proper language

models. If limited English-proficient parents only speak to their children in English, they may limit language development that can occur. The lack of appropriate models in English and lack of exposure to their first language can contribute to significant language loss as well as present social communication problems that interfere with the relationship.

Students in school must have a high level of linguistic competence in at least one language to be communicatively and academically successful. In the case of limited English proficient students, for example, a child who has moved here from India and is in first grade and has only been exposed to Hindu, the family's native language provides the foundation on which English competence is built. This implies that students who are limited English proficient must be given the opportunity to develop interpersonal communication skills and academic language proficiency in the native language (Cummins, 1986). However, a student whose native skills are significantly deviant from those of age-level peers from the same speech and language community is likely to have a speech and language disorder. The student who is not fluent in English may appear hyperactive, distractible, or passive in unfamiliar situations because she is not comfortable or cannot comprehend the language (Ortiz, 1986). How would you react if your instructor provided all the information about this topic in a language you did not understand? Would you leave, become frustrated, maybe even resistant to staying in class? Would you talk to your neighbor, frequently go to the bathroom, look out the window, or engage in other off-task behaviors because you are bored or frustrated? These types of behaviors then cannot be considered as clearly indicative of a language disorder although they are comparable to those often presented by children who are described as having attention-deficit disorder (ADD) or attention-deficit disorder with hyperactivity (ADHD) or those described as having learning disabilities.

There are many challenges in determining if an English-language learner has a language disorder. There is much to consider given what we now know about second-language learning processes. However, several factors contribute to the difficulty in distinguishing differences from disorder. Many teachers and specialists are not aware of this

knowledge base or how to apply it to individuals they work with. There is a shortage of appropriately trained bilingual professionals across all of the disciplines (Barrera, 1993). There is a need for nonbiased assessment tools and procedures that can render results that do not discriminate against an individual who has limited knowledge of English and the culture from which test items are derived (Hamayan & Damico, 1991). There are also many sociopolitical issues to consider given the marked differences of popular opinion regarding how English-language learners should be taught (Kushner & Ortiz, 2000). There is certainly a need for more research to determine the effectiveness and efficacy of programs intended to support English-language learners, and decisions should be made based on multiple factors described in this chapter rather than popular or sociopolitical opinion alone (Barrera, 1993). There are many myths that influence our opinions about individuals who are learning English as a second language. You might have heard comments from teachers or others such as: "my grandparents learned English quickly and without any language support" or "the sooner students are transferred out of native language instruction the better" or "teaching children to read in their native language hinders learning to read in English" or "younger children find it easier to learn a second language." Are these myths or realities? For more than 25 years the issue of how to best address the educational needs of English-language learners has been vigorously debated. The issues are complex and each situation needs to be examined according to multiple factors based on research by linguists, educators, and SLPs about ways to support the learning of a second language.

IMPLICATIONS FOR PRACTICE

There are many resources and references concerning implications for practice. Second-language acquisition is a topic that is being researched and discussed by many professionals across disciplines. There are several professional organizations (e.g. American Speech-Language-Hearing Association [ASHA], National Association for the Education of Young

Children [NAEYC], NABE etc.) that have addressed this topic in their scope of practice and have developed position statements regarding working with culturally and linguistically diverse populations. ASHA is one such organization that recognizes the workforce is not always adequately prepared to address these issues in depth. ASHA has developed a division in its national office to address this issue on an ongoing basis. It also has earmarked cultural competence as a special initiative needing to be addressed. ASHA recognizes that there is a definite shortage of well-prepared bilingual professionals in the speech-language pathology and audiology professions. Only about 7% to 8% of members of the national association self-identify as being representative of traditionally underrepresented populations. This issue goes beyond language difference to one of cultural competence in meeting the needs of the many individuals from different cultures or groups who need services related to speech, language, and hearing problems. You can explore ASHA position statements and obtain many resources regarding this topic from http://www.professional.asha.org, ASHA's Web site, or contact the multicultural affairs office of ASHA for additional resources that address cultural differences.

As seen in Figure 6-2, there are several general implications for practice that you may want to consider given the likelihood of your working with patients, clients, or students and their families who speak other languages or have backgrounds different from your own. Development of cross-cultural competency is a worthwhile objective. Strategies suggested by Lynch and Hansen (1998) and Tabors (1997) include developing self-awareness and recognizing that everyone has a culture and acknowledging and respecting differences rather then minimizing them. Sanchez (1999) discusses learning about other cultural perspectives from books, travel, and interactions with others and gathering information from families by listening to family stories in a nonjudgmental way. It is important to learn about the expected ways to communicate with others from backgrounds or cultures different from your own, including use of nonverbal communication strategies such as eye contact, hand shaking, proximity, and touching. What is acceptable and what is offensive? Communicate your attitude through words and practices. According to Lynch and Hansen

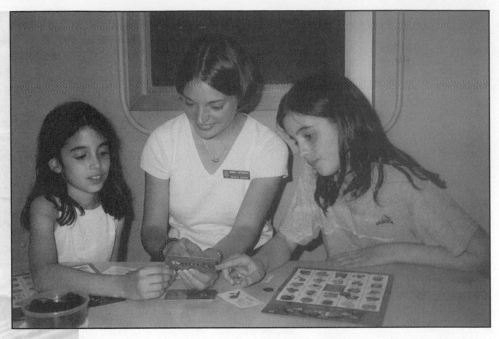

Figure 6-2 An SLPA at work with students who speak English as their second language.

communication effectiveness is significantly improved when providers use strategies such as showing respect for other cultures and making continued and sincere attempts to understand the world from another's point of view, are open to new learning and are flexible. It is also important to use humor appropriately and to be careful not to offend. It is always important to approach others with a desire to learn about their culture. Moore, Beatty, and Perez-Mendez (1995) focus on working with appropriately trained cultural mediators, interpreters, and translators when there are linguistic differences to address.

Given the information about second-language learning in this chapter, there are also several factors to consider when you are involved in providing services to young children, other individuals, and their families. Responding to linguistic and cultural diversity can be challenging. At times the challenges can be complicated further by the specific needs of the child, individual, the family, or the intervention

KEYS TO UNDERSTANDING DIFFERENCES AND INTERACTING WITH INDIVIDUALS FROM DIFFERENT CULTURES

There are a number of factors to consider that can increase your understanding of differences and enhance your skills when interacting with individuals from different cultures. These include:

- Recognizing that when you are lacking in knowledge about a culture and seeking information appropriately

- Recognizing there is a need for native speakers in the provider workforce

- Understanding that health care and education systems are often difficult to access for individuals from cultures different from your own

- Understanding that many of the tools and procedures used to identify developmental challenges or communication problems may be biased and inappropriate for use with certain populations

- Recognizing that there are differences in cultural expectations and not assuming they apply to all individuals even if they come from a similar background

- Understanding that individuals and family members may have had prior negative experiences that influence their interactions with professionals

- Avoiding acceptance of stereotypes or judging family members regarding their participation in an intervention program

- Recognizing that cultural conflicts can exist and need to be negotiated in order to improve service and support for individuals with communication challenges

program providing services. Recognition that all children are cognitively, linguistically, and emotionally connected to the language and culture of their home and acknowledging that children can demonstrate their knowledge and capabilities in many different ways is recommended by the NAEYC (1995). It is obvious that without comprehensible input, second-language learning can be difficult. The NAEYC also suggests active involvement of families in the child's early learning program and setting, encouraging, and assisting all parents in becoming knowledgeable about the cognitive value for children of knowing more than one language is important. Discuss with your SLP how services can provide families with strategies to support, maintain, and preserve home-language learning. NAEYC reminds us to recognize that parents

and families must rely on caregivers and educators to value and support their children in the cultural values and norms of the home in a culturally consistent way.

Can the intent of these ideas be applied to interactions and support for all individuals and families who speak a language other than English? It makes sense that providers receive personnel preparation and information specific to the areas of culture, language, and diversity. There is a recognized need by ASHA to recruit and support personnel who are fluent in languages other than English. Many professionals recognize that children can and will acquire the use of English even when their home language is used and developed, thus there is a need to support and preserve home language usage, even if children have an identified disability.

Yolandra Torres (1993) discusses the need for cultural consistency between home, school, or childcare settings. In a video developed by the West Ed Program for Infants and Toddlers, she says, "The child's culture is tied to self-esteem. This is what we are looking at right from the beginning. We want a child to feel good about himself. If you shame a child because he is using his own language, or if you shame the parents of the child and say his mother shouldn't do that and the child knows that this is very important to the mother, that's terrible because what you have done is tell the child that his parents don't know how to raise him." When working with individuals from linguistically or culturally diverse backgrounds, it is important to recognize the connections between culture and language and culture and self-esteem. Respecting parental decisions regarding use of language(s) is critical to the support of second-language learners with and without disabilities. Actions, activities, and work with children and individuals from culturally and linguistically diverse backgrounds need to be viewed from the perspective of culture and be consistent with it.

CONCLUSION

This chapter has asked you to explore your own culture as you learn about the cultures of others. It provides a cursory

overview of the multiple factors to consider when working with individuals from different cultural or linguistic backgrounds. It is important to recognize that we all may come to the table with bias, opinions, and even prejudice, but it is important to set these biases aside as we work with individuals from cultural and linguistic backgrounds different from our own. The information regarding cultural competence, and moving beyond stereotypes, will be helpful as you examine your own biases and prejudices, which could potentially interfere with your work.

The information provided about language development in L1 and L2 is directly relevant to your work with your supervising SLP. You will most likely be asked to collect information or organize data that involve accurate language sample transcriptions and other information that is critical to the process of determining a language difference from a language disorder. Your understanding of these issues and challenges will increase your usefulness to your supervising SLP. Review of the resulting implications for practice will hopefully peak your interest in learning more about different cultures and lifeways that affect the lives of individuals you work with regardless of your setting.

DISCUSSION QUESTIONS

1. Review the stages of second-language acquisition and the information presented on bilingual processes. Discuss how these relate to your own or your peers' real-life experiences. Are these stages evident in the stories told by your instructor or others in your class who have attempted to learn another language? How many of your peers are bilingual? At what level are they functioning—incipient, passive, active, or balanced? Are they bicultural as well? Are they bicultural without being bilingual? Do you see evidence of bilingual processes in their expressive language?

2. Discuss your knowledge about different cultures in terms of common beliefs, child-rearing practices, values, religions, and lifeways. Are there unfair stereotypes evident in your thinking or do they only become

stereotypes if you assign them to all individuals who may come from that background?

3. Discuss the many considerations to be shared with parents who are questioning whether they should speak their native language to their children at home. What resources can you provide them? What factors should they consider as they make a decision? Review Almir's story. Did his pediatrician share valid information with his mother?

SUGGESTED ACTIVITIES

1. If you are interested in finding out more about cultures and linguistic differences and how they affect perspectives, read books about specific cultures. Some suggestions are included in the references cited at the end of this chapter and include the book about collision of two cultures by Fadiman (1997).

2. Do this activity as a process in self-reflection. It is about lifeways and cultural continuity. Think about the family in which you grew up. What were some of the common beliefs about certain aspects of child rearing, such as letting children cry or how to discipline a child. Was it acceptable for toddlers to play with their food? What was thought about children with disabilities? Did they belong at home, in institutions, or special classrooms? What do you believe now? Have your beliefs changed? What does this tell you about culture and change? Can you compare the beliefs of your cultural background with those of others?

REFERENCES

Anderson, P. P., & Fenichel, E. (1989). *Serving culturally diverse families of infants and toddlers with disabilities.* Arlington, VA: National Center for Clinical Infant Programs.

Bateson, M. C. (2000). *Full circles, overlapping lives.* New York: Random House.

Barrera, I. (1993). Effective and appropriate instruction for all children: The challenge of cultural/linguistic diversity and young children with special needs. *Topics in Early Childhood Special Education,13*, 461–487.

Bernstein, D. K., & Tiegerman-Farber, E. (1997). *Language and communication disorders in children*. Needham Heights, MA: Allyn & Bacon.

Bloom, L., & Leahy, M. (1978). *Language development and language disorders*. New York: Wiley.

Colorado Department of Education. (1993). *Colorado Child Identification Process, birth–five years: Screening and evaluation process guidelines*. Denver: Colorado Department of Education, Child Find Project.

Colorado Department of Education. (2001). Retrieved from http://www.cde.state.co.us

Cummins, J. (1986). The role of primary language development in promoting educational success for language minority students. In J. Cummins (Ed.), *Schooling and language minority students: A theoretical framework*. Los Angeles: California Association for Bilingual Education.

Cummins, J. (1989). Towards anti-racist education: Empowering minority students. In J. Cummins (Ed.), *Empowering minority students* (pp. 35–50). Sacramento: California Association for Bilingual Education.

Cummins, J. (1992c). The role of primary language development in promoting educational success for language minority students. In C. Leyba (Ed.) *Schooling and language minority students: A theoretical framework*. Los Angeles: California State University.

Damico, J., & Hamayan, E. (1991). *Multicultural language intervention: Addressing cultural and linguistic diversity*. New York: EDUCOM Associates.

Fadiman, A. (1997). *The spirit catches you and you fall down*. New York: Farrar, Straus, and Giroux.

Hamayan, E., & Damico, J. (1991). *Limiting bias in the assessment of bilingual students*. New York: Basic Books.

Kayser, H. (1993). Hispanic cultures. In D. Battle (Ed.) *Communication disorders in multicultural populations*. Stoneham, MA: Butterworth-Heineman.

Kayser, H. (1995). *Bilingual speech-language pathology: An Hispanic focus*. San Diego: Singular.

Krashen, S., & Terrell, T. B. (1983). *A natural approach to language acquisition in the classroom*. Hayward, CA: Alemany Press.

Kushner, M. I., & Ortiz, A. A. (2000). The preparation of early childhood education teachers to serve English language learners. In National Institute on Early Childhood Development and Education, U.S. Department of Education, *New teachers for a new century: The future of early childhood professional preparation* (pp. 125–154). Washington, DC: U.S. Government Printing Office.

Lynch. E., & Hanson, M. L. (1998). *Developing cross-cultural competence: A guide for working with young children and their families.* (2nd ed.). Baltimore: Paul H. Brookes.

Moore, S. M., Beatty, J. & Perez-Mendez, C. (1995). *Developing cultural competence in early childhood assessment.* Boulder: University of Colorado at Boulder.

National Association for the Education of Young Children (1995). *Responding to linguistic and cultural diversity: Recommendations for effective early childhood education; A position statement.* NAEYC; Washington DC.

Ortiz. A. (1986). Recognizing learning disabilities in bilingual children: How to lessen inappropriate referrals of language minority students to special education. *Journal of Reading, Writing and Learning Disabilities International, 2,* 43–56.

Ortiz, A. (1994). *Second language acquisition, assessment and instruction.* Paper presented to Boulder Valley School District, Boulder: CO.

Roseberry-McKibbon, C. (1995). *Multicultural students with special language needs,* Oceanside, CA: Academic Communication Associates.

Sanchez, S. (1999). Learning from the stories of culturally and linguistically diverse families and communities. *Remedial and Special Education, 20,* 351–359.

Tabors, P. O. (1997). *One child, two languages.* Baltimore: Paul H. Brookes.

Thorpe, E. (2000). Increasing opportunities for partnership with culturally and linguistically diverse families. *Intervention in School and Clinic, 32,* 261–269.

Torres, Y. (1993). Essential connections [Motion piture]. (Available from the West End Center for Child and Family Studies Program for Infant Toddler Caregivers, Sacramento, CA)

U.S. Census Bureau. (1996). Retrieved from http://www.census.gov/main/wwwcen1996.html

U.S. Census Bureau. (2000). Retrieved from http:// www.census.gov/main/wwwcen2000.html

U.S. Census Bureau. (2000). Retrieved from http://www.quickfacts.census.gov.gfd

Valdez, G. (1996). *Con Respeto: Bridging the distance from culturally diverse families and schools.* New York: Teachers College Press.

Professionalism and Ethical Issues

Key Concepts

■

Ethics are a part of everyday life and are shaped over time based on maturation, culture, values, religious beliefs, and experiences.

■

ASHA has a Code of Ethics that governs the ethical behavior of the profession.

■

SLPAs are part of a profession that has specific guidelines for professional behavior.

■

Conflicts in ethics happen on a regular basis, and an SLPA needs to use the ASHA Code of Ethics as a resource to help solve those conflicts.

■

It is required by law that the SLPA report suspected child abuse and knows how to identify possible abuse.

■

We all have different cultural backgrounds and the SLPA needs to learn how to recognize those cultural differences and integrate that understanding into his ethical perspective.

Overview

■

Definition and Description of Ethics

■

Professional Behavior

■

ASHA Code of Ethics

■

Other Professional Issues

INTRODUCTION

As an SLPA, you are joining a large health care team made up of many professionals. You are entering the health care and educating professions that are made up of other practitioners, individuals you serve, and the community at large. "The honoring of this social compact will require a commitment to excellence in clinical practice and a commitment to a set of appropriate moral, ethical, and social behaviors" (Edge & Groves, 1999, p. 1). Along with a scientific basis of communication difficulties, you will learn how to apply this knowledge in practice. You will not be functioning in a vacuum, and when interacting with other professionals, individuals, and the community, you may be faced with ethical dilemmas.

ETHICAL DILEMMAS

Think about the following ethical dilemmas you or your colleagues could be faced with once you begin your career as an SLPA (Edge & Groves, 1999)

- When is it permissible to take a gift or gratuity from an individual?

- When is it okay to break a patient's confidence?

- Can you lie to an individual if it is for his own good?

- Can a school SLP refer an individual to a private practice where she works part time?

- What must I do if a therapy technique appears inappropriate but does not seem to harm the individual?

- What obligation do I have to report a colleague who may be abusing alcohol or appears chemically impaired?

- What if I come upon a practice that is legal, but personally I feel it is unethical?

DEFINITION AND DESCRIPTION OF ETHICS

Unlike scientific matters that follow the scientific method of levels of evidence, health care **ethics** are in the arena of human values, morals, individual culture, intense personal beliefs, and faith. People tend to filter situations and information through their own **worldview** to make ethical decisions. The field of SLPAs is filled with an abundance of value

questions that must be dealt with on a daily basis. Even though an ethical situation may arise that you feel very strongly about, it is important that you remain constructive and appropriate in your actions. Always consult with your SLP mentor as needed when these situations arise.

When defining ethics, people usually think of the "golden rule" as well as behavior that is right, moral, or good. "For many of us ethics is simply doing the right thing according to accepted standards of our specific community, culture, or profession" (Seymour, 1994, p. 62). The *American Heritage Dictionary* defines an ethic as "A principle of right and good conduct or a body of such principles" and ethics as "The study of the general nature of morals and of specific moral choices." Some think that the words *morals* and *ethics* mean the same thing. Morals tend to refer to the rules that society imposes on people and expects them to obey, whereas ethics deals more with the philosophical concepts. According to White (1988), ethics is a part of philosophy and uses reason, logic, concepts, and philosophical explanations to analyze its problems and find answers. Harris (1986) compared the meanings of morals and ethics and explains that morals implies complying with the general accepted standards of goodness in conduct or character. In contrast, ethics implies conformity with an elaborate, ideal code of moral principles. Ethics tends to be a higher standard than the federal and state laws that are in place. It is important to distinguish ethical behavior or guidelines from that associated with obeying the law. Sometimes there is an overlap.

One criterion for a profession is that it is self-regulating, and a major part of that regulation is a professional code of ethics. The **ASHA Code of Ethics** is the basic standard for our profession, which includes SLPs, SLPAs, and audiologists. Refer to Appendix C of this text for the complete ASHA Code of Ethics.

Health professionals work with people who hold many different roles: individuals, family members, students, supervisors, colleagues, support staff, spouses, and vendors. Everyone comes to these relationships with their own set of personal values, religious beliefs, and moral beliefs. Because of the individual nature of values and beliefs, people have differences of opinion, conflicting goals, and beliefs.

Learning to work with these differences is a rewarding part of being an SLPA. "Professional ethics incorporate those values, principles, and morals into professional decision making" (Kornblau & Starling, 2000, p. 14). As an SLPA, you will need to synthesize your personal ethical code as well as the professional ethical code to make decisions in situations that will arise on your job.

Professional Code of Ethics

Professionals draw from their training and professional obligations as a source of ethical values. Many professions have their own codes of ethics. A professional code of ethics puts together specific ideals that each profession holds of value in professional behavior. Often licensing boards or credentialing agencies adopt the profession's code of ethics into their regulations. Thus, even those who are not members of the professional association are also subject to the code of ethics. Many codes of ethics help describe ethical terms in ways people can understand. Many health professions are in the business of helping people and a significant focus of their ethics is on helping people and looking out for people's well-being. "First, do no harm" is the principle that guides many professions in their efforts to put the interests of the consumer ahead of all others. Competency and confidentiality are also common themes. These codes of ethics do not define absolutes in behavior but provide guidelines.

When dealing with ethics, one must also consider unethical practices. These are practices that do not conform to set professional standards. "This includes practices that range from unreasonable, unjustified, and ineffective to immoral, questionable, and (knowingly) harmful or wrong" (Kornblau & Starling, 2000, p. 15). Unethical behavior may be defined differently from person to person because we all use separate social, religious, and cultural perspectives to arrive at what we consider ethical. Some people see things as black and white, whereas others see things as shades of gray. Unethical practice in speech-language pathology does not just affect the individual who is responsible, but it affects the patient, family, the team, professional organization, insurance providers, and even the community or society at large.

Foundations of Ethics

The shaping of our ethics began when we were children. Our morals, values, and religious beliefs form a foundation for us at an early age. First we are taught a list of do's and don'ts, such as be nice to others, don't lie, don't steal, and obey your parents. As we grow, we pick and choose what we want in our belief system and we realize that ethics is a system of values and principles. We determine as we grow how we want others to view us, which is the beginning of our reputation. Children learn from those in authority and allow them to shape their worldview. These authorities may include social norms, authority figures, religious orientation, traditional popular culture and contemporary popular culture (Kornblau & Starling, 2000). Authorities in a child's life are the major influences on his development of an ethical system. As people mature they take pieces from all of these sources to make their own individual belief system.

Changes in Society

Health care professionals have always had to face ethical dilemmas. That is one major reason that most health professionals belong to national organizations that have codes of ethics or standards for their profession. The world is constantly changing and with those changes brings new ethical issues that you may need to face. The main changes have occurred in managed care, cultural diversity, societal and political values, and technology advances.

Managed Care

Managed care has made dramatic changes in the health care system. According to ASHA, "Managed care is an organized system of health care services in which financial, clinical services, and management are combined. Health plan members (enrollees) are directed to specific health care providers and their access to and a gatekeeper controls use of health care services. The gatekeeper, usually a primary care physician, works with enrollees to determine what types, amounts, and frequency of health care services are appropriate. Primary care physicians are those who practice family medicine, internal medicine, obstetrics/gynecology, and pediatrics. Health care providers are rewarded for offering necessary, quality services while containing costs" (ASHA, 1996, p. 31).

HALLMARKS OF MANAGED CARE

Managed care has the following hallmarks (ASHA, 1996):

- Services are provided by a specified group of professionals.
- Providers are paid by the managed care plan (salary or contract)
- Organizations offer a continuum of services emphasizing primary care, prevention, and health education
- Services for specialists must be authorized.
- Hospitalization is de-emphasized.
- Management of resources is the means to keep costs down.
- Information systems monitor costs processes of care and outcomes.

Managed care is always changing and, ASHA has taken proactive steps to look at implications for practice. It is important to keep informed regarding the changes that can affect your work with your supervising SLP in both education and health settings, especially because school districts are now pursuing additional reimbursement for services from Medicaid. One way to stay informed about these changes is to investigate rules and regulations within the state in which you practice as well as at the national level. The ASHA Web site, http://www.professional.asha.org, may be an excellent resource.

Some of the challenges that have come to the surface include professionals being forced to cross-train (OT and PT) to help keep hospital costs down. For example, what if only one motor therapist, either an OT or PT, has been hired to provide service in a specific facility? An OT usually works on functional skills and hand and finger movements like dressing, eating, and writing. A client comes into this setting and needs help learning to walk after a hip replacement. The

therapist is required to do the work of a PT because one is not available to do this type of therapy. This kind of cross-training or multiskilling is viewed negatively, because it may force therapists to perform tasks that they have not been trained to do. Therapists also report their caseloads are increasing, as is the use of therapy aids. This is of concern given the need to maintain quality of service. Other challenges include "caps" on services so services are not paid for after a certain number of sessions. The increased competition for the limited funds that are available from insurance agencies has forced companies to provide therapy services the least expensive way possible. However, this could mean referrals are driven by reimbursement instead of the patient's needs. These changes have brought up many ethical questions about how health care is provided.

Cultural Diversity

Another factor to consider in ethics is cultural diversity. With rapid demographic changes in our country, many different cultures are now represented in our population. SLPs are now being asked to provide services to individuals from varied cultural and linguistic background and also are being asked to learn to work with these culturally diverse individuals as colleagues. Ethical issues can arise when an SLP or SLPA who works with language is asked to work with an individual who speaks a language different from his own. One consideration is whether it is in the individual's best interest to work in English or with an interpreter. Questions of preservation of home language and culture affect the language of instruction as well as who should be working with the individual. These considerations have been addressed in Chapter 6.

Cultural diversity also includes individuals with differing abilities. With the passage of the Individuals with Disabilities Act (IDEA) and the Americans with Disabilities Act (ADA), more individuals with disabilities are being trained to work in many different fields; one is speech pathology. The workplace now has more people from different backgrounds, including different cultures as well as different abilities. However, there remains a shortage of health

care and education providers with the expertise to work with the many different languages and cultures represented in our population.

Science and Technology

Scientific advances always bring up ethical issues in the use or misuse of concepts and technology. People now survive accidents and illness that once would have been fatal. Now controversies in cloning and genetic mapping are familiar to many people when once they sounded like science fiction. Other advances in technology bring up issues of confidentiality with the use of computers in record keeping. Consumers can now educate themselves on many issues with easy access to the Internet. This may lead to conflicts in how intervention proceeds due to consumers' misinformation or exposure to alternative approaches. A positive aspect of technology and family-centered practice is that families may want to research all the options or get a second opinion before following the recommendations of a professional. As described in Chapter 4, parents need to be respected as the key decision maker for their family member and need to have access to all pertinent information. For example, a family member may have heard about an augmentative communication device on television that has many "bells and whistles." The parents may demand that their child be trained in using that device to communicate when another system is more appropriate for the child. It is thus critical that they are provided with all the information needed to make an informed decision. Changes in technology bring up many ethical issues that the medical professions and society are going to have to solve.

PROFESSIONAL BEHAVIOR

Throughout your time in your training program, you may have opportunities to represent yourself as an SLPA, as well as your department and school in general. For example, you plan to do an observation with a school SLP. You make the call and set up the time to observe. You then arrive 10 min-

utes late and interrupt the small group of second graders working on listening activities. The SLP might be less likely to agree to an observation with another student from your program because of your disruptive arrival. Your behavior, if appropriate, can help you develop a positive reputation that will follow you into the start of your career. Another example would be if you use inappropriate language when working with students at a high school. You are not only causing problems for yourself, but it may also decrease the opportunity of other SLPA students going to that same location after you. You want to demonstrate appropriate and acceptable professional behavior, which, like your knowledge of SLPA responsibilities, begins long before you start your first job. Honesty, integrity, respect for others, and a desire to help characterize appropriate professional behavior. This type of behavior is very important for individuals who conduct themselves in a professional manner.

ASHA gives specific guidelines to define your role, as well as your behavior and responsibilities. These guidelines also hold up high standards of service to protect those you work with. One of the foundational standards for an SLPA's behavior is not to cause harm to the individuals with whom you are working. If you are helping a 3-year-old learn how to say final sounds, you want him to make progress and learn new skills, and not make him feel self-conscious about his speech difficulties. The documents that include this information are the ASHA Code of Ethics (see Appendix C), ASHA's Preferred Practice Patterns, Scope of Practice for the SLPA, Technical Reports, and the Consumer Bill of Rights.

General rules of professional behavior include punctuality, working cooperatively, assuming responsibility, being well prepared, and maintaining appropriate dress and demeanor. Punctuality includes being on time for meetings, clinic appointments, and clinic deadlines as well as submitting paperwork in a timely manner. Working cooperatively is a way of working that does not challenge authority or purposefully "make waves." It is an attitude of helping and cooperating that makes work go smoothly. Taking responsibility for clinic or school property and equipment is a sign of maturity and professionalism. You want to take the time to be

ready for interactions with individuals as well as meetings with your supervisor. For example, you are meeting with your SLP supervisor and she expects you to have the files up to date as well as a language sample completed and your regular therapy schedule followed. You will want to get the paperwork ready and review your notes on therapy so you can talk with her without having to look up information. You may also want to think of questions you may have concerning therapies or the paperwork. Getting ready ahead of time for meetings, taking responsibility for equipment, and turning in paperwork in a timely manner are a few signs that you are well prepared. Professional demeanor refers to behaviors such as appearing confident in your abilities; communicating clearly and appropriately with the client, supervisor, and families; presenting yourself as a mature adult; following prescribed instructions and rules; and using your time effectively. Regular attendance and learning new procedures quickly will also affect your professional demeanor and influence those you work with in positive ways.

During your clinical experiences both at the program you attend and off site, you will interact with many different people. A good impression is very important even though you may be nervous when you first talk to them. The initial interaction sets the stage for future interactions and may determine how willing individuals and their families are to work with you. You want the people you work with to see you as self-confident and as a well-trained SLPA. Those individuals need to believe that you will provide quality services. Your professional demeanor will make an impact on how others you work with perceive you, with your goal always being to be respected as a competent service provider.

Malpractice Insurance

Another aspect of professionalism is to maintain malpractice insurance. In some academic institutions malpractice insurance is required before going out on clinical fieldwork. Some settings provide it as an employment benefit. Malpractice insurance provides financial resources for lawyers and court costs if anyone decides to sue you for fraudulent or inade-

quate services. You will want to discuss this issue with your instructor or look up the state regulations in your area for more specifics.

Dress Code

People's first impressions or judgment of you may affect your interactions with them in the future. You want to quickly establish a degree of trust, and that can be done through your professional demeanor, attire, and general appearance. Neat appearance and appropriate clothing will be a positive influence on those first impressions. No universal dress code exists, but where you work may have specific guidelines for how you dress. Appropriate dress means wearing clothes that do not draw undue attention or distract those you are helping; for example, very short skirts, or concert tee shirts might not be appropriate in your work setting. You will not have to buy an entirely new wardrobe, but, typically, shorts, jeans, tee shirts, sandals, and strapless dresses are not considered appropriate. A good rule of thumb is if you wonder if your clothes are appropriate, then wear something else.

When you are doing your off-site training, you may want to check if there is a specific dress code. You also may need to think about the environment you will be working in. If you are going to be on the floor playing with 1- and 2-year-olds, high-heeled shoes and a miniskirt would not be appropriate. But if you are working with adults in a rehabilitation center, a nice dress or a tie may be required. You may want to notice what the other professionals around you have on and dress similarly to them. You always want to dress with the thought that you want to appear professional.

ASHA CODE OF ETHICS

ASHA has a code of ethics that has been adopted by the profession as its ethical standard. The latest revision was made by the Legislative Council in November 2001, and can be found at http://www.professional.asha.org/resources/ethics_index.cfm. "The ASHA Code of Ethics gives guide-

lines of professional behavior for individuals providing clinical services in speech-language pathology or audiology. There is no legal basis for enforcement of the Code of Ethics except in states that have adopted the code as part of licensure requirements" (Hegde & Davis 1995, p. 59). Many other professions (law, medicine, engineering, social work, accounting, etc.) also have codes that help keep the public's confidence in their services. According to Schmeiser (1992, p. 5), "these codes deliver a clear message that the professions want their members to recognize the ethical dimensions of their work and to adhere to ethical standards in their practice on behalf of the public, individuals, and the profession itself."

The main reason for founding the American Academy of Speech Correction (later ASHA) in 1925 was to establish scientific standards and codes of ethics to assure patients/clients that practicing members of the organization offered a consistent level of behavior and quality of service. They were concerned that individuals in speech-language pathology may have no values or would trick people and that would undermine public confidence and destroy the profession's reputation. Individuals were accepted into the academy if they had a good professional reputation and had a high level of integrity. The first constitution of the academy included how new members would be accepted and guidelines for those already members. In 1952, the Code of Ethics was separated as its own document apart from the by-laws of the association. ASHA has only made few revisions of the code, but the Legislative Council of ASHA can amend the code at any time (Seymour, 1994).

If you choose to take part in the ASHA national registry, you will sign a document that states you will follow the Code of Ethics in your clinical interactions. This may also be required by certain states for licensure. If you do not follow this code of ethics, you may lose your registration with ASHA as an SLPA. Your supervisor may help you with ethical dilemmas, but you need to understand what the Code of Ethics says. If your value system is dramatically different from ASHA's Code of Ethics, you may want to consider a different career because you will need to abide by the Code of Ethics in your practice. As stated before, to maintain your registry

in ASHA, you must uphold the Code of Ethics. Many employers will require that you be registered with ASHA before they will hire you. In some states you have to be registered with ASHA to fulfill local laws licensure for SLPAs.

Board of Ethics

The Board of Ethics (BE) of ASHA is the group that works out the interpretation, administration, and enforcement of the Code of Ethics. The Board of Ethics first hears the allegations of violations of the Code of Ethics. Then the BE determines if an investigation is needed. They contact the alleged offender in writing about the charges and they give the alleged offender 45 days to respond to the allegations. The respondent's status with membership and certification does not change while the case is pending. The BE considers all the information obtained in the investigation and ends the process if there is not enough evidence. If there is sufficient evidence, the BE determines the nature of the violation, penalties for the offender, and the amount of information to be released beyond the respondent. For example, decisions from the BE are usually published in the *ASHA Leader*. The BE may decide not to publish the information and the details around the proceedings. They then contact the offender and ask him to stop the practice that violates the Code of Ethics. If the respondent does not agree with the decision of the BE, he may appeal to the Executive Board of ASHA. The Executive Board's decision is the final step in the process. The ultimate liability for client care rests on the supervising SLP (ASHA, 2001; Hegde & Davis, 1995).

The 2001 Code of Ethics is made up of a Preamble, four Principle Ethics and a number of Rules of Ethics. ASHA's philosophy of delivery service is included in the Preamble as well as an introduction to the rest of the code. The Principles of Ethics outlines basic ethical behavior and included under each Principle, the Rules of Ethics give the detail around professional behavior. The Code of Ethics is a guide for behavior and does not include every possible ethical issue you may face. The complete Code of Ethics is found in Appendix C. You should familiarize yourself with this code because it governs your professional behavior.

SIDELIGHT: *Emily's Story*

Emily just started her career as an SLPA in a hospital outpatient clinic. She was very nervous the first few weeks, especially when Harold, a new patient, asked if she was the SLP and she agreed without clarifying she was an assistant and describing the difference. She continued to let him believe that she was an SLP and when asked several months later about a previous assessment, she described the procedures and the meaning of the results with Harold and his wife, Joan. Joan was talking informally to Emily's supervising SLP a year later and said they appreciated the time that Emily had spent with them describing the assessment when they started therapy and how helpful that information had been in understanding what was going on with Harold's communication. The supervising SLP discussed the issues with Emily and reported her to the BE for misrepresentation. She immediately stopped the misrepresentation and explained her error to Harold and Joan. Emily received a formal reprimand and was placed on probation for a year. Her supervising SLP made it clear with all new patients with Emily present that Emily was an SLPA.

Principle of Ethics I

Principle I of the Code of Ethics is very straightforward and puts the patient's welfare as most important. As you grow in your professional skills and abilities, you will learn what is the best for the patient and begin to think of his needs and desires first. Under this principle it also states that the SLPA may not misrepresent himself as an SLP. The SLP may not transfer to a noncertified individual any responsibility that is not within the scope of practice of that individual (ASHA, 1994). They also added in the revised code is that individuals might provide services by telecommunication if they use the correct methodologies that best meet the needs of the client.

ASHA CODE OF ETHICS: PRINCIPLE 1

Individuals shall honor their responsibility to hold paramount the welfare of persons they serve professionally (ASHA, 2001, p. 1)

Preparation

The Code of Ethics insists that all SLPAs be competent in their service delivery. One way you can demonstrate competence is by being well prepared through training and practical experiences. In some situations you may be required to take certain coursework before working with a certain type of disability (e.g., completing a stuttering class before seeing an individual who stutters). To be prepared for your clinical interactions, you may need to spend time looking over the SLP's session plans, familiarize yourself with a particular screening tool, or assemble materials for a session with a client. You may need to do additional research before working with some individuals to prepare yourself with their specific needs or learn more about their disability. Your supervisor can help direct you to resources if you need that assistance. Keeping current in your field by attending conferences or even taking some university courses will help keep your skills sharp. Maintaining professional competence is an ongoing process that will continue through your entire career. See Chapters 1 and 2 for more information on the requirements for the SLPA.

SIDELIGHT: *Taking the Initiative*

Francis just met with his supervising SLP. He worked very hard to get all of the materials that are needed for the meeting ready before the meeting. He learned that he would be starting intervention with a middle school student who has Fragile X syndrome. In his training he was introduced to this syndrome, but after practicing for 5 years, he had forgotten the details of the syndrome. He decided to do a search on the Internet to find out the current information about that specific syndrome before seeing this student. Once he did his search, he felt prepared to work with this specific individual.

Your supervising SLP needs to hold a Certificate of Clinical Competence from ASHA. This means that your clinical supervisor will have current clinical certification in the area in which he provides clinical supervision. Your supervisor has been trained to do speech-language assessment and intervention with individuals; for example, when you are working in a rehabilitation center, your supervising SLP has had specific training to work with adults.

If you struggle with substance abuse or major health issues (including mental health issues), ASHA recommends that you do not interact with individuals and that you receive help for your difficulties. You cannot be adequately prepared if you struggle in these areas. Recognizing and doing something about these issues will not preclude you from practicing as an SLPA in the future.

Referral

You or your supervising SLP cannot provide services for everyone because the field of speech pathology is very diverse. To follow the guideline that you will only provide services to those you are qualified for, your supervising SLP may need to refer individuals to other professionals to receive the best care available. A **referral** is a recommendation that an individual seek specialized help from another professional like another SLP, medical doctor, audiologist, etc. If an individual is struggling with fine motor tasks, he may be referred to an occupational therapist. If some type of physical problem is uncovered, he may be referred to his doctor. When a referral is made, the SLP will provide several names of qualified professionals so the individual can make the choice of who to see. Once the referral is made, the SLP may follow up to see if he can be of any more help, especially if the individual is no longer seeing the SLP for services.

SIDELIGHT: *Janice's Story*

Janice had been working for about 3 months with a second grader who stutters. She noticed that the student's voice quality had changed over that time and was becoming more raspy and hoarse. She told her supervising SLP her concerns and the SLP listened to the child during therapy one day. The supervising SLP decided she needed to refer this child to an otolaryngologist, an ear, nose, and throat specialist (ENT). She called the student's mother and she quickly took him to see the ENT. They discovered that his vocal folds were damaged and had nodules. The ENT referred them back to the school SLP to provide therapy for vocal abuse to hopefully avoid surgery. Janice had received training on this type of therapy but had never actually done it herself. With the help of her supervising SLP, she learned the new techniques and after a recheck with the ENT, the child's vocal folds received a clean bill of health.

Discrimination

Discrimination is prohibited by the ASHA's Code of Ethics. Decisions related to delivery of service must not be based on "race or ethnicity, gender, age, religion, national origin, sexual orientation, or disability." You will come in contact with and provide services for a wide range of individuals. You may work better with certain individuals than others or you may decide to work primarily with a specific population (children, adults, severe disabilities, nursing homes, or early intervention programs). If you specialized in the area of geriatrics care, it would not be discrimination to decline to work with a group of children. However, you cannot decide not to work with a specific individual because you do not like the color of the skin, gender, age, religion, national origin, sexual orientation, or disability. Clinical judgment must guide your decisions, not unrelated issues.

Misrepresentation

The revised Code of Ethics (2001) includes misrepresentation as part of the ethical code. One needs to be very clear about his position as an SLPA. You may not allow individuals to have the impression that you are an SLP. That would misrepresent your position as an SLPA. This concept is covered in depth in Chapter 2 and the story about Emily earlier in this chapter.

Informed Consent

Informed consent is the ability to make choices and give your consent after receiving the proper information to help in your decision. Your SLP supervisor is required to give enough information so an individual or his family can understand all the relevant aspects of clinical services. That gives the individual the ability to make a decision to seek treatment or not. Individuals need information on both the benefits and drawbacks of therapy and they need to understand what may happen if no therapy is provided. Many schools, hospitals, and rehabilitation centers require that individuals

sign a statement that this information has been given to them, whether or not they decide to pursue therapy.

For their own protection, and for your own protection and that of your SLP supervisor, individuals need to be given complete information regarding the nature and possible effects of services. The SLP also must provide information regarding the prognosis (or future results) of the therapy performed. The Code of Ethics forbids therapists to guarantee treatment results. That is different from providing a patient and his family with a clinical judgment about a prognosis or what the patient will be able to do after therapy is completed. For example, the SLP could not say "You child will speak clearly in 3 months after therapy." But the SLP could say, "I have worked with this type of problem before and the treatment was effective with problems similar to yours. Based on the information I received through the testing and with your child's motivation, your child's potential for improvement is strong." These statements can be made with complete, accurate information, but if there are holes in the information, the fact that information is missing must be communicated with the individual.

An individual must be told if his therapy is part of a research program, and a complete description of the research must be provided. Then the client must be given a choice whether or not to participate in the research project. Individuals who agree to participate in experimental therapy have the right to withdraw at any time without any negative consequences.

Individuals must also be fully informed about who is providing the speech-language services and what that person's qualifications are. If you are providing services to an individual, he must understand that you are an SLPA and you are under the supervision of a certified SLP. You may never misrepresent your position, because it is unethical. In many settings you will be required to wear a name tag that gives your name and your title for both your protection and that of the individuals you work with. The name tag clearly states your position, and this will help your clients know you are an assistant as well as some of the boundaries that come with being an SLPA. Your setting may also require consent forms to be signed before any services are provided.

Treatment Efficacy

Individuals who are not expected to benefit from therapy may not be given speech-language services. The Code of Ethics addresses this issue, focusing on treatment efficacy and forbidding starting or continuing unnecessary treatment. The positive effects or changes made as a result of intervention are defined as treatment efficacy. This area may be made more complicated by an insurance plan defining whether therapy would be efficacious with different disabilities. This is especially significant given maximal concerns regarding fraudulent billing practices in the Medicare-Medicaid system. The SLP may determine that therapy with an individual who stutters would be beneficial, whereas the insurance company disagrees even if there is coverage available in the insurance plan. If the individual goes forward with treatment, the insurance company may not pay for these services. The SLP has acted ethically in recommending treatment even though the insurance company will not pay for those services.

Financial pressures of certain agencies, hospitals, or clinics, may try to put the SLP in compromising situations. A therapist may be required to see a certain number of individuals a day. If those individuals are not available, a therapist may be tempted to treat individuals who do not need therapy to meet the business's standard for productivity. The therapist is not providing effective treatment because the treatment will not benefit the individual. Another situation may arise between two SLPs disagreeing on who benefits from treatment. For example, therapists may disagree if treatment is effective with an individual with severe cognitive delays where progress may be made, but it may be very slow. It is crucial with individuals who make slow, steady progress to keep detailed records to help prove that therapy is effective.

Maintaining inadequate records is also considered unethical. Adequate records consist of information that documents little or no change as well as changes over several treatment sessions. If you continue therapy when no changes are being made, it would be considered unethical. Your supervising therapist may not have to dismiss the client, but definitely needs to change the treatment approach you are using.

A growing concern has been addressing Medicare and Medicaid fraud. This happens when an SLP bills for more therapy than what was given, individuals are put on a caseload when they do not need therapy, one type of therapy was provided and another type of therapy was billed at a higher rate, and individuals are not dismissed when treatment goals have been met. This issue has been added to the Code of Ethics (2001) to clarify that SLPs need to follow the Medicare and Medicaid guidelines for treatment and billing. Although reason dictates that these behaviors are unethical, the Code of Ethics now also helps protect patients and insurance companies from unethical behavior.

Confidentiality

A client's rights to privacy are protected under the Code of Ethics. You must maintain your client's **confidentiality** except when you need to give out information to protect your client or community's welfare, or because you must do so according to the law. Federal and state laws also protect the client's right to privacy.

When you are in your training program, you need to be especially careful about maintaining confidentiality. Because most learning comes from sharing experiences and information with your supervisor, one must be aware that there are special ways of sharing information that keep the individual's rights of confidentiality as a priority. You will not want to catch a supervisor in the copy room with many other people around and talk about details of a therapy session or aspects of family dynamics that concern you. A private room is a great place to discuss client issues. Also be careful not to discuss an individual with friends, family, or other students. Special permission needs to be obtained when doing a presentation on a specific individual to a class. The other aspect of training programs is that people who are not directly involved in the treatment of a client may observe individuals. Information seen and heard in a therapy session must be kept confidential. If you have questions about what you have observed, catch the therapist or supervisor at a time and place where confidentiality can occur. In all of these situations, you need to be aware of maintaining a client's rights to privacy.

Three different types of consent are discussed by Flower (1984) that relate to disclosure of confidential information. They include implied consent, written consent, and consent that are part of the private areas of a client's life. "Implied consent means that individuals seeking services implicitly approve access to their record by staff or support personnel without the need for written authorization. For example, it is not necessary for the clinic secretary to obtain written authorization before accessing a client's record because reviewing the client records is typically a part of a secretary's duties" (Hegde & Davis, 1995, p. 65). Another example of implied consent is when you are assigned an individual to follow for therapy and you need to discuss the therapy session with your supervising SLP. It is up to the supervising SLP if written consent must be obtained or if implied consent is sufficient.

The next form of consent is the written consent in which a client signs a form that allows the individual providing treatment to contact inside or outside agencies for information about the client. This type of written consent is called a release of information. For example if a child has just been evaluated by an early intervention team, an SLP may wish to request that information from them so another evaluation does not need to be performed. Another example of written consent involves an elderly man who has just sustained a stroke and was released from the hospital and intensive rehabilitation. Those records would be requested through a written consent form or release of information from the hospital, his personal doctor, a neurologist, and from those who did the rehabilitation work. Another example may be two professionals who are working with the same client and need to communicate to coordinate their services and discuss progress. A written consent is needed before any professionals may discuss a client. As an SLPA, you may be responsible for tracking the paperwork that follows a written consent.

Inherent consent is the third type of consent. It deals with the private interests of the client and is assumed when sharing of information is in the best interest of the client. This usually takes place between a professional and the client's family, especially when the client is a child or an adult under the care or guardianship of his family.

SIDELIGHT: *Written Consent*

Jim is working with Colin, who has had a significant hearing loss and wears bilateral hearing aids. On a regular basis, Colin goes to an audiologist to test his hearing, monitor the function of the hearing aid, or make repairs or adjustments to the hearing aids. Before Jim is able to call the audiologist to find out about Colin's most recent visit, he must have Colin's parents sign a release of information giving him permission to talk to the audiologist.

Other rules about the importance of client welfare are discussed in the Code of Ethics. You are not allowed to charge for services that were not provided. Adequate records need to be maintained and a client may not be treated only by correspondence.

GUIDE TO MAINTAINING CONFIDENTIALITY

The following is a list of precautions to help you maintain confidentiality, especially with your speech language pathology supervisor (Hegde & Davis, 1995).

■ Do not discuss your client by name.

■ Do not discuss your client in public areas.

■ Do not mention your client's name in presentations or discussions.

■ Do not leave client reports, lesson plans, or other written information unattended.

■ Follow all the office rules regarding checking out and returning client files.

■ Do not take client files home and do not remove information from the files.

■ If you have to make copies of the information for your own working files, black out the name to keep the information confidential.

■ Do not discuss your client with others.

■ Remind any observers that they should respect a client's rights to privacy.

■ Obtain written consent to make videotapes or take photographs of individuals.

■ Comply with your work setting's rules regarding release of information.

Principle of Ethics II

One of the highest levels of professional competence is for an SLP to hold a Certificate of Clinical Competence in Speech-Language Pathology (CCC-SLP). For SLPAs, the highest level of professional competence is to be registered with ASHA and their state licensure or regulation board. These levels are the minimum standard, and additional training may be needed to ensure competence in service delivery. You will also need to know your state's specific requirements to be employed as an SLPA.

ASHA CODE OF ETHICS, PRINCIPLE II

Individuals shall honor their responsibility to achieve and maintain the highest level of professional competence (ASHA, 2001, p. 1).

Scope of Competence

The field of speech-language pathology is growing all the time. Services include more aspects of client care and are provided to individuals of every age. Some SLPs work with newborns in the hospital, whereas others work with elderly people in the nursing home, and there are levels and types of care for every age in between. SLPs can specialize in certain areas of speech and language disabilities: stuttering, **articulation**, swallowing and feeding, augmentative alternative communication (AAC), deafness and language, individuals who have had a stroke or head injuries or professional voice issues. Your SLP supervisor will be competent to provide services to certain areas within speech-language pathology. You will also have areas that you are competent in as an SLPA. The Code of Ethics encourages you to work in the area you have received training. For example, you may have received training working with preschool children; therefore, it would not be ethical to work with adults in an acute care setting. You may have training in treatment with individuals with aphasia; which means you should not work with learning disabled students in a middle school. There are many areas in the field of speech-language pathology and you may want to pick certain areas to develop specialized skills. Competence is far above the minimal requirements necessary for registration. ASHA registration means that you have met the entry-level requirements to practice as an SLPA. These requirements include completing specific coursework, and fulfilling observation, screening, and intervention hours.

Continuing Education

Your learning as an SLPA does not stop after you graduate from your program. You will need to continue your education to help maintain the high standard of professional skill. Researchers and clinicians in the field are continually producing new and relevant information about the field. To keep up on the current information and practices, you will need to do independent study, read journals, and attend conferences that present the most recent information. Some view the SLPA as one step in a "career ladder" toward continuing professional preparation to a bachelor or eventually a master's degree. Whether you see being an SLPA as a "stepping stone" toward continued educational preparation or as a career choice, your commitment to lifelong learning is required.

Supervision

The Code of Ethics requires that clinicians be well prepared for the services they provide. The speech-language pathology supervisors are also responsible for ensuring that support personnel (SLPAs) are well prepared and work only in those areas of competence. Positive relationships with your supervising SLP are critical to your success as an SLPA. Supervision from an SLP is an ongoing process.

Principle of Ethics III

Principle III mandates that the SLP and SLPA do not misrepresent their ability, education, credentials, or experience. No misrepresentation of services or products is tolerated. The information you give needs to be clear and accurate, especially when presenting your services to potential clients or patients. This principle also addresses the need for clarity in roles when working with individuals and their families. They need to understand that you are an SLPA, a very vital part of their intervention, and not an SLP. In the 2001 Code of Ethics it was added that an SLP may not make any agreements that they will receive referrals for any type of reimbursement of any kind.

ASHA CODE OF ETHICS, PRINCIPLE III

Individuals shall honor their responsibility to the public by promoting public understanding of the professions, by supporting the development of services designed to fulfill the unmet needs of the public, and by providing accurate information in all communications involving any aspect of the professions (ASHA, 2001, p. 1).

Principle of Ethics IV

As an SLPA, you represent the profession as well as SLPs. As you interact with SLPs and other professionals (teachers, psychologists, occupational therapists, physical therapists, and doctors), you need to remember that interpersonal relationships are part of the Code of Ethics. Effective professional relationships are important because they are the foundation for your services.

Boundaries for relationships, especially sexual ones, are limited to individuals who are not students or colleagues over whom one exercises professional authority. The other aspect of this principle that was more clearly defined recently was in relation to clearly referencing the source when using another person's ideas, research, presentations, or products in any form (written, oral, or any other media presentation).

ASHA CODE OF ETHICS, PRINCIPLE IV

Individuals shall honor their responsibilities to the professions and their relationships with colleagues, students, and members of allied professions, maintain harmonious interprofessional and intraprofessional relationships, and accept the professions' self-imposed standards (ASHA, 2001, p. 2).

Supervisor

A supervisor is responsible for those who work under his direction. That would include you as an SLPA. During your training, supervisors are responsible for making sure that your behavior is professionally acceptable. Professional behavior is made up of adequately preparing for clinical sessions, protecting the client's confidentiality, maintaining

effective working relationships with other professionals, and so on. See Chapters 3 and 4 for SLPA roles and relationships with other professionals. Review your scope of practice to help you define your role as an SLPA and the role of your SLP supervisor. Your supervisors will be evaluating your professional skills as well as your technical and academic skills during your clinical assignments. When you are out working, your supervising SLP will be ultimately responsible for you and what you do. According to ASHA's current guidelines for SLPAs, you need to be supervised at least 20% of the time you are working strictly with a client, student, or patient. This ensures continuity of service and provides you with valuable feedback on your performance.

Assigning Credit

Everyone who contributes to a written work must be given proportional credit. Reports you submit for academic or clinical coursework must contain references and credit other individuals involved in the work. If two professionals were working with the same individual and write the report together, both should sign the report. Your supervising SLP will be writing most of the reports and signing most documents, but there may be instances when your signature is appropriate.

Professional Judgment

Your supervising SLP will be using his professional judgment regarding who would benefit from treatment. This judgment must be unclouded by financial or business pressures. Those decisions must be made on clinical data, not what insurance companies, hospitals, clinics, or schools think is best. In schools, a specific criterion is used to determine whether or not children receive speech-language services. Most of these criteria are based on standardized testing, but some are based on the professional judgment of the SLP. If you have questions regarding how individuals are placed on a caseload, ask your supervising SLP.

Upholding the Standards of the Profession

The Code of Ethics is the standard that clinicians must abide by according to ASHA. One more standard that is outlined in the Code is the matter of discrimination. You are not allowed to discriminate in relationships with others (including other professionals, families, individuals, or other SLPs) on the basis of race or ethnicity, gender, age, religion, national origin, sexual orientation, or disability. If you feel that someone has violated the Code of Ethics, you have the responsibility to discuss it with your supervisor/mentor and report the individual to the Board of Ethics (previously named Ethical Practice Board). If you are still in your training, you need to report these issues to your instructors. The instructors and department chair will decide the next steps to be taken.

OTHER PROFESSIONAL ISSUES

Scope of Practice

As an SLPA, it is important for you to understand your scope of practice and how it differs from a certified SLP. Two sections of the Code of Ethics specifically relate to SLPAs. Principle of Ethics I states "Individuals shall honor their responsibility to hold paramount the welfare of persons they serve professionally," and Principle of Ethics II, Rule D states that "Individuals shall delegate the provision of clinical services only to persons who are certified or to persons in the education or certification process who are appropriately supervised. The provision of support services may be delegated to persons who are neither certified nor in the certification process only when a certificate holder provides appropriate supervision."

The SLPA may assist the SLP in providing services. The supervising SLP is directly responsible for the services provided by the assistant and the decisions related to the client's welfare in all phases of assessment and intervention. The SLPA may not independently diagnose, treat, or advise indi-

viduals of their progress or prognosis (ASHA, 1994). An SLP may not delegate these responsibilities to an SLPA because it goes against the Code of Ethics and because it puts the patient/client/student's level of care at risk.

SLPAs are a vital part of many settings and SLPs rely on their services. SLPAs must be very careful not to misrepresent themselves as SLPs. An SLP who only provides minimal supervision over an assistant because of the responsibility for too many assistants is in violation of the Code of Ethics requiring the SLP to hold paramount the welfare of persons he serves.

Reporting Suspected Abuse

Every state has laws that govern disclosure of information to protect the well-being of the individual or of the public. One responsibility you have as a professional working with people is reporting suspected abuse. The SLPA cannot leave the reporting to the agency he works for (Flower, 1984). Abuse can be physical, emotional, financial, sexual, or it can result from neglect. When people think of abuse, most think of child abuse, but abuse can happen to anyone. Harm to children or adults can come from physical injury; constant criticism, insults, or the withholding of love; rape, fondling, or incest; failure to provide food, clothing, shelter, or medical care; or stealing from an individual's finances. Most children and elders are abused in the family home or by those they know such as parents or caregivers, siblings, relatives, or family friends (American Association of Retired Persons [AARP], n.d.; Prevent Child Abuse America, n.d.; The Elderly Places, n.d.). Elder abuse in nursing homes makes up only 4% of the reported cases (American Psychological Association [APA], 2001; Clearinghouse on Abuse and Neglect of the Elderly, n.d.). While child abuse has received significant attention by the media, government, law enforcement, and advocacy groups, elder abuse is becoming more understood (Administration on Aging, 1998). According to the Executive Summary of the Third National Incidence Study of Child Abuse and Neglect (National Clearinghouse on Child Abuse and Neglect Information), in 1993 over 1.5

million children in America were abused or neglected. It is reported that approximately 2.1 million older Americans are victims of abuse (Woolf, n.d.). For every case of elder abuse and neglect that is reported to the authorities, experts estimate that there may be as many as five cases that have not been reported (APA, 2001). Elder and child abuse comes in many different forms—physical, emotional, sexual, financial, or neglect (Administration on Aging, n.d.; Elder Abuse Prevention, 2001).

You do not have to wait until you can prove abuse before you report it. You should talk to your supervisor immediately. Make a report when your worries or concerns about the safety of a child or elder turn into suspicions that the child or adult is being abused or neglected. You need to organize the facts (times, names, places, specific suspicions of abuse or neglect, and other details) before you call the appropriate agency. The sooner you call, the more likely the evidence will be preserved for the authorities to investigate. To report suspected abuse, call your local Child Protective Service Agency, Department of Social Services, the Department of Children and Families (DCF), Eldercare locator 800-677-1116, or the National Center on Elder Abuse. You will receive specific information regarding policies from your SLPA training or at your employment setting. Most employers make training about abuse and neglect part of their orientation trainings. See Appendix H for more detailed information on recognizing the signs and symptoms of elder and child abuse.

Cultural Differences and Abuse

As an SLPA you will need to be aware of cultural differences and be able to distinguish those differences from abuse. Demographics are rapidly changing, with increased diversity, language differences, and many cultures represented in each setting. Many people in the United States have differing backgrounds: African, Asian, European, Hispanic, and Native Americans, to name a few. "Over the past 20 years, the United States has experienced a great influx of immigrants from all over the world: Afghanistan, Cambodia, Cuba, El Salvador, Ethiopia, India, Iran, Mexico, Nicaragua,

Philippines, Thailand, Vietnam, and so on" (National Clearinghouse on Child Abuse and Neglect Information, p. 8). With this increase in diversity among immigrants, you will be likely to come in contact with many different cultural backgrounds in your work that makes your own cultural sensitivity critical for your professional success. Becoming culturally sensitive will help you distinguish between child-rearing practices that are different and others that are defined by law as abusive.

When you come across parents who hold values and customs different from your own, you may want to ask the parents to explain these values or customs, rather than just making judgments about them. Child-rearing practices vary from family to family, as well as between cultures and ethnic groups. Some cultures require a child to look at the adult when the adult is talking to him, whereas others feel that looking at adults is disrespectful. Some cultures encourage children to participate in adult conversations, while others feel that children should be seen and not heard. This list could go on and on covering every aspect of child rearing. Knowing the inflexible legal definitions of child and elder abuse will help you determine differences and actual abuse.

Client Bill of Rights

A major protection for individuals receiving services is the Client Bill of Rights. In 1994, ASHA's Task Force on Protection of Client's Rights published a technical report that outlined the Model Bill of Rights for People Receiving Audiology or Speech-Language Pathology Services. This is a general document that relates to children and adults across all different service delivery settings. You can find a copy of the Protection of Rights of People Receiving Audiology or Speech-Language Pathology Services in Appendix D.

CONCLUSION

Ethics are part of our everyday life. You started developing your belief system when you were a child. Your ethical development was influenced by those around you such as your

parents, teachers, siblings, friends, and relatives. Religious training may be a part of your ethical training growing up. In your training as an SLPA, you are learning about another standard, a professional ethical standard for you to work by.

As an SLPA you have a specified Code of Ethics developed by ASHA to follow in your professional life. These are minimum standards that apply when you are working as an SLPA. The first is to always consider the welfare of the individual you are working with as top priority. This could be a child, teenager, parent, grandparent, or an entire family. The second is to honor the profession and achieve a high level of competence. Learning is a lifelong process. To keep your skills current and develop new skills, you will need to continue your education after you graduate. This may be a requirement of specific states for licensure and registry. The third discusses providing the public with information about the profession of speech-language pathology and ensuring you provide other professionals with accurate information about individuals you are working with and descriptions about your screening and therapy. The fourth principle outlines the responsibilities of the profession and learning and maintaining skills in working with other people. Ethics and professional behavior provide a foundation that the profession is built on.

DISCUSSION QUESTIONS

The following ethical scenarios are provided for discussion with your peers and instructor. Use the ASHA Code of Ethics and the information presented on professionalism as a resource in determining solutions.

Scenario 1: Your supervising SLP is running out of time to perform an evaluation. She asks you to give 2 subtests of a standardized evaluation tool. What do you do? Why?

Scenario 2: A few therapists in your department treat home health individuals after work hours for a private home health agency. On several occasions, you have seen the therapists taking supplies from work and not returning them. Do you share this information with anyone?

Scenario 3: Mrs. Brown is referred to therapy for treatment. She is 89 years old and has made statements that she is waiting to die and does not want therapy. Your supervising SLP has told you to work with her on feedings to maintain her quality of life. What questions do you have?

Scenario 4: You are an SLPA in a pediatric clinic. You notice that every Monday morning, Stephen, a 7-year-old patient, comes to therapy with bruises all over his arms and small round marks that look like cigarette burns on his legs. When his mother is out of the room you ask Stephen about the bruises and he replies, "I fall a lot." Do you take him at his word?

Scenario 5: Your SLP supervisor has called in sick and there is a very important IEP scheduled. You were a part of obtaining a language sample on a child and he is in a classroom where you spend part of your day. The principal asks if you would be able to share the results of the evaluation with the parents and special education team. How do you respond?

Scenario 6: You are an assistant in a rural school district where there are no therapists in other disciplines. The district has been unable to get therapists from other disciplines despite numerous recruiting efforts and a current open position. Clara, a kindergarten student, has mild cerebral palsy. She is bright but not yet walking and her language is delayed. Her parents request that you focus more on motor skills instead of language skills. What do you do?

Scenario 7: Your speech-language supervisor asks you to work with a 40-year-old client. As you read his chart, you discover that he has AIDS. You are 8 weeks pregnant and you do not want to work with him. What do you do?

Scenario 8: You are assigned to treat Bob Smith, the mayor of your town. Later that evening you mention to your spouse that Bob Smith is your new patient. Your spouse asks you what you are doing with Bob Smith. In the past you have discussed this sort of information about nameless individuals with your

spouse. How do you respond to your spouse's questions?

Scenario 9: You are very busy at work so you decide to catch up on some of your work at home. You are writing your therapy notes in clients' charts and you have to answer a phone call. When you return, you find your teenager reading through your clients' charts. You live in a small community where everyone knows everyone else. How do you respond to the situation?

Scenario 10: You work for a therapy company that contracts with long-term health care facilities. Your company has just obtained a new contract with a nursing home that you have been assigned. After some time there, you realize that all the individuals seen in therapy are wearing the same clothes and the clothes have the same dirt marks they did the last time you saw them. The men you see will go weeks without being shaven and the individuals have an odd odor to them. Because you do not work directly for the nursing home, you do not feel comfortable saying anything. You have indirectly made comments, but nothing has changed. You decide to talk to your supervisor about the conditions and she tells you to "stay out of this one" because it does not affect your therapy with individuals. What do you do?

Scenario 11: You work in a large therapy department in a large hospital. You find out that assistants in another discipline are being paid higher salaries than the assistants in your discipline, even though the billing rates and charges for both therapy services are the same. What do you do?

Scenario 12: You attend an important regional therapy conference. You decide to show your support for your supervisor by going to her session to hear her present a paper for which she is listed as the sole author. As you listen, you discover that your supervisor's presentation sounds almost identical to training given by another SLP almost 7 months ago. How do you react? What do you do?

Scenario 13: Your state has recently instituted a continuing education requirement for SLPAs. You attend a workshop with a large attendance. Several of your coworkers are also attending the workshop. At the workshop, after about 1 hour, one of your coworkers leaves and then returns about 1 hour before the workshop ends, with shopping bags from the mall. She receives her certificate of attendance for the full 6.0 hours. What do you do?

Scenario 14: You have been working at a hospital for about 6 months. A couple of weeks after a patient was discharged he comes in to talk to you about how much he was charged for therapy services. You call your supervisor, who tells you to tell the client not to worry about it because Medicare will pay for it. How do you respond?

Scenario 15: You work in a nursing home and you are sharing a therapy room with a nurse's aide. He is working with an older adult who is severely developmentally delayed. During therapy you notice that he pinches this individual when he does not respond. As the individual leaves, you notice a bruise on his arm. What do you do?

Scenario 16: You receive a call from an SLP who is now seeing a client you used to work with. She wants to know about your therapy and what type of progress the client made under your care. She said that she is planning to get written permission for release of information the next time she sees the client, but she needs the information as soon as possible to plan her sessions. Since that time your supervising SLP has moved to another state and is not available. How do you respond?

Scenario 17: A parent walks up to your session with her son in a private setting. She wants to know how the child is doing in your practice sessions and how long the child will need services because she needs to make financial plans tonight to pay for therapy. What do you tell her?

Scenario 18: Your SLP supervisor is running behind in her care of adults in a rehabilitation hospital. She asks you to see a client who has been having difficulty swallowing. She asks if you would join the client for lunch and watch for any choking or signs of difficulty swallowing. What do you tell her?

Scenario 19: You are working at a hospital where you see an adult stroke patient for therapy. The client's son brings him in for the therapy and is very charming. After about 3 months of seeing the client, the son asks you out for a date. What do you do?

Scenario 20: You are asked to do an observation of a 10th grader in a high school and document the number of interactions the student has with her peers. The SLP then asks your impressions of what you saw and to make some judgments about the student's social functioning. How do you respond?

SUGGESTED ACTIVITIES

1. Take the opportunity to talk or interview an SLP regarding common ethical concerns. How do the ASHA Code of Ethics and scope of professional responsibilities compare to the examples she provides?

2. Given your scope of responsibilities as an SLPA, think through how you would develop a code of ethics specific to your practice. What principles would you emphasize and how would you include information that would provide appropriate guidelines for individuals with communication disabilities?

3. Research another code of ethics from a related discipline such as occupational therapy or physical therapy. Compare and contrast principles that guide professional behaviors and interactions with the ASHA Code of Ethics.

REFERENCES

American Association of Retired Persons. (n.d.). *Avoiding abuse.* Retrieved January 15, 2002 from http://www.aarp.org/confacts/ health/avoidabuse.html

Administration on Aging. (n.d.). *Elder abuse prevention.* Retrieved January 15, 2002, from http://www.aoa.dhhs.gov/factsheets/ abuse.html

Administration on Aging. (1998, September). *The National Elder Abuse Incidence Study: Final Report.* Retrieved January 15, 2002, from http://www.aoa.gov/abuse/report/default.htm

American Psychological Association. (2001). *Elder abuse and neglect: In search of solutions.* Retrieved January 15, 2002, from http://www.apa.org/pi/aging/eldabuse.html

American Speech-Language-Hearing Association. (n.d.). *Frequently asked questions about speech-language pathology assistants.* Retrieved March 12, 2002, from http://www.professional.asha.org/ certification/faq_slpa.cfm#us

American Speech-Language-Hearing Association. (1994, March). ASHA policy regarding support personnel. *ASHA, 36*(Suppl. 13), 24.

American Speech-Language-Hearing Association, (1996). *Curriculum guide to managed care.* Rockville, MD: Author.

American Speech-Language-Hearing Association. (2001). *ASHA Code of Ethics.* Rockville, MD: Author.

American Speech-Language-Hearing Association Professional Services Board. (1994, January). The protection of people receiving audiology or speech-language pathology services. *ASHA, 36,* 60–63.

Child Abuse Prevention Network. (n.d.). *Reporting child abuse and neglect.* Retrieved August 25, 2001, from http://child-abuse.com/ report.html

Clearinghouse on Abuse and Neglect of the Elderly. (n.d.). *The basics: What is elder abuse?* Retrieved January 15, 2002, from http://www.elderabusecenter.org/basics/index.html

Edge, R. S., & Groves, J. R. (1999). *Ethics of health care: A guide for clinical practice* (2nd ed.) Clifton Park, NY: Delmar Learning.

Elder Abuse Prevention. (2001, August 30). *Recognizing elder abuse.* Retrieved November 28, 2001, from http://www.oaktrees.org/ elder/recog.shtml.

The Elderly Place. (n.d.). *Possible causes of elder abuse and prevention: In family members.* Retrieved November 28, 2001, from http://www.geocities.com/~elderly-place/abuse8.html

Flower, R. (1984). *Delivery of speech-language pathology and audiology services.* Baltimore, MD: Williams & Wilkins.

Harris, C. E., Jr. (1986). *Applying moral theories.* Belmont, CA: Wadsworth.

Hegde, M. N., & Davis, D. (1995). *Clinical methods and practicum in speech-language pathology* (2nd ed.) San Diego, CA: Singular.

Kornblau, B. L., & Starling S. P. (2000). *Ethics in rehabilitation: A clinical perspective*. Thorofare, NJ: Slack.

National Clearinghouse on Child Abuse and Neglect Information. (2001, April 6). *Recognizing child abuse and neglect*. Retrieved August 25, 2001, from http://www.colib.com/nccanc/Pubs/usermanuals/caregive/section2/cfm

National Clearinghouse on Child Abuse and Neglect Information. (n.d.). In A. Sedlak & R. Broadhurst, *Executive summary of the third national incidence study of child abuse and neglect 1993*. Retrieved August 25, 2001, from http://www.calib.com/nccanch/pubs/statinfo/nis3.cfm

Prevent Child Abuse America. (n.d.). *Child abuse and neglect: What you should know*. Retrieved August 25, 2001, from http://www.preventchildabuse.org

Prevent Child Abuse America. (n.d.). *Recognizing child abuse: What parents should know*. Retrieved August 25, 2001, from http://www.preventchildabuse.org

Prevent Child Abuse America. *Ten Ways to Help Prevent Child Abuse*. Retrieved August 25, 2001 from http://www.preventchildabuse.org

Schmeiser, C. B. (1992, Fall). Ethical codes in the professions. *Educational measurement: Issues and Practice*, 5–11.

Seymour, C. M. (1994). Chapter 6: Ethical considerations. In R. Lubinski, & C. Frattali (Eds.), *Professional issues in speech-language pathology and audiology: A textbook* (pp. 61–74). San Diego, CA: Singular.

White, T. I. (1988). *Right and wrong: A brief guide to understanding ethics*. Englewood Cliffs, NJ: Prentice-Hall.

Woolf, L. M. (n.d.). *Elder abuse and neglect*. Retrieved on January 15, 2002, from http://www.webster.edu/~woolflm/abuse.html

Legislation

Key Concepts

■

Applicable legislation and case law help provide protections and define rights for people with disabilities.

■

IDEA transformed public education access and educational opportunities for children with disabilities.

■

Section 504 offers protections regarding discrimination that may have an impact on practices in public institutions.

■

The Americans with Disabilities Act is considered civil rights legislation for individuals with disabilities.

■

Federal and state funding options include SSI, SSDI, Medicare, and Medicaid.

Overview

■

Individuals With Disabilities Educational Act (IDEA)

■

Programs and Services for an Adult

■

Americans With Disabilities Act (ADA) of 1990

■

Government Benefits

■

Technology Public Law 100-407

INTRODUCTION

The laws protecting individuals with disabilities have set many standards for speech pathology treatment and services over the past 20 years. The speech-language pathology assistant (SLPA) needs to be aware of these laws so she can work with her supervising speech-language pathologist (SLP) to provide the most appropriate services. Some laws deal with free and appropriate education for children, long-term planning for a child's future, accessibility in the community, and financial and medical assistance. This chapter, however, is primarily concerned with federal laws, including **Individuals with Disabilities Education Act (IDEA)**, Section 504, and **Americans with Disabilities Act (ADA)**. State and local laws need to be investigated by the reader. To learn more about the laws in your community, you may contact the national offices of the ARC (formerly the Association for Retarded Citizens) or your local or state affiliate of the ARC, your Department of Health and Human Services, and the United States Department of Education. Most state departments currently have active Web sites that will update your knowledge regarding applicable state laws and policies. One example is the Colorado Department of Education at http://www.cde.state.co.us.

INDIVIDUALS WITH DISABILITIES EDUCATION ACT (IDEA)

During the middle of the last century, schools started providing educational services for children with disabilities. Before that time, children with disabilities were sent to residential schools, homes, and institutions where their needs were met but minimal education was provided. According to Budoff and Orenstein (1988), traditionally "slow" children were given intelligence quotient tests and placed in classrooms for the mentally retarded without parental knowledge. Once placed, they were targets of verbal abuse from peers and school staff. In the 1960s, state and federal governments started to work toward providing educational services to children with disabilities. In 1975 major changes in education came after what is now called the Individuals with Disabilities Education Act (IDEA) was passed (Kaplan & Moore, 1995). This law, originally called the Education for All Handicapped Children Act of 1975, was better known as **Public Law 94-142**. Along with recent amendments, the IDEA has dramatically improved educational opportunities for most children with disabilities. An updated version of IDEA was "reauthorized" in 1990 under Public Law 101-476, with the most recent "reauthorization" passed in 1997 (Kaplan & Moore, 1995; Turnbull, Rainbolt, & Buchele-Ash, 1997). The 1997 amendments have several areas of significant impact and may be found in Figure 8-1.

SIDELIGHT: *Assessing Penny*

A young family has a 3-year-old girl named Penny. She was a little slow in developing most of her developmental milestones, but overall Penny is a happy and social child. The one thing her mother was concerned about is that she could not understand what Penny was trying to say most of the time. Her pediatrician recommended that Penny receive a speech and language evaluation. Her mother contacted the preschool team in their local school district. There were several individuals who provided the play-based assessment, including an SLP, special education teacher, psychologist, social worker, and occupational therapist (OT). Penny's mom learned that Penny had a few additional areas that she needed some extra help with along with her speech. Penny had difficulty with fine motor activities like coloring, cutting, and picking up small objects. She also had trouble playing with toys beyond what an 18-month-old would play with. Because eligibility was determined based on the results, the team set up a meeting with Penny's mom to write an individualized education plan (IEP) and discuss the results of the testing. At the meeting they discussed what Penny's needs were and how to meet those needs, and they wrote goals and objectives to guide their treatment plan. Penny then was enrolled in an inclusive preschool program that could provide for her special needs. Her mom was so excited to find support for Penny and she looked forward to watching her daughter grow up and develop with the team's help.

The federal government under IDEA, provides funding for state special education programs to ensure that the education of children with disabilities meets federal standards. To qualify for these funds, states must demonstrate a thorough and detailed plan that ensures all children with disabilities have access to a free appropriate public education

IDEA 1997 Amendments

1.
Evaluation and Placement: IDEA connects evaluation to programs and placement, creating a more databased process for decision making.

2.
Least Restrictive Environment: Least restrictive environment is the access a child has to the general curriculum and peers. IDEA has strong support for least restrictive environment.

3.
Outcome-Based Special Education: The IDEA revisions made special education more outcome-based and require performance goals with performance indicators and biennial reports to be filed on the student's progress.

4.
Discipline: IDEA reflects current laws around order as well as school safety concerns. If a child is expelled, he must be provided a free appropriate public education, and ending special education services is illegal.

5.
Positive Behavioral Support and Functional Assessment: IDEA specifically mentions positive behavioral support and functional assessments for prevention for students whose behavior makes them subject to school discipline.

6.
Parents' Rights: IDEA grants parents new rights to be a part of all-educational decisions and decision–making processes.

7.
Mediation: Mediation is strongly encouraged through IDEA before going to a due process hearing.

8.
School Reform and Special Education: IDEA encourages schools to have special education students be included in school reform efforts. It also requires states to develop alternative assessments for those who are exempt from the regular assessments.

Figure 8-1 Amendment made during the reauthorization of IDEA in 1997. *Note.* From *Individuals With Disabilities Education Act: Digest and Significance of 1997 Amendments,* by R. Turnbull, K. Rainbolt, and A. Buchele-Ash, 1997, Beach Center on Families and Disabilities, Lawrence: University of Kansas. Adapted with permission. (continues)

IDEA 1997 Amendments (continued)

9.

Service Coordination and Other Entitlements: Services like health, mental health, social service, and disability-entitlement programs will not offset, but must complement other benefits the student is receiving through IDEA.

10.

School Capacity Building: A school's capacity to serve special education students is linked to student development and school improvement. It also requires state and local agencies to develop new capacities to serve students.

11.

Flexible Funding: The schools receive great flexibility in using federal funds to respond to student rights, school capacity building, and school reform needs through IDEA.

12.

Attorney's Fees: IDEA stipulates that parents may no longer recover funds for a lawyer's services at an IEP meeting.

13.

Early Intervention: Part C is now the early intervention program. Transition services must be provided a child going from early intervention to early special education. Part C also emphasizes services in the child's natural environment. Head Start and childcare agencies must be represented on the Interagency Coordinating Council.

14.

Empowerment: IDEA encourages student/parent–school interaction at all levels and desires a systems-based approach to special education.

Figure 8-1 (continued)

(Kaplan & Moore, 1995). As an SLPA it is important to understand how a free and appropriate education looks.

Free Public Education

"Free" means that every part of a child's special education program must be provided at public expense through taxes, regardless of the parent's ability to pay. If a child needs a special cushion on his chair to help him focus, the school cannot ask the parents to pay for the cushion. A free education is usually achieved by placing the child in public school and modifying or adapting the curriculum or services provided to meet the child's needs. If no suitable public program is available, the school district must pay for all necessary services a child will receive through a private program. For example, if the child needs a residential facility to meet emotional needs, the school may contract with a private agency to provide that service. Or if a child needs vision therapy and the district does not have a vision specialist on staff, the family might be sent to a private vision specialist or optometrist who provides vision therapy. The school, however, does not have to pay for private services that they do not deem necessary for the child. Most districts have specialists available to meet the needs of their students. Some of these specialists may include an SLP, OT, physical therapist (PT), vision specialist, audiologist, psychologist, social worker, behavior specialists, and special education teachers. Whatever the financial situation may be for the family of a child with disabilities, federal laws ensure that an education will be provided to that child at no cost to the family.

Appropriate Public Education

"Appropriate" education does not necessarily guarantee the best education money can buy. Children with disabilities have access to specialized education services that benefit them. The services must directly address the needs of the child with disabilities and relate to their educational or academic functioning. "The Supreme Court has ruled on IDEA that 'free appropriate public education' need not enable a child with disabilities to maximize her potential or to develop self-sufficiency" (Kaplan & Moore, Jr., 1995, p. 228). Part of an appropriate education may include services beyond the regular school year. For example, a child may need a year-

round school to maximize her abilities, but she may not be given summer school if she does not qualify by the school district's standards (usually "**regression**" or losing a certain amount of information over a break time). This is usually measured over a winter holiday vacation. Decisions about summer school are made at the IEP meeting. Both parents and educators are encouraged to work together and form a partnership to design an IEP for students 3 to 21 years old and an individualized family service plan (IFSP) for children from birth to 3 years old. If disagreements occur over the planning process, there are dispute resolution provisions in the law. A mediation or a due process hearing may be part of this process if resolutions cannot be reached before this point. At times families and school personnel may disagree on what is appropriate education for a child. Appropriate education meets the specific needs of a child.

Legal Cases

The following two legal cases address the issue of free and appropriate education.

Case 1:

Issue: What is the minimum federal standard for determining what constitutes appropriate education?

Case: *Board of Education of the Hendrick Hudson Central School District v. Rowley*, 458 U.S. 116 (1982).

Description: The parent of a child with a hearing impairment claimed she had a right under Public Law 94-142 to the services of a sign language interpreter as part of her free appropriate public education.

Outcome: Supreme Court ruling:

- Public Law 94-142 does not require schools to provide the best possible education, but only to provide child with disabilities "access" to an appropriate education.
- Services provided must be sufficient to provide "some educational benefit" or a "basic floor of opportunity."

Case 2:

Issue: All students with disabilities are entitled to a free appropriate public education.

Case: *Timothy W. v. Rochester N.H. School District*, 875 F.2d 954 (1989).

Description: Timothy W. had vision and hearing impairments, cerebral palsy, frequent seizures, mental retardation requiring pervasive care, and no discernible communication skills. He had made no observable educational progress in the school year, and the school district sought to exclude him from special education services by contending that he was not capable of benefiting from special education.

Outcome: First Circuit Court ruling:

- IDEA was designed for every child with disabilities; especially the most severely handicapped and the severely handicapped are given priority.
- "Zero-reject policy is at the core of the Act, and … no child, regardless of the severity of his or her handicap is to ever again be subjected to the deplorable state of affairs which existed at the time of the Act's passage in which millions of handicapped children received inadequate education or none at all" (*Timothy W. v. Rochester N.H. School District*, 1989, pp. 960–961).

Special Education and Related Services

One part of IDEA under "appropriate" education is "special education and related services." **Special education** instruction is specifically designed to meet the unique needs of the child with disabilities. The school, at the public's expense, provides special education teachers who have specialized training to meet the needs of children with disabilities. A child may need help in math or reading that is beyond the scope of the regular education teacher; thus a special education teacher takes the responsibility for providing services for the child in the areas of reading and math. A special educa-

tion teacher may provide materials or adaptations to the regular curriculum to the regular education teacher so that the child can stay in the regular education classroom. "**Related services**" are defined as transportation and other developmental, corrective, and supportive services necessary to enable the child to benefit from special education. Under IDEA and related services, the services of a speech-language therapist, OT, PT, psychologist, social worker, school nurse, aide, or other qualified person may be required. Medical services (doctor or hospital services) and immunizations are not included under related services. Other medical services that may be provided by the school district under IDEA are nursing assessment, monitoring, catheterization, administration of medication, gastrostomy tube feeding, lifting and positioning, and teaching self-care in the school setting. However, typically a formalized "individualized health plan" needs to be in place in order to implement these types of specialized services (Rutledge et al., 1997)

Least Restrictive Environment

The IDEA requires that children with disabilities must be educated in the **least restrictive environment**. The least restrictive environment is the educational setting that provides the most exposure or time with children without disabilities (Long & Chapman, 1996). The law states that public agencies must ensure that, " to the maximum extent appropriate, children with disabilities ... are educated with children who are not disabled and that special classes, separate schooling or other removal of children with disabilities from the regular educational environment occurs only when the nature or severity of the disability is such that education in regular classes with the use of supplementary aids and services cannot be achieved satisfactorily" (20 U.S.C. § 1412 [5][B]). This means that a quadriplegic boy who relies on a ventilator to breathe can have someone, like a paraprofessional, help him work on his self-help skills and still participate in the regular education classroom. He may need adaptations or modifications to help him function well in that situation, including recording class notes or administering tests orally, but by being in the "regular" classroom he is learning in the least restrictive environment.

Other Aspects of IDEA

The IDEA also outlines other procedural rights and safeguards for the benefit of the caregiver. It also specifically singles out autism and brain injury in its classification of disabilities.

Procedural Rights and Safeguards

One critically important aspect of IDEA is that it involves parents directly in the education of their child. This law requires procedural rights and responsibilities to be fully explained to a parent or guardian as part of the special education process. Parents' informed consent must be in writing at the time their child is referred for special assistance before any testing occurs. Parents are the major information source during the evaluation; if parents do not like the educational plan, they have the right to contest it, first before an impartial hearing examiner and ultimately in court. Before IDEA was passed, parents had no say in the education of their child (Montgomery, 1994). Including parental involvement in this process is threfore a dramatic change.

Newly Defined Disabilities

Two disabilities are singled out under the classification of disabilities under the IDEA. The first is "autism" and the second is "brain injured." Brain injured includes brain injury due to trauma or another source, such as near drowning. It is the hope of lawmakers that singling these disabilities out will help educators provide more focused programming and placement for children with these disabilities.

Full Inclusion

IDEA has brought the issue of inclusion of children with disabilities with peers without disabilities to people's attention. This law was intended to discourage the practice of segregating or isolating children with disabilities by placing them in

separate schools or in secluded, out-of-the-way classrooms where there was little to no opportunity to interact with the **mainstream** school population. Segregated schools prepare children to function only in segregated environments. The world is not segregated and only an integrated setting can expose children to experiences they will have in their everyday lives. It is also important for nondisabled peers to learn from their peers who have disabilities. To date, researchers have looked at the impact on achievement scores of students without disabilities when students with disabilities are educated in their classrooms. No negative impacts on achievement have been reported (Project Choices, n.d.). Many teachers report an increase of sensitivity in peer interactions throughout the school when students with disabilities are educated in general education classroom (Educational Resources Information Center, 1998; Project Choices, n.d.). Parents and educators of children without disabilities express concerns that inclusion will take away from the direct instruction of other students. When appropriate supports, aids, and modifications are provided to the student with disabilities, inclusive education will not take away from the direct instruction of nonlabeled students (Project Choices, n.d.). In Illinois, researchers are noticing that regular education teachers are using ideas from the appropriate aids, supports, and modifications of disabled students to enhance their overall teaching skills (Educational Resources Information Center, 1998; Project Choices, n.d.). The greatest benefit for children with disabilities is in the area of learning social skills and how to interact with typical peers (Worley & Wilbers, 1994). For inclusive childcare centers that serve infants and toddlers, reimbursement may be at a higher rate from public agencies; therefore, increasing the resource base and improving the quality of care for all children (O'Brien, 1997). "In general, students with disabilities in inclusive settings have shown improvement in standardized tests, acquired social and communication skills previously undeveloped, shown increased interaction with peers, achieved more and higher-quality IEP goals, and are better prepared for postschool experiences" (National Early Childhood Technical Assistance Center [NECTAS], 1998, p.1). Many benefits come from full inclusion.

Some schools, especially middle schools and high schools, have developed "peer assistance programs" where nondisabled peers help the disabled student in a particular classroom or with homework. Children with disabilities have the right to attend their neighborhood school. IDEA recognizes that the regular classroom may not be the ideal place for all children to receive their educational training. There is a provision in the federal regulations that acknowledge that separate classroom and schools may be necessary to meet the individualized educational needs of some children. Excellent resources for inclusion are http://www.nectas. unc.edu, http://www.ericec.org/digests, and http://www. projectchoices.org.

Transition Services (Part B)

Planning for transitions from one service system to another is one of the provisions under Part B of IDEA designed to protect the child and family. One major transition occurs when a young adult transitions from school services to adult living. After high school an individual may seek postsecondary education, **vocational training**, integrated employment, continuing and adult education, adult services, independent living, and community participation. Planning for this major transition starts at early adolescence.

Procedural Safeguards (Part E)

A process to ensure that families of children with disabilities are involved in education decisions affecting their children is included in E of IDEA (Gerry, 1987). Parents have several options under the guidelines set out by IDEA when they have disagreements with the school district, including (Hurth & Goff, 1996):

- Requesting an administrative due process hearing or mediation to appeal an IEP
- Filing a complaint with the state's Department of Education to complain formally of violation of IDEA and its regulations
- Filing a complaint with the U.S. Department of Education Office for Civil Rights (OCR)

■ Appealing a hearing officer's court decision

Families and students have the right to an impartial hearing on any matter related to identification, evaluation, placement, and the provision of a free appropriate public education. States are required to offer a two-step program for due process, mediation, and a **due process hearing** (Turnbull, Rainbolt, & Buchele-Ash, 1997). The case is heard at the local level and then if there are still disagreements, appeals can be made to the state education agency (Budoff & Orenstein, 1988; Gerry, 1987). Other states only offer due process hearings at the state level. These can be appealed to the state or federal court. Mediation is also an alternative that states have implemented consistent with the federal requirement. This process is less formal than a due process hearing and is often initiated parallel to filing of a due process request. Mediation is an option for a family but not required. Mediation involves a mediator who is a trained neutral person. The mediator hears both sides of the disagreement and tries to facilitate a compromise. The families and the school district, not the mediator, make final decisions. However, mediation is an option, not a requirement. Participation cannot be mandated, but development of this option by the state is considered a compliance requirement of the federal law. Teamwork described in previous chapters will help families and school personnel work together so they can avoid a due process hearing.

IDEAS FOR TEAMING

1. Communicate openly and frequently.
2. Recognize the need to establish good rapport, which helps collaboration and respect.
3. Share reports between agencies.
4. Discuss possible dilemmas in planning meetings.
5. Talk about what every person expects from the child.
6. Consider all options and suggestions.
7. Ask advocates to attend meetings.
8. Stress that professionals and family members are equal members of the team.
9. Start with areas of agreement and then discuss the difficult issues.

Section 504 of the Rehabilitation Act of 1973

Congress enacted other safeguards to protect the rights of all persons with disabilities from discrimination by passing the Rehabilitation Act of 1973 (Rehabilitation Act of 1973). **Section 504** of this act is a civil rights statute for persons of all ages who have disabilities or "handicapping conditions." This differs from IDEA, which focuses solely on education. Any agency such as a state-funded university or public schools that receive federal funding must prove to the government that they are following the requirements of Section 504. They need to provide equal access to the services, programs, activities, and so forth for all recipients. For example, if a school district provides a summer school program, it must allow children with disabilities to enroll in the program as well as nondisabled children. Equal opportunity or equal access is the emphasis of Section 504 (Long & Chapman, 1996).

So how is Section 504 used practically? In an educational setting where a student does not fall into the narrow definition of a disability under IDEA, she may still be able to obtain education-related supports from the local school district. Personnel outside of the special education staff may provide services to an eligible student. The school district is required to meet the needs of a student with a handicapping condition in the educational setting. A specific example of a child who does not qualify for services under special education may include a student with asthma, HIV/AIDS, or seizure disorder. The student would qualify for services under Section 504. A student with a temporary disability, such as one recovering from surgery or an automobile accident could qualify for special services such as home tutoring, adapted homework assignments, or alternative testing, for as long as these services are needed. The school usually writes a plan to follow so the individual receives the special services needed. Because a special education team or other school personnel is not specifically assigned to monitor the 504 plan, the individual or her parents have the responsibility to make sure that the plan is being followed.

One major drawback of Section 504 is that no federal funds are specifically set aside to carry out Section 504.

Although funds do come through the general flow of funding for educational services, these funds are unspecified and are usually used in the school's general budgets. No extra money is provided for Section 504. This is very different from IDEA, where states are given a funding formula based on the state's population, disability statistics, and state matching dollars in order to fund a variety of special education services to children who qualify under the IDEA.

Handicapping Condition

Compared to the definition of disability under IDEA, the definition of "handicapping condition" under Section 504 is much broader. Handicapping condition is comprised of three major components: (1) an individual who has physical or mental impairment, which substantially limits one or more major life activities, (2) an individual who has a record of such impairment, and (3) an individual who is regarded by those around her as having such an impairment.

Part C—Public Law 102-119

In 1986, Congress amended IDEA and required all states to begin providing special educational services from birth through the age of 2 years, 11 months (Long & Chapman, 1996). Originally, Part C was called **Public Law 99-457** or Part H. The law was reauthorized as Public Law 102-119 in 1991. The law was then strengthened and reauthorized with the 1997 IDEA amendments (Turnball, Rainbolt, & Buchele-Ash, 1997). See the summary of early intervention changes in Figure 8-1. **Part C of IDEA** initially gave states several years to develop early intervention services, and each state was able to design a unique program to fit its state's needs. These services and qualifications for services vary dramatically from state to state but can be found in every state. The intent of Part C of IDEA is to enhance families' abilities to meet the special needs of their infants and toddlers by strengthening their authority and encouraging their participation in meeting those needs. It also aims to provide services for children with disabilities as early as possible. Providing children speech and language therapy, occupation-

al therapy, physical therapy, and early educational opportunities during those formidable developmental years is vital. **Early intervention** is key in preventing or reducing the impact of disabilities on later learning and academic performance.

Part C offers funding to states helping to implement early intervention services for children from birth through age 2 years, 11 months. In order for a state to participate in this program, it must guarantee that early intervention services will be available to every eligible child and its family. Each state chooses a lead agency to receive the grant and administrate the program. The state also appoints an interagency coordinating council (ICC), which includes parents of young children with disabilities as well as service providers, to advise and assist the lead agency (NECTAS, n.d.).

Parents, day care providers, and doctors who have contact with infants and young children and suspect that a child is at risk for developmental delays can refer the child for testing and early intervention services. Most evaluations are done by a multidisciplinary team to determine eligibility for early intervention services. The requirements for eligibility are met by children under the age of 3 "with developmental delays or with a diagnosed physical or mental condition (e.g., cerebral palsy, Down syndrome) or who are at risk of having substantial developmental delays if early intervention services are not provided (e.g., low birth weight, mother addicted to cocaine). This particular criterion is at the discretion of each state" (Rutledge et al., 1997, p. 20). Service coordination is also an integral part of Part C of IDEA. A **service coordinator** is an individual who helps a child and family receive the rights, procedural safeguards, services, and supports.

Individualized Family Service Plan

Families with children from birth through the age of 2 use a different plan than the IEP. Their plan is called an **individualized family service plan (IFSP),** and it has an early intervention focus. Unlike an IEP, which focuses primarily on the needs of the child, the IFSP focuses on services for the family. The law recognizes that families with young chil-

dren with special needs often have special needs themselves. IFSPs specify services for the child as well as services to help parents learn how to use daily activities to teach their child and help siblings learn to cope with having a brother or sister with special needs. IFSPs are reviewed every 6 months because a child changes so much between birth and 3 years of age. A family may see decreasing a child's frustration in communication as a need. The IFSP will then delineate how to address this need. This need may be addressed in the home setting, so pictures may be placed around the house so the child can point to them to express her desires. This may decrease temper tantrums because the child is able to communicate her wants and needs. Another child may need help in articulating words correctly. The way to meet this need may include providing home practice activities for the family to use daily to practice specific sounds.

The written plan, a legal document, is called an IFSP and is developed by a team of individuals made up of parents and professionals. The assessment pages and signature page from an IFSP can be found in Appendix E. The sample does not include any outcome pages or transition pages. IFSP must contain the following components (Rutledge et al., 1997):

- The child's level of development
- The family's strengths and needs as they relate to the child's development
- Major outcomes expected for the child and accompanying time lines
- Early intervention services that are to be provided and the environment where services will be delivered
- The dates on which services are expected to start and how long they will last
- The name of the case manager who will be responsible for implementing and coordinating the plan
- The steps to be taken to support the transition of the toddler to school programs

The IFSP looks at the child in the context of her family and looks at needs and how to meet them effectively.

Identification and Evaluation

IDEA only applies to children with disabilities, thus a child must first receive a multidisciplinary assessment to determine if she qualifies for special education services. The law requires each state to develop assessment procedures to identify and evaluate the needs and abilities of each child before recommending placement in a special education program. IDEA requires that the process include parental input. Some states have a Child Find Team that works through the school district to provide the evaluation and identification services for children 3 through 5 years of age, and then when the child reaches kindergarten, a school-based team performs the evaluations. The teams may be made up of parents, SLP, OT, PT, psychologist, nurse, regular education teacher, special education teacher, and social worker. The team is encouraged by the law to perform developmentally appropriate evaluations often called play-based assessments for the younger children. These assessments are the primary tool determining a child's qualification for special education services.

Individualized Education Plan

Every child is unique and IDEA provides a way to make an individualized plan for each child to address her specific needs. Based on a child's evaluation, a program is specifically designed to meet each child's needs. It is then written down in a legal document called an **individualized education plan (IEP)**.

An IEP is used for children 3 to 21 years of age. If a child is under 3, an **IFSP** (described below) is written. The IEP is written during a meeting or series of meetings between the parents, teachers, therapists, and representatives from the school district. When a child gets older, it is recommended that the child be a part of these meetings. An IEP is reviewed at least once a year by the special education team or parents, and the meeting is called an annual review. It can be reviewed or modified as often as is necessary. It is important for the IEP to contain goals that help promote the most independence and self-help care. The team of professionals can provide important information about the scope and sequence needed for a particular child to achieve goals toward independence.

IEP COMPONENTS

■ The child's current level of functioning or level of development

■ Annual and short-term goals of the special education program

■ The specific services the child will receive

■ The date the services start and the duration of those services

■ A statement of transition services needed to prepare the student for life after leaving school

■ Standards for determining if the goals of the education program are being met or that instructional objectives are being met

■ The extent that the child will participate in the regular education classroom

Under the federal guidelines, the educational program should be based on the IEP and not vise versa. The child's individualized needs dictate the services, not what services or programs are available in the school district; a "one size fits all" mentality is not appropriate when developing an IEP. School districts are required to have committees make placements and program decisions, and these teams are sometimes called child study teams or administrative placement teams. An IEP is a personalized plan to meet the specific needs of the individual regardless of special classrooms or programs a school district offers.

SIDELIGHT: *Susie's Story*

Susie was born with a profound hearing loss and has worn hearing aids since she was 6 months old. She will be starting kindergarten in the fall. Susie has spoken some words, but primarily communicates using American Sign Language. She lives in rural Montana and the district school only uses Signed Exact English in its instruction. The team brainstorms options on how to best meet Susie's individual needs.

Ideally, writing an IEP is a cooperative effort between families and school professionals. The role of parents in this

process cannot be overemphasized because they are the experts on their child. Parents are also advocates for their children and may need to push for the appropriate services for their child. For example, if parents feels that a program using augmentative alternative communication methods is the best for their child, they might need to demonstrate that failing to provide these services would not be appropriate for their child's specific needs. If parents want an academic-oriented program for their child, they might need to demonstrate that a program that emphasizes only vocational or functional skills is not appropriate given that child's specific abilities and needs.

IEPs need to be very detailed in their definition of each child's education plan. The teachers and parents set specific goals for every area of development and detail how each of these goals must be met. The amount of detail may seem tedious, but it helps everyone involved monitor the child's education and makes sure that she is receiving all the prescribed services in the IEP. You need to be familiar with IEPs because you may be involved in implementing activities that are designed to meet these goals. A general goal for a child may be to improve functional communication. The objectives to meet this goal may delineate different methods of achieving this goal. Objectives must also be measurable. For example: The child will use signs or an augmentative communication device to answer questions during group time from 2 times in 30 minutes to 5 times. The law requires that IEPs be reviewed and revised at least once a year. It can be done more frequently if needed (for example, a child is transitioning from preschool to kindergarten or middle school to high school). These annual meetings ensure that an educational plan continues to meet a child's changing needs. A few pages from an IEP can be found in Appendix D.

Part of the IEP process is to determine whether a child qualifies under IDEA for special education services. The following is a list of disabilities:

- Preschool Disability
- Significant Limited Intellectual Capacity
- Significant Identifiable Emotional Disability
- Perceptual or Communicative Disability

- Hearing Disability
- Vision Disability
- Physical Disability
- Speech-Language Disability
- Multiple Disabilities

Each of these disabilities has a very specific set of guidelines that a child must meet before placement is assigned. The primary focus of qualification is how a child's disability affects her ability to learn in a school setting and if it is significant enough to need special accommodations and modifications to help her learn effectively. A sample IEP may be found in Appendix E. The information on the following disabilities was adapted from Individualized Education Program Boulder Valley School District Division of Special Education (10/30/98) from the determination of disability section of the IEP. The following descriptions include the legal Boulder Valley School District (Colorado) definitions of each particular disability. You need to find out the specific qualifications and disability definitions in your area. Some are easily defined, whereas others have many intricacies. Some of the disabilities require a doctor's diagnosis of the disability (autism and head injured) to qualify for services whereas others lean greatly on the testing provided by the special education team. In Colorado, autism and head injured fall under physical disability so specific information on each disability is not included. As an SLPA working in the schools, you may be working with individuals who have the following disabilities and you can use these definitions to gain vital information about those with whom you will be working.

Preschool Disability

A preschool disability is a category for children ages 3 through 5 years. The schools, however, are not required to specify the disabling condition until they are 6 years of age. At age 6 the child is retested (before a **triennial review**) to help determine a disability other than preschool disability. To qualify they have to be 2 standard deviations below the mean in two or more areas: speech, language, fine motor, gross motor, cognitive abilities, or educational abilities.

SIDELIGHT: *Matthew's Story*

Matthew was a slow talker. His mother had been told not to worry; he will talk when he is ready. Finally when he was 3 ¹/₂, she called Child Find and scheduled an evaluation. The social worker took the background information and, with the team, planned the play-based evaluation. Matthew demonstrated difficulties in both speech and fine motor skills and qualified to receive support under the preschool disability.

Significant Limited Intellectual Capacity

Significant limited intellectual capacity is used for a child with reduced general intellectual functioning that prevents the child from receiving reasonable benefit from general education. All three of the following indicators must be present for a child to qualify under this condition. A child must have a score of more than 2.0 standard deviations below the mean on individually administered measures of cognition, evidence that the level of independent adaptive behavior is significantly below the culturally imposed expectation of personal and social responsibilities, and a deficiency in academic/preacademic or developmental achievement, as indicated by scores 2.0 standard deviations below the mean in measures of language, reading, and math.

Significant Identifiable Emotional Disability

Significant identifiable emotional disability is used for children with emotional or social functioning that prevents the child from receiving reasonable educational benefit from general education. This is a challenging disability to define because it has to be an emotional disability, not a behavior problem. The child must fit either of the two following categories: (1) Academic functioning: an inability to receive reasonable educational benefit from regular education, which is not primarily the result of intellectual, sensory, or other health factors, but due to the identified emotional condition, or (2) Social/emotional functioning: an inability to build or maintain interpersonal relationships that significantly interferes with the child's social development. Social development is defined as those adaptive behaviors and social skills

that enable a child to meet environmental demands and assume responsibility for her own and others' welfare. The following criteria must be met:

- Several strategies have been tried within regular education and the child is still unable to benefit from it. His presence is detrimental to the education of others.
- There are indicators that social/emotional dysfunction exists to a marked degree (above peers and cultural norms).
- Indicators are observable in at least two environments (one must be school).
- Indicators have existed for a period of time and are not isolated incidents.

Emotional or social functioning could mean one or more of the following:

- Exhibits an overall sad affect, depression, and feelings of worthlessness; cries suddenly and frequently
- Displays atypical affect for a situation (very angry, hurt, sad, etc.)
- Excessive fear and anxiety
- Continual physical complaints not causd by a medical condition
- Has behaviors of withdrawal, avoidance of social interaction, or lack of personal care to an extent that personal relationships cannot be maintained
- Out of touch with reality—hallucinations, disorientation, or delusions
- Has trouble getting her mind off of certain thoughts or ideas
- Consistently aggressive toward objects or others
- Oppositional, defiant, or noncompliant responses
- Significantly limited self-control
- Exhibits persistent patterns of stealing, lying, or cheating
- Patterns of bizarre or exaggerated behavior in routine environments

The significant identifiable emotional disability has many components to separate children who qualify for this disability and those who have behavior problems.

Perceptual or Communicative Disability

Learning disability can be either perceptual or communicative. It is defined as a disorder in one or more of the psychological processes involved in understanding or in using language, which prevent the child from receiving reasonable educational benefit. The criteria for a perceptual or communicative disability include two main items and one or more of several others. The first two are a significant discrepancy between estimated intellectual potential and actual level of performance and difficulty with cognitive or language processing. The other factors include significantly impaired achievement in prereading or reading skills, reading comprehension, written language expression (problems in handwriting, spelling, sentence structure, and written organization) or comprehension, and application and retention of math concepts. The child's reading problems may not be caused by any other disabling condition. The perceptual or communicative disability may also be defined as a learning disability and translates into a discrepancy between the cognitive potential and actual performance. This definition is currently being reviewed. It is expected that criteria will change with the reauthorization of IDEA in the next year or two. This is a perfect example of how the focus of the law or regulations can change with each reauthorization. It is necessary to continually update your information in this area because definitions and regulations can change.

SIDELIGHT: *Justin's Story*

An eighth grader, Justin, was having difficulty keeping up in his history class. He was social and intelligent, but just couldn't keep up in that class. His teacher referred him to the special education team where he was evaluated. His scores showed a discrepancy between his performance and verbal abilities due to difficulties in auditory processing. He qualified for special education and speech-language services. Juanita, the school SLPA, started working with Justin after the SLP had written relevant goals, objectives, and treatment plans.

Hearing Disability

A hearing disability is defined as having a deficiency in hearing sensitivity, as demonstrated by an elevated threshold of auditory sensitivity to pure tones or speech where, even with the help of amplification, the child is prevented from receiving reasonable benefit from general education. The child must have one or more of the following to qualify for a hearing disability.

- Sound-field word recognition (unaided) of less than 75% in quiet as measured with standardized open-set audiometric speech discrimination tests presented at average conversational speech (50 to 55 decibels).

- **Receptive** or **expressive language** delay as determined by standardized tests:
  - Under 3: less than one half of the expected development for chronological age
  - 3 to 8 years: 1 year delay or more
  - 9 to 13 years: 2 years delay or more
  - 14 to 21 years: 3 years delay or more

- An impairment of speech articulation, voice, or fluency

- Significant discrepancy between verbal and nonverbal performance on a standardized intelligence test

- Delay in reading comprehension due to language deficit

- Poor academic achievement

- Inattentive, inconsistent, or inappropriate classroom behavior

A deficiency in hearing sensitivity includes one of the following:

- An average pure tone hearing loss in the speech range (500 to 2000 Hz) of at least 20 decibels in the better ear that is not reversible within a reasonable period of time (this disqualifies someone who has an ear infection)

- An average high-frequency, pure tone hearing loss of at least 35 decibels in the better ear for two or more

of the following frequencies: 2000, 4000, or 6000 Hz
- A unilateral hearing loss of at least 35 decibels that is not reversible within a reasonable period of time

A hearing disability involves the child's ability to hear information that is presented in a classroom setting. If the disability is significant, it will interfere with a child's ability to learn in a regular classroom without adaptations to the curriculum.

Vision Disability

A child with a vision disability shall have a deficiency in visual acuity or visual field or visual performance where, even with the use of lenses or corrective devices, she is prevented from receiving reasonable educational benefit from general education. The criterion starts with a child who needs Braille or educational materials or needs specialized methods, aids, or equipment for learning, literacy, or mobility. Visual disability does not include children who have learning problems as a result of visual perceptual or visual motor difficulties. A vision disability shall be one of the following:

- Visual acuity of no better than 20/70 in the better eye after correction
- Visual field restriction of 20 degrees or less
- A physical condition of the visual system, which cannot be medically corrected, and, as such, affects visual functioning to the extent that specially designed instruction is needed

A visual disability is another disability that relates to the sensory system. Most of the curriculum in schools is presented visually and cannot be accessed by a child with a visual disability. See Figure 8-2 for a preschooler with a visual disability.

Physical Disability

A child with a physical disability has a sustained illness or disabling physical condition that prevents her from receiving

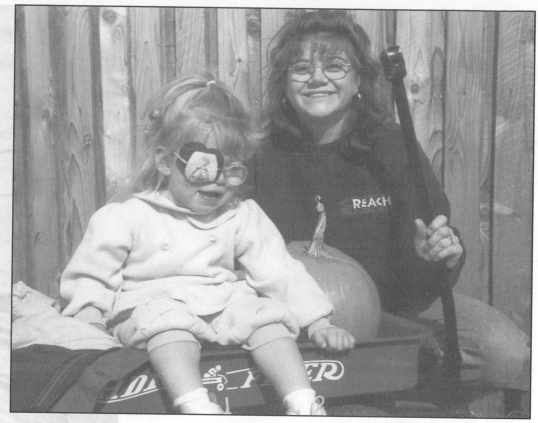

Figure 8-2 Visually impaired preschooler on a field trip

reasonable educational benefit from general education. Criteria may include any of the following:

1. A chronic health problem or sustained illness that requires continual monitoring, intervention, or specialized programming. A sustained illness means a prolonged, abnormal condition requiring continued monitoring characterized by limited strength, vitality, or alertness due to chronic or acute health problems.

2. The child's physical disability interferes with:
   - Ambulation
   - Attention

- Hand movements
- Coordination
- Communication
- Self-help skills
- Other activities of daily living

A disabling condition means a severe physical impairment. Conditions such as, but not limited to, traumatic brain injury, autism, attention-deficit disorder, and cerebral palsy may qualify as a physical disabilities if they prevent a child from receiving reasonable educational benefit from general education. Sensory integration difficulties do not constitute a physical disability.

Speech-Langauge Disability

A child with a speech-language disability shall have a communicative disorder that prevents her from receiving reasonable educational benefit from general education. The criteria for speech-language disability includes any of the following:

- Interference with oral or written communication in academic and social interaction in the child's primary language
- Demonstration of undesirable or inappropriate behavior as a result of limited communication skills
- The inability to communicate without the use of assistive, augmentative alternative communication devices or systems

Speech-language disorders may be classified under the following categories:

1. Receptive or expressive (oral or written) difficulties (syntax—word order, form, and developmental level; semantics—vocabulary, concepts, and word finding; and pragmatics—purposes and uses of language)
2. Auditory processing problems (sensation or acuity, perception-discrimination sequencing, analysis and synthesis, and auditory attention)

3. Deficiency of structure and function of oral mechanism

4. Articulation difficulties (substitutions, omissions, distortions, or additions of sounds)

5. Voice disorders (problems with respiration, phonation-pitch, intensity and quality, or resonance)

6. Problems with fluency (hesitant speech, stuttering, cluttering, and related disorders)

7. Problems with auditory perceptions (discrimination and memory)

A speech or language disability is the one that an SLPA will be working with in the schools. This disability centers around the ability to communicate clearly with others and the breakdowns may occur anywhere along the process: hearing the message, processing the message, formulating a response, and then articulating the response.

SIDELIGHT: *Jose's Story*

Jose and his family moved to the United States from Central America when he was 6 years old. He was now 8 and enjoying going to school and learning. He sometimes had difficulty saying words or thoughts in English and they came out stuttered. The teacher referred him to the SLP, and after obtaining parental permission, she performed a speech-language evaluation. Jose demonstrated strong language skills, but demonstrated difficulty in the area of fluency. Because his difficulties were significant, he qualified to receive speech and language services through the schools. Because Maria, an SLPA, was bilingual in Spanish, she worked with Jose on his fluency goals.

Mulitiple Disabilities

A child with multiple disabilities needs to demonstrate two or more areas of significant impairment; one must be a cognitive impairment except in the case of deaf-blindness. A cognitive impairment is defined as significant limited intellectual capacity (2 standard deviations below the mean on a standardized cognitive test). Other areas of significant

impairment include physical, visual, auditory, communicative, or emotional. The combination of these impairments prevents the child from receiving reasonable educational benefits from regular education. Other areas that are considered when determining a multiple disability include: inability to comprehend and use instructional information, inability to generalize skills consistently, inability to communicate fluently, and inability to demonstrate problem-solving skills when information is presented in a traditional academic curriculum.

PROGRAMS AND SERVICES FOR ADULTS

Some children with developmental disabilities grow up and need special services after they graduate from high school (usually at the age of 21). To achieve community living and employment skills, some adults need specialized training. These services include employment, job training, and residential or community-living programs. Typically, these programs have long waiting lists and are underfunded. Thousands of children receive education and training that equip them to live independently and productively, only to be sent home after graduation with nowhere to go and nothing to do.

One job-training program that is supported by federal funding is through the states' Department of Vocational Rehabilitation. Sometimes the Department of Vocational Rehabilitation is called DVR or "Voc Rehab." Adults must fulfill two requirements to qualify for job-training services: (1) they must have a physical or mental disability that constitutes a "substantial handicap to employment"; and (2) they must be expected to benefit from vocational services. These services are not just for developmentally delayed adults, but for any adult needing vocational training. It could be an adult who has had a stroke or head injury and is unable to do her job. Recent amendments to the IDEA require that services and training be provided to people even if what they achieve is "supported employment." **Supported employment** means employment in a setting where services such as

a job coach or special training allows an individual to work productively. Job training through vocational rehabilitation gives adults with disabilities an opportunity to work.

AMERICANS WITH DISABILITIES ACT (ADA) OF 1990

The ADA prohibits discrimination against people with disabilities. The ADA is a law that operates like other federal laws that outlaw racial, religious, age, and sex discrimination. ADA applies to most private employers, public and private services, **public accommodations**, businesses, and telecommunications.

Employment

An employer cannot discriminate against qualified individuals with a disability "in regard to job application procedures, the hiring or discharge of employees, employee compensation, advancement, job training, and other terms, conditions, and privileges of employment," according to the ADA. A "qualified individual with a disability" is a person with a disability who, with or without reasonable accommodation, can perform the essential functions of a job. The law defines "reasonable accommodation" as accommodations that an employer makes to remove obstacles from the job, the terms and conditions of employment, or the workplace that would prevent an otherwise qualified person from working because she has a disability. Accommodations can include job restructuring, schedule shuffling, modified training and policies, and access to readers, interpreters, or other technology. An employer who does not make an effort to make these accommodations would be in violation of this law. A blind individual working on computers may need a screen reader to use her computer effectively. The employer would be expected to provide this adaptation. This law, however, only applies to companies that have more than 15 employees because smaller businesses may not be able to handle the potentially higher costs of hiring an individual who needs adaptations to do a job effectively.

This law does not require employers to hire people with disabilities or to make accommodations if an "undue hardship" will result for the employer. If an individual feels that she has been discriminated against by a potential employer, she may contact and file a complaint with the federal Equal Employment Opportunity Commission (EEOC). This agency is responsible for resolving employment discrimination complaints.

SIDELIGHT: *Jessie's Story*

Jessie needed to find a job. She had been on many interviews but no one had offered her a job. She wondered if her blindness kept her from being hired. She was great at researching information on the World Wide Web, but she needed a screen reader to do it effectively. She wondered if her special needs disqualified her from being hired. How would she know? The next day she had an interview and it seemed to go well. They were very interested in the adaptations she would need to do this job. She was hired the following day, and her employer provided her with a computer with a screen reader.

Public Accommodations

One of the most well-known aspects of the ADA involves making public accommodations for individuals with disabilities. The ADA states that no discrimination may occur in any public place, including hotels and motels, restaurants and bars, theaters, stadiums, convention centers; bakeries, grocery stores, gas stations, pharmacies, and other retail businesses; doctors' or lawyers' offices; airports and bus stations; museums, libraries, parks, and zoos, any schools; day care centers; homeless shelters; and so forth. Any place open to the public must be accessible to any person with a disability. This, however, does not apply to private residences. Many new building codes have been adopted beccause of the ADA. For example, a movie theater may not restrict where individuals with disabilities sit, what time they come, or separate them from their family. An individual with a hearing disability must be provided special hearing devices called assisted listening devices (ADLs) at a movie theater so they can hear the movie.

SIDELIGHT: *Frank's Story*

After an accident 4 years ago, Frank's left leg had to be amputated above the knee, and his right leg was paralyzed. He was very athletic and was great at getting around in his wheelchair. Today he had a business meeting and he knew that the building was very old. He was concerned how he would get to the second floor office. He took a taxi to the building. Frank was glad to see a wheelchair ramp next to the long flight of stairs to the front door. He had to get to the second floor and was able to find an elevator at the back of the building and get to the office. His meeting ran long but went smoothly. As he was leaving he needed to use the restroom. It was easy to use the adapted stall, sink, and door. He was thankful for the changes they had made to this building so he could get to where he needed to go.

The ADA is like many other civil rights laws and also requires integration of individuals with disabilities with those without disabilities. The law prohibits the exclusion of people with disabilities on the grounds that there is a separate "special" program available for them. For example, if an individual with a prosthetic leg wants to play volleyball on a city league, the city could not exclude him from playing just because there is a volleyball league for people with disabilities. If someone feels that she has been a victim of discrimination, she can file a lawsuit. If the U.S. Department of Justice brings a lawsuit against a public facility to halt a pattern and practice of discrimination, monetary damages and civil penalties may be imposed.

Legal Cases for ADA

Case 1:

Issue: Is a school system in violation of ADA if it does not allow children with severe to profound hearing loss the right to choose the type of signing used by interpreters provided by the school?

Case: *Petersen v. Hastings Public Schools*, 831 F. Supp. 742f (1993)

Description: Several parents of students with severe to profound hearing loss requested that the school system allow

them to choose the type of signing interpreters used with students.

Outcome: U.S. District Court ruling:

- If the auxiliary aid that is requested is more than what is needed for effective use, the law does not require the use of the superior aid. (831 F. Supp at 752 [D. Neb., 1993])
- Students were not able to prove the superiority of the system they devised and thus failed to demonstrate any discrimination on the part of the school.

Case 2:

Issue: Is a university in violation of ADA when a student with disabilities, requiring a personal care attendant, does not have a roommate randomly assigned as is the case for other students attending the university?

Case: *Coleman v. Zatechka*, 824 F. Supp. 1360 (1993)

Description: A college student, who required a personal care assistant, applied for student housing and requested a roommate who did not smoke. The university assigned the student a room but not a roommate. The student repeated her request that the university randomly assign her a roommate.

Outcome: U.S. District Court ruling:

- The university's blanket policy of excluding students who use attendant care from the roommate assignment program violated both the ADA and Section 504 of PL 93-112.

Olmstead Decision

The Supreme Court issued the *Olmstead v. L.C.* decision in July 1999. The Olmstead decision interpreted Title II of the ADA that states must run their services, programs, and activities in the most integrated setting appropriate to the needs of qualified individuals with disabilities (Health Care Financing Administration [HCFA], 2001). Medicaid may be a resource that states use to fund their programs, but it should not be limited to those who receive Medicaid. HCFA

is working with states and individuals with disabilities to make sure that the ADA and the Olmstead decision are being implemented.

GOVERNMENT BENEFITS

Financial assistance is available from a wide variety of federal, state, and local programs for people with disabilities. Everyone who has worked is probably familiar with social security; when paychecks come, certain percentage of money is taken out for taxes, retirement, and social security. When you reach 65, you are eligible to start receiving an income from the Social Security Administration based on your previous earnings. In 2027 you will have to be 67 years old to qualify for retirement benefits (Social Security Administration, 2001). But government benefits provide for more that just retirement income—they also provide for disability income and insurance.

During the 1930s social security was developed as a retirement benefit for everyone over a certain age. Currently, according to the American Association of Retired Persons (AARP, 2001), 44.5 million Americans receive social security benefits (retirees and their spouses, 30.5 million; disabled workers and their spouses, 5.0 million; children of retired deceased or disabled workers, 3.8 million; and widows and widowers and parents of deceased workers, 5.2 million). Since the 1930s, the Social Security Administration has expanded substantially to include social security, Aid to Families and Dependent Children (AFDC), Temporary Assistance for Needy Families (TANF), social security income (SSI), **social security disability insurance (SSDI)**, **Medicare**, and **Medicaid** (Social Security Administration, 2001). Each one has its own set of eligibility requirements. You will probably not work directly with these government benefits, but it is good to become familiar with them. The main forms of assistance include monthly payments and medical insurance. SSI and SSDI help provide financial support for those with disabilities, whereas Medicare and Medicaid are the two main forms of medical assistance available from the government (AARP, 2001). Hospitals, clinics,

and some schools are able to bill Medicaid and Medicare for services. Both Medicaid and Medicare cover speech-language services so, as an SLPA, you may be seeing individuals with this type of insurance and you may be assisting your SLP to complete the paperwork around therapy and billing these insurance providers.

Social Security Insurance (SSI)

What you may not know is that SSI also covers individuals with disabilities. Monthly checks are mailed from SSI to senior citizens and to children and adults with serious disabilities. A disabled adult will receive a monthly check from SSDI, with the amount based on her past earnings. An individual who was disabled before the age of 18 or children of deceased or retired persons who earned social security coverage also receive money from SSDI (Kaplan & Moore, 1995). Both SSI and SSDI are administered by the Social Security Administration. Other programs that may provide financial assistance to individuals with disabilities include children of deceased federal employees, military personnel, and railroad employees (AARP, 2001).

Qualifying for SSI

One has to meet two qualifications to receive SSI. First, the individual must prove that she or her child is disabled. The SSA has a specific set of tests that helps determine qualification, which are different for children and adults. An individual's condition must be so disabling that she cannot engage in "substantial gainful activity." This means that the disability interferes with basic work-related activities and one cannot be retrained and compensated to do another type of job (Social Security Administration, 2001). An individual may also be required to provide documentation from medical personnel to prove that she has a disability. It is a strict definition and does not include short-term or partial disabilities. A disability must be expected to last for at least 1 year or potentially result in death. If an individual is working and making more than approximately $750 a month, she cannot be considered disabled (Social Security Administration,

2001). The Social Security Administration (2001) has a list of medical conditions that are so severe such as a coma, quadraplegia, or lymphoma that would automatically qualify someone as disabled.

The second qualification an individual must meet is financial. In 2001, the maximum benefits an individual could receive was $534 and the maximum for a married couple was $796. An individual's income cannot exceed a certain amount or SSI benefits are cut off. In 2001, this was $1147 a month for an individual, $1943 for a family with one child, and $2209 for a family with two children. This increases with the number of children in a family. For a child with disabilities to qualify, the SSA takes into account the parents' income. A parent's income must be very restricted to have her child with disabilities qualify for SSI. However, in 1990 the U.S. Supreme Court ruled that the guidelines for children to qualify for SSI were too restrictive, and today more children are allowed to qualify as disabled (Social Security Administration, 2001).

It has been a challenge for disabled adults to hold a job and continue to receive SSI. Many people have to choose between the two: job or SSI. Moore & Kaplan (1995) explain a work incentive program called Plans for Achieving Self-Support (PASS). It allows a recipient to receive an income or assets in her own name as long as they are used for the SSI recipient to work in the future or to establish a business or occupation that would allow her to be employed. During the time they are on the PASS program, they may continue receiving some SSI benefits. Many issues affect how families plan their estates for their disabled children. To find out current information from the Social Security Administration call their toll free number at (800)772-1213.

Social Security Disability Insurance (SSDI)

SSDI is available to individuals with disabilities. According to the Social Security Administration (2001), a 20-year-old worker has a 3-in-10 chance of becoming disabled before reaching retirement age. The same criterion for "disability" is used for SSDI and SSI. Unlike SSI, SSDI does not have a financial component to qualify. To be eligible for SSDI, an individual must qualify on the basis of her own work record for social security purposes, or she must be unmarried, have a disability that began before the age of 18, or be the child, under 18, of a parent covered by social security who has retired or died.

SIDELIGHT: *Robin's Story*

Robin delivered soda for a local bottling company. One day a loose can of pop slid off the top off her load and hit her in the throat and damaged her vocal cords. Because of the injury, she had to have surgery and a lot of speech therapy. She was unable to work during that time due to the extreme pain she was in. She applied for social security disability income and with some red tape came a check. She had been worrying about how to pay her bills. Hopefully she will have a complete recovery and can return to work soon.

If a person works and makes more than a certain amount a month, she is no longer considered disabled and can no longer qualify for SSDI. There is a program through SSDI that allows a person to work for 1 year on a trial basis without losing eligibility to determine her ability to work (Social Security Administration, 2001). Individuals can receive SSDI benefits if they qualify under the guidelines for disabled, and individuals on SSDI can qualify to receive medical insurance through Medicare.

Medicare

Medicare is a federal health insurance program that helps with medical expenses. People who are eligible for SSDI benefits also qualify for Medicare. Also those who are 65 years or older qualify for Medicare. The Social Security Administration (2001) explains that Medicare has two parts. The first is Part A, hospital coverage, that comes automatically for those who have SSDI after they have been on SSDI for 24 months. The second part is called Part B, medical coverage, and those on SSDI may get this coverage for a premium. If someone qualifies for Medicaid (described next), it

will pay for Part B of Medicare. Individuals who do not qualify for Medicare can purchase it like any other health insurance through a parent, relative, or charities called "third party buy-in." Medicare does not include outpatient medications or short-term stays in nursing homes (Social Security Administration, 2001).

Medicaid

Medicaid is medical coverage for those who cannot afford medical insurance. If an individual qualifies for SSI, she automatically qualifies for Medicaid in 39 states. It pays for medical care for people who do not have private health insurance or who cannot pay for medical care. It also pays for residential services for many people with disabilities. It is funded partly by the states and partly by the federal government, and the states administrate Medicaid.

In each state there are Medicaid waiver programs that provide Medicaid benefits for a specific population that has to meet special qualifications. This is one way to qualify for Medicaid for individuals with disabilities. In Colorado, for example, 10 Medicaid waiver programs are available for individuals with disabilities (Colorado Department of Health Care Policy and Financing, 1999). See Figure 8-3.

All but one of the waiver programs described in Figure 8-3 requires that an individual (or family for the children's waivers) have limited resources to qualify. In 1999, the applicant's income must have been less than $1500 per month and his total assets less than $2000. Some waiver programs have long waiting lists because a certain number of spots are designated and funded by the states. To be disqualified from many of these waivers, an individual either has to be older than the qualifying age, or has passed away so those on the waiting list may have to wait a long time. (Colorado Department of Health Care Policy and Financing, 1999).

Many are familiar with welfare reform and how social security has started emphasizing personal responsibility, incentives, and a new limit on entitlements for benefits. Some of the welfare reform touched SSI and SSDI. For example, in 1996, all people who qualified as disabled through drug addiction and alcoholism were eliminated from

Colorado Medicaid Waiver Programs

- **Children's HCBS Waiver (formerly Katie Beckett): birth through 17**

  Disabled children in the home at risk of nursing facility or hospital placement. Enrollment 430 children. Waiting list.

- **Children's Medical Waiver: Birth through 17**

  Children in the home at risk of nursing facility or hospital placement. Children, birth through age 4, must have a developmental delay. Children 5 through 17 must have a developmental disability. Enrollment 200 children. Waiting list.

- **Children's Extensive Support Waiver: Birth through 17**

  Children with intensive behavioral or medical needs who are at risk of institutionalization. Children, birth through age 4, must have a developmental delay. Children 5 through 17 must have a developmental disability. Enrollment 152 children. Waiting list.

- **Children's Habilitation Residential Program Waiver: Birth through 21**

  Children, birth to 21 years of age, who are placed through the County Departments of Social Services, have a developmental disability and extraordinary service needs, and for whom services cannot be provided at the county negotiated rate. Enrollment 343. No waiting list.

- **Brain Injury Waiver: Ages 16 through 64**

  Persons with brain injury within an approved range of diagnosis codes. Must be in the process of discharging from a hospital, rehabilitation hospital, or rehabilitation facility. Enrollment 400 persons. No waiting list.

- **Mentally Ill Waiver: Age 18 and older**

  Persons diagnosed with a major mental illness. Enrollment 2,040. No waiting list.

Figure 8-3 Summary of Colorado Medicaid waivers. *Note.* From *Home and Community-Based Services (HCBS) Medicaid Waivers*, by Colorado Department of Health Care Policy and Financing, 1999, Denver, CO: Author. Adapted with permission. (continues)

Colorado Medicaid Waiver Programs (continued)

- **Persons Living With AIDS Waiver-:All ages**

  Persons with a diagnosis of HIV/AIDS. Enrollment approximately 155. No waiting list.

- **Elderly, Blind, and Disabled Waiver: Age 18 and older**

  Elderly persons with a functional impairment (aged 65+), blind persons, or physically disabled (aged 18–64). Enrollment 13,500 persons. No waiting list.

- **Supported Living Services Waiver: Age 18 and older**

  For persons who can either live independently with limited supports or who, if they need extensive supports, are already receiving that high level of support from other sources, such as family. Enrollment approximately 2,800. Waiting list.

- **Developmentally Disabled Waiver: Age 18 and older**

  Persons who require extensive supports to live safely, including access to 24-hour supervision, and who do not have other resources for meeting those needs. Enrollment approximately 3,200 persons. Waiting list.

Figure 8-3 (continued)

the rolls. The other major piece of legislation was the Personal Responsibility and Work Opportunity Reconciliation Act (PRWORA) of 1996. PRWORA changed the Aid to Families with Dependent Children (AFDC) program from an open-ended entitlement program into a grant. Temporary Assistance for Needy Families (TANF) set time limits for the receipt of benefits and strict work requirements. PRWORA also had stricter eligibility for children and narrowed eligibility for noncitizens receiving benefits (Social Security Administration, 2001).

Ticket to Work and Work Incentives Improvement Act of 1999

In 1999, Public Law 106-170 was passed (HCFA, 2001). This landmark legislation is called the Ticket to Work and Work Incentives Improvement Act of 1999 (TWWIIA) and allows millions of Americans with disabilities to join the workforce without fear of losing their Medicare and Medicaid coverage. The TWWIIA provides improved access to employment training and placement services for people with disabilities who want to work. It also improved access to health care coverage under Medicaid and Medicare for individuals with disabilities, and ensures that more Americans with disabilities have the chance to work and lessen their dependence on public benefits (HCFA, 2001). The Tickets program began in 2001 once the regulations were published. During the first year, 2001, this voluntary program was only available in 13 states: Arizona, Colorado, Delaware, Florida, Illinois, Iowa, Massachusetts, New York, Oklahoma, Oregon, South Carolina, Vermont, and Wisconsin. It expanded during the next few years, and by January 1, 2004, every state should have access to the Ticket program. Once an individual gets a Ticket, she may take it to an employment network, private organizations or public agencies including Vocational Rehabilitation Agency, and receive employment services. Through the Ticket, the earning limitations for Medicaid and Medicare are lifted so the individual is not disenrolled from her insurance benefits.

The other advantage of the TWWIIA is that health benefits will be extended to those with disabilities who work. On October 1, 2000, the law extended Medicare A premium free coverage for 4 1/2 years beyond the current limit (39 months) for disabled people who work. The law also gives states the option of providing Medicaid to more people 16 to 64 years old with disabilities who work. States may also permit working individuals the opportunity to purchase Medicaid coverage if their income is 250% of the federal poverty level. A Work Incentives Advisory Panel within Social Security is made up of 12 members appointed by the president and Congress. This advisory panel reports to Congress on the implementation of the Ticket program. At least half of the panel members must be individuals with disabilities or represent an individual with a disability (HCFA, 2001).

SIDELIGHT: *Juan's Story*

Juan, 20, was about to graduate from high school. He was so excited to get out on his own and get a job. He was not able to completely take care of himself, but he wanted to try. His parents decided to look into a group home for Juan. He would live with four other men in a home where they would get some extra help with daily living skills such as cooking, cleaning, and dressing. Juan was thrilled with the idea and moved into Evan's house later that summer. The next hurdle was to find a job, but he was concerned about losing his SSI and medical benefits. He was good at things he could repeat. Through a vocational rehabilitation center and the Ticket to Work program, he found out that a local company needed someone to staple, fold, and put papers into envelopes. It sounded like something Juan could do. He went out with a job coach for the first few weeks to help him learn the job. Then he was on his own. He liked being independent and doing things for himself. It made him feel good to be out in the community. He met a few friends at his new job and Juan enjoyed watching football with them at his new house.

TWWIIA also requires Social Security to establish community-based work incentives planning, as well as assistance programs to give out accurate information about the work incentives, to provide more choices to those with disabilities. Social Security is required to share information about the protection and advocacy services to the beneficiaries. Work incentive specialists work in Social Security offices and provide up-to-date accurate information about SSA's employment support programs for those who want to work.

TECHNOLOGY PUBLIC LAW 100-407

In 1988, Congress passed PL 100-407, the Technology-Related Assistance for Individuals with Disabilities Act, which was amended and became the Technology-Related Assistance for Individuals with Disabilities Act of 1998 (Cohen, 1999). Currently, all 50 states, the District of

Columbia, and the Trust Territories have an assistive technology project funded under this act. The Tech Act requires projects to examine barriers to accessing and obtaining assistive technology in its state and then work to eliminate those barriers. The Tech Act encourages partnerships between the public and private sectors as well as consumers of technology products. Augmentative alternative communication is a part of the technology resources the states provide. Initially, states primarily provide training on the technology that is available to individuals with disabilities, and some states use their money to help fund the technology (Rocky Mountain Resource and Training Institute, 1989). In the past 10 years, "projects have focused on changing legislation, policies, practices, and organizational structures to overcome barriers in three areas: access to assistive technology, availability of assistive technology, and funding for assistive technology" (Cohen, 1999, p.1).

CONCLUSION

The federal government has passed several key laws that have dramatically changed the lives of individuals with disabilities. IDEA has made public education available for children with disabilities. Children are also encouraged to be in classes with their peers, while also receiving specialized services to meet their individual needs. An individualized education plan or an individualized family service plan is written to document a child's functioning levels, services she needs and adaptations or modifications that are needed to help her learn effectively. The law has specified what it takes to qualify as disabled in the schools with nine specific handicapping conditions. ADA prohibits discrimination against people with disabilities and applies to employment, public and private services, public accommodations, businesses, and telecommunications. The government also provides financial and medical benefits for those with disabilities and with recent legislation, they have a ticket to work. It is important to keep in mind that laws are constantly changing, and as an SLPA you will need to understand new legislation that affects individuals with disabilities with whom you work. It is also

important to look at applicable state mandates because these specify how the federal legislation is implemented in any given state. It is important to know how differences in implementation can affect who is eligible to receive services under IDEA in a given school district or program. Legislation is a critical part of the SLPA's life because it gives boundaries and guidelines for practice.

DISCUSSION QUESTIONS

1. What are the applicable state mandates in your state? How do they affect access to services for individuals with communication challenges? (For example, Nebraska has had a state law that mandates services from birth to 21 for children identified as eligible under their provisions for many years. In contrast, Colorado has state laws that mandate services for children 3 through 21, although they have developed a system of early intervention that complies with federal law.)

2. Compare and contrast the protections provided to consumers under Section 504 and ADA. Are protections clearly defined across settings and situations? How does case law clarify any confusions or illustrate implementations?

3. Do you think differences in eligibility definitions affect access to services for children from birth to 3 years old? What happens if a young child and her family move to another state? Will the intensity of services and supports change?

4. Your supervising SLP has asked you to look into resources that might help her support the grandmother of a young man with developmental disabilities being seen at your center. She has been told that he may qualify for a part-time job, but is concerned that he will lose his insurance benefits if he becomes employed. What information or resources can you share with your supervising SLP that will help her?

5. One of your peers has a self-identified learning dis-

ability and is concerned about needing extended time for the final in this course. Do any of the laws or mandates discussed in this chapter apply to her situation?

SUGGESTED ACTIVITIES

1. Explore and research how the Technology Act has been implemented in your state. Has it increased access to technology for individuals with disabilities? Does your state have a lending library or a loan system for current devices? Are there systems in place in your state that provide updated training and education regarding the use of technology for people with disabilities?

2. Working with your peers and instructor, complete an IFSP or IEP for a specific child or family. Role play the different processes and procedures that might apply. Create a sticky situation that involves a conflict regarding the least restrictive environment for services delivered to a child with significant communication challenges.

3. Investigate and find out the specifics regarding any waiver programs for a 36-year-old individual with a recent head injury receiving services in your setting for which he could apply. What services, if any, would be covered for this person who needs speech-language intervention, physical therapy, and psychological services. Is he eligible for vocational rehabilitation services?

4. In Appendix E, you are given a sample IEP. Locate an IEP form that is used in your state. How does it compare with the one provided? Fill out the form for a specific child.

REFERENCES

American Association of Retired Persons. (2001). *What is social security and what does it do for me?* Retrieved August 19, 2001, from http://www.aarp.org/socialsecurity/facts/question1.html

American Association of Retired Persons. (2001). *Who receives benefits from social security?* Retrieved August 19, 2001, from http://www.aarp.org/socialsecurity/facts/question2.html.

American With Disabilities Act of 1990, Pub. L. 101-336, 42 U.S.C. § 12101 *et seq.*

Board of Education of the Hendrick Hudson Central School District v. Rowley, 458 U.S. 116 (1982).

Boulder Valley School District Division of Special Education. (10/30/98). Determination of disability: Significant limited intellectual capacity, *IEP*, Form 51.10334, p. 10.

Boulder Valley School District Division of Special Education. (10/30/98). Determination of disability: Significant identifiable emotional disability, *IEP*, Form 51.10314, p. 11.

Boulder Valley School District Division of Special Education. (10/30/98). Determination of disability: Perceptual or communicative disability, *IEP*, Form 51.10318, p. 12.

Boulder Valley School District Division of Special Education. (10/30/98). Determination of disability: Hearing disability, *IEP*, Form 51.10348, p. 13.

Boulder Valley School District Division of Special Education. (10/30/98). Determination of disability: Vision disability, *IEP*, Form 51.00104, p. 14.

Boulder Valley School District Division of Special Education. (10/30/98). Determination of disability: Physical disability, *IEP*, Form 51.00105, p. 15.

Boulder Valley School District Division of Special Education. (10/30/98). Determination of disability: Speech/language disability, *IEP*, Form 51.00106, p. 16.

Boulder Valley School District Division of Special Education. (10/30/98). Determination of disability: Multiple disabilities, *IEP*, Form 51.00107, p. 17.

Budoff, M., & Orenstein, A. (1988). *Due process in special education: On going to a hearing.* Cambridge, MA: Brookling Books.

Cohen, C. (1999, Spring). *Technology-related assistance for Individuals with Disabilities Act of 1998.* Office of Special Education and Rehabilitative Services, U.S. Department of Education. Retrieved on March 12, 2002, from http://www.ed.gov/offices/OERI/ECI/newsletters/99spring/early5.html

Coleman v. Zatechka, 824 F. Supp. 1360 (D. Neb. 1993).

Colorado Department of Health Care Policy and Financing. (1999). *Home and community based services (HCBS) Medicaid waivers.* Denver, CO: Author.

Education for All Handicapped Children Act of 1975, Pub. L. 94-142, 20 U.S.C. § 1401 *et seq.*

Education for the Handicapped Act Amendments of 1986, Pub. L. 99-457, 20 U.S.C. § 1400 *et seq.*

Educational Resources Information Center (ERIC). (1998, November). *Long-term effects of inclusion—FAQ.* Retrieved March 12, 2002, from http://www.ericec.org/faq/I-long.html

Gerry, M. (1987). Procedural safeguards insuring that handicapped children receive a free appropriate public education. *NICHCY News Digest, 7,* 1–8.

Health Care Financing Administration. (2001). *Americans with Disabilities Act/Olmstead Decision.* Retrieved August 19, 2001, from http://www.hcfa.gov/medicaid/olmstead/olmshome.htm

Health Care Financing Administration. (2001). *TWWIIA Fact Sheet.* Retrieved August 19, 2001, from www.hcfa.gov/medicaid/twwlla/factsh01.htm

Hurth, J. L., & Goff, P. E. (1996). *Assuring the Family's Role on the Early Intervention Team: Explaining Rights and Safeguards.* Chapel Hill, NC: The National Early Childhood Technical Assistance System (NEC*TAS).

Individuals with Disabilities Education Act (IDEA) of 1990, Pub. L. 101-476, 20 U.S.C. § 1401 *et seq.*

Individuals with Disabilities Education Act Amendments of 1991, Pub. L. 102-119, 20 U.S.C. § 1400 *et seq.*

Kaplan, K. E., & Moore, R. J., Jr. (1995). Eight: Legal rights and hurdles. In K. Stray-Gundersen (Ed.), *Babies with Down syndrome: A new parents' guide* (2nd ed., pp. 223–264). Bethesda, MD: Woodbine House.

Long, M. J., & Chapman, R. (1996). *Handbook of rights to special education in Colorado: A guide for parents,* (2nd ed.). Denver, CO: The Legal Center for People with Disabilities and Older People.

Montgomery, J. (1994). Chapter 16: Federal legislation affecting school settings. In R. Lubinski, & C. Frattali (Eds.), *Professional issues in speech-language pathology and audiology: A textbook.* San Diego, CA: Singular.

National Early Childhood Technical Assistance Center. (n.d.). *Overview of part C under IDEA.* Retrieved March 12, 2002, from http://www.nectas.unc.edu/partc/ptcoverview.asp

O'Brien, M. (1997). *Inclusive child care for infants and toddlers: Meeting individual and special needs.* Baltimore, MD: Paul H. Brookes.

Peterson v. Hastings Public Schools, 831 F. Supp. 742 (D. Neb., 1993).

Project Choices. (n.d.). *Benefits and impact.* Retrieved March 12, 2002, from http://www.projectchoices.org/faq-benefits.htm

Rehabilitation Act of 1973, Pub. L. 93-112, 29 U.S.C. § 794 *et seq.*

Rocky Mountain Resource and Training Institute. (1989, February). *Public Law 100-407.* Denver, CO: Author.

Rutledge, J., Beyer, H. A., Schwab, N., Anderson, B., Caldwell, T. H., & Harrison, J. (1997). Legal Issues in the education of students with special health care needs. In S. Porter, M. Haynie, T. Bierle, T. Caldwell, & J. S. Palfrey (Eds.). *Children and youth assisted by medical technology in educational settings: Guidelines for care* (2nd ed., pp. 19–39). Baltimore: Brookes.

Social Security Administration. (2001). *Benefits for disabled children.* Retrieved August 19, 2001, from http://www.ssa.gov/diplan/dqualify10.htm

Social Security Administration. (2001). *Fact sheet: Ticket to work and work incentives improvement Act of 1999*. Retrieved August 19, 2001, from http://www.ssa.gov/work/ ResourcesToolkit/ geisregfact.html

Social Security Administration. (2001). *Frequently asked questions*. Retrieved August 19, 2001, from http://www.ssa.gov/planners/ faqs.htm

Social Security Administration. (2001). *How we decide if you are disabled*. Retrieved August 19, 2001, from http://www.ssa.gov/ dibplan/dqualify5.htm

Social Security Administration. (2001). *The effect of welfare reform on SSA's disability programs*. Retrieved August 19, 2001, from http://www.ssa.gove/cgi-bin/cqcgi/@ssa.env? CQ_SESSION_KEY= GNLEJMHGSXSK&CQ_CUR_DOCUMENT=13&CQ_RESULTS _DOC_TEXT=YES.

Social Security Administration. (2001). *Ticket to Work Program questions and answers*. Retrieved August 19, 2001, from http://www.ssa.gov/work/ResourcesToolkit/legisregQA.html

Social Security Administration (2001). *What we mean by disability*. Retrieved August 19, 2001, from http://www.ssa.gov/dibplan/ dqualify4.htm

Technology-Related Assistance for Individuals with Disabilities Act of 1988, Pub. L. 100-107. Rep. No. 100-438.

Timothy W. v. Rochester N.H. School District, 875 F.2d 954 (1st Cir. 1989).

Turnbull, R., Rainbolt, K., & Buchele-Ash, A. (1997). *Individuals with Disabilities Education Act: Digest and Significance of 1997 Amendments*. Beach Center on Families and Disabilities, Lawrence: University of Kansas.

Wolery, M., & Wilbers, J. S. (1994). Introduction to the inclusion of young children with special needs in early childhood programs. In M. Wolery, & J. S. Wilbers (Eds.), *Including children with special needs in early childhood programs*. Washington, DC: National Association for the Education of Young Children.

CHAPTER 9

Health and Safety

Key Concepts

■

Prevention of transmitting infection is a critical part of the SLPA's job.

■

Infection is spread when enough germs are present, contact the right part of the body, and the individual's resistance is low enough that the germs overwhelm his immune system.

■

Hand washing is the cornerstone to infection control.

■

The universal precautions were designed to prevent the spread of bloodborne pathogens.

■

First aid and CPR are the first care that an individual receives after an accident or injury. They keep individuals safe and alive.

■

Medical procedures take place in many settings where an SLPA will work, and awareness of those procedures is important.

Overview

■

How Infection Spreads

■

Hand Washing

■

Materials

■

Universal Precautions

■

First Aid and CPR

■

Other Medical Issues

INTRODUCTION

You are out to dinner with your family and as you walk into the public restroom, there are signs on the paper towel holders and mirrors "Employees must wash their hands before returning to work." Signs like these have become very common, especially because hand washing has been proven to decrease the spread of infections and **disease**. Infections can be spread through the air, by direct contact with someone with the infection, indirect contact where the individual with the infection has touched a surface and another person then touches the same surface, or by intimate contact. The Centers for Disease Control and Prevention (CDC) is continually researching and updating the precautionary measures for controlling infection spread. A main focus of the CDC has been how to stop disease through fluids that contain blood. These precautions, which have been passed into law, are called the universal blood and body fluid precautions (1987). They are defined as a "set of precautions designed to prevent transmission of **human immunodeficiency virus (HIV)**, hepatitis B virus (HBV), and other bloodborne pathogens when providing first aid or health care. Under **universal precautions**, blood and certain body fluids of all patients are considered potentially infectious for HIV, HBV, and other blood borne pathogens" (Hospitals Infections Program: Centers for Disease Control and Prevention, p. 1).

For many years, hospitals were one of the few places that practiced strict disease prevention. Now with the entrance of medically fragile individuals in schools and other public facilities, these practices have become much more widely used. Individuals—from toddlers in preschool settings to elderly persons, both of who may need speech intervention—can carry infections. Recent federal legislation has made it a right of disabled individuals to have a free, appropriate public education. This means that children with lower **resistance** to infections may need speech or language services. So as an SLPA, you need to be as aware of infection control as those who work with high-risk populations in the hospital. Because SLPAs work so closely with people, any situation that brings you in direct contact with body fluids mandates precautions. You need to protect yourself, but you

also need to protect others if you are the source of an infection such as the flu or a cold. A cold to you may mean bronchitis or pneumonia to a frail, elderly person in a nursing home.

HOW INFECTION SPREADS

Infections are spread from one person to another in many different ways. For a germ to get into an individual's system and cause the start of a infection, four specific conditions must be present (American Red Cross, 1993):

1. A pathogen (germ) is present.
2. There is enough pathogen to cause infection.
3. A person is susceptible to the pathogen.
4. The pathogen passes through the correct entry site.

If one of these conditions is not present, then infection cannot be spread. People who are more susceptible to infection include infants, the elderly, individuals with chronic infection (diabetes, cancer, or asthma), people who have just had surgery, and people with medical devices (catheters, IVs, etc.).

Germs enter the body in the following four ways: direct contact, indirect contact, airborne, and vector borne. Direct contact transmission of a germ occurs when an individual touches the body fluids of an infected person. This could be from someone sneezing on you or from holding someone's improperly washed hand. Indirect contact transmission occurs when a person touches objects that have touched the blood or body fluid of an infected person. This could be from touching soiled dressings, equipment, or work surfaces that an infected person's body fluids have come in contact with. It can also come from needles from an infected person that are handled carelessly and can puncture the skin of an uninfected person. Airborne transmission occurs when a person breathes in droplets of infected fluids that become airborne when an infected person coughs or sneezes. If a tissue or handkerchief is not available, it is a good practice for you and those around you to sneeze into an arm sleeve instead of

your hand. This decreases the number of droplets entering the air or depositing on your hand to be spread to other surfaces or other people. Vector transmission occurs when an animal (dog or raccoon) or an insect (tick or mosquito) transmits germs through a bite. Rabies and Lyme infection are transmitted this way. A bite from an infected human is also considered vector-borne transmission that you may need to be aware of in preschool or early elementary settings.

The infection process begins when a germ (pathogen) enters the body. The germs sometimes overwhelm the body's defenses and cause illness. There are six types of pathogens, the most common of which are bacteria and viruses. Bacteria are everywhere and they do not depend on other organisms to live. Most do not affect humans. Some, however, may cause serious illness, including scarlet fever, meningitis, and tetanus. When the body has difficulty fighting a bacterial infection, a doctor may prescribe antibiotics. Viruses rely on other organisms to live and reproduce and, unlike bacteria, they can cause many infections, including the common cold. When they become established in a body, they may be difficult to destroy because few medications are effective. The body's **immune system** is the main defense against them and once you catch a virus, you may have to just let it run its course. The rule of thumb for either bacterial or viral infection is that if you or someone you are caring for has a fever, you are considered contagious. After you have been on antibiotics for 24 hours, you are much less likely to spread the bacterial infection.

The body's immune system is good at fighting infection. The main component to our immune system is white blood cells. These move throughout the body and identify and release antibodies to weaken or destroy pathogens. Another main defense the body has is the skin. It is an excellent block that keeps pathogens from entering the body. If you have a break in your skin such as a cut or a sore, you are much more susceptible to germs.

Another way to fight infection, especially childhood diseases, is through immunizations. In your childhood memories, you may recall going to the doctor and getting a few shots and drinking a bitter liquid. What you probably do not remember or did not realize is that this was to keep you from contracting a wide range of potentially damaging, even fatal, diseases. The diseases targeted through immunizations include diphtheria, pertussis, tetanus (DPT), polio, hepatitis B, measles, mumps, rubella (MMR), and now influenza (flu).

HAND WASHING

Hand washing is the cornerstone of infection control and the most effective step in preventing infections (*American Journal of Infection Control [APIC]* & Larson, 1995). The goal of hand washing is to get rid of as many potentially contaminating germs off the hands as possible (Centers for Disease Control and Prevention, 1988). See Figure 9-1 to learn about the steps to effective hand washing. To wash your hands thoroughly you need running water and soap. Using friction to wash all surfaces of your hands is essential. Then you need to rinse under a stream of water and then dry your hands. Another tip to washing hands is to turn off the running water with the paper towel you used to dry your hands. Taking off jewelry is also recommended. If water and soap are not available, wet towelettes or a waterless skin antiseptic may be used. These are temporary and cannot be used as a substitute for hand washing.

WHEN TO WASH YOUR HANDS

Good practice mandates the SLPA to always wash his hands (Kemp, Roeser, Pearson, & Ballachanda, 1996):

- Upon arrival at work
- After using the toilet
- After helping a child or adult with toileting or diapering
- Before and after contact with clients
- After wiping runny noses
- After blowing or wiping his nose
- When preparing to assist with eating or feeding with children and adults
- After removing gloves or other personal protective equipment
- After accidental contact with blood or blood-tinged fluids
- Before leaving the work setting

Hand washing dramatically decreases the chances of spreading germs to other people (American Red Cross, 1993). Our hands touch many things throughout the day and we pick up unwanted germs. When we wash our hands, those germs die thus stoping the spread of infection. Procedures for washing hands may be found in Figure 9-1.

SIDELIGHT: *Taking the Initiative*

Ron used musical instruments during his therapy time with three toddlers. He noticed that one toddler was wiping his nose on his sleeve and another was coughing fairly regularly during the therapy time. Ron tried to wipe one toddler's nose before he wiped it on his sleeve. He washed his hands after each time he wiped the child's nose, but he made a mental note to make sure he washed his hands thoroughly after the session and wipe the toys down with a bleach solution so as not to spread the germs to other children he saw.

The Stop Disease Method of Handwashing

- Use SOAP and RUNNING WATER
- RUB your hands vigorously
- WASH ALL SURFACES including:
    - backs of hands
    - wrists
    - between fingers
    - under fingernails
- RINSE well
- DRY hands with a paper towel
- Turn off the water using a PAPER TOWEL instead of bare hands.

Figure 9-1 Hand washing techniques. *Note.* From *Rules and Regulating Child Care Centers*, by Colorado Department of Human Services, Division of Child Care, 2001, Denver: Author. Adapted with permission.

Materials

As an SLPA you may be asked to maintain all materials used in sessions. This is not just busy work. It is necessary to thoroughly clean the therapy items you use, especially toys or therapy tools. Clean and disinfect all items that clients touch and use during therapy. These items can pass germs from one client to another if not properly washed. It is recommended that you use therapy materials that can easily be wiped or washed clean. Avoid furry or fabric dolls and stuffed animals. Toys or therapy items that have been put in a child's mouth should be immediately isolated and then washed and disinfected before using with other children. Disinfect therapy materials that may be put in an individual's mouth. Oral motor speech therapy may require use of straws, whistles, tongue depressors, toothettes, and washcloths. Some of these items are disposable, such as the tongue depressors and toothettes, but the specialized straws and whistles must be disinfected. According to Sara Rosenfeld-Johnson (2002), you can make a bleach and water mixture to disinfect your therapy materials. The ratio is 96% water to 4% bleach. This mixture may also be used to disinfect tables, chairs, doorknobs, and other furniture in your therapy setting. The Colorado Department of Human Services (2001) recommends a solution composed of 1 tablespoon bleach and 1 gallon of cool water to disinfect toys and food surface areas. In hospital and health clinics, you may be required to use a specialized solution to disinfect your therapy materials as well as frequently used surfaces. A dishwasher may also be an option for disinfecting toys that can withstand the heat without melting. Figure 9-2 demonstrates a good time to wash hands.

UNIVERSAL PRECAUTIONS

To help decrease the spread of infection, the Centers for Disease Control and Prevention (CDC) designed precautions that have been accepted throughout the United States called "universal blood and body-fluid precautions." They were initially proposed during the summer of 1987 and were accepted by the medical board in November 1987. In May

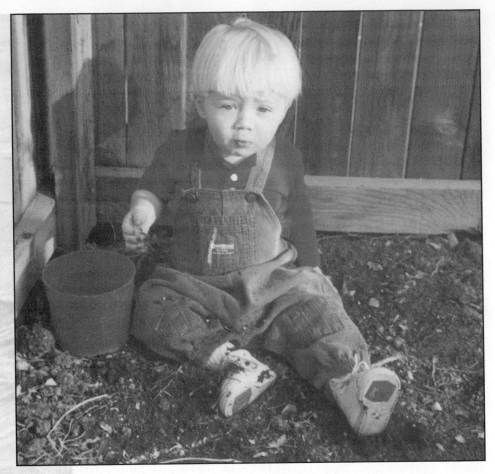

Figure 9-2 A little boy having fun in the dirt. Good hand-washing practice is important when he is finished.

1989, the Occupational Safety and Health Administration (OSHA) of the Department of Labor issued its own advisory that these precautions needed to be implemented as soon as possible. The final OSHA standard was issued in December 1991, making it a federal law ("Occupational Exposure to Blood-borne Pathogens: Final Rule," 1991). These precautions directly relate to the protection from blood-related modes of transmission. Two diseases that are passed through contact with blood include HBV and HIV. Because it is difficult to tell which people harbor bloodborne pathogens, these precautions were designed to protect health care work-

ers. The universal precautions include (Centers for Disease Control and Prevention, 1987; U. S. Department of Health and Human Services, 1988):

1. Wearing latex gloves when coming into contact with blood, skin, and mucous membrane cuts, or any open skin lesion

2. Using gloves only for the care of one individual, then discarding the gloves

3. Washing hands after discarding the gloves

4. Properly disposing of contaminated materials exposed to blood, such as needles

When you follow these guidelines carefully, the universal precautions help to prevent exposure to **bloodborne pathogens**, including HIV and HBV. This is an especially important task when working in a hospital or nursing home.

HIV transmission concerns many individuals. HIV is one of the diseases contracted from a bloodborne pathogen transmitted only through intimate contact, use of contaminated needles, or contact with blood. HIV is not transmitted through nasal secretions, saliva, sputum, sweat, tears, urine, vomit, and feces unless they contain visible blood (National Pediatric and Family HIV Resource Center [NPHRC], n.d.). Casual contact between infected and uninfected individuals does not transmit HIV. Several studies have shown that family members of an individual who has HIV do not acquire it (Rustein, Conlon, & Batshaw, 1997). With modern advances in medicine, fewer individuals with HIV are contracting **acquired immune deficiency syndrome (AIDS)**. People may be concerned that donated blood may be contaminated with HIV. "Since 1985, all donated blood in the United States has been tested for HIV antibodies. As a result, the blood supply is considered extremely safe. The risk of becoming infected through a blood transfusion is very low" (American Red Cross, 1992, p. 11). As an SLPA, you may be working with an individual who is HIV positive or has AIDS, and knowing and using the universal precautions will protect you and the individual you are working with. Few family members of individuals with HIV or AIDS have contracted the disease by casual contact of living together. (Rustein et al., 1997). If you are working with children as an SLPA, you need to understand that 90% of the children who were newly diagnosed with HIV infection in 1997 acquired it from their mothers during gestation, at birth, or postnatally (Rustein et al., 1997). See the story of Laura and her baby.

SIDELIGHT: *Laura's Story*

Laura is a 25-year-old woman who contracted HIV from an intimate relationship with a man who was HIV positive. She is now 39 weeks pregnant and concerned about her baby. She just met with her doctor and at this time it does not look like the HIV has crossed the placenta. The first hurdle has passed. The next is labor and delivery. She has decided to take AZT during labor and delivery to decrease the chances of her baby contracting HIV to 8% instead of 26% without it. She will then have to give AZT to her newborn for 6 weeks. She feels it is worth the risk of developing mild transient anemia. She wants her baby to be healthy, just like other mothers want their babies to be healthy. Hopefully no complications occur during labor and delivery. She was told that they would not do an automatic cesarean section because it has been proven not to decrease the chances of the disease to be spread. She also knows that if her baby does develop HIV, the later the child gets it, the longer her child will live. Prenatal HIV children tend to live 3 to 5 years, whereas children who contract HIV at birth have a median survival of more than 9 years. Children who develop HIV after birth are living into their teens. She is so thankful for the advances in medicine that have decreased the chances of her baby acquiring HIV, but she is still concerned. Eight days later Laura has a healthy 7-pound baby boy with no complications. She is very thankful. Now she must continue giving her son his medication for 6 weeks (Rustein et al., 1997).

In an emergency, you will rarely know the details of a person's lifestyle or health history. The only physical danger to you occurs when you feel so secure in a situation that you neglect to take the safety precautions that prevent infection transmission. The other danger to you as a person exists when you allow preconceptions and prejudices to interfere with those qualities that are an important component of giving first aid.

Blood-borne Pathogens

In 1991, the Occupational Safety and Health Administration (OSHA) issued final regulations on job exposure to bloodborne pathogens. These are bacteria and viruses present in human blood and body fluids that can cause infection in humans. The specific pathogens may include HBV and HIV. HBV causes hepatitis B, a serious liver infection. HIV causes AIDS. OSHA designed some provisions for employers to implement to reduce the spread of bloodborne pathogens.

Personal Protective Equipment

The use of personal protective equipment helps reduce the risk of contact with blood and other potentially infectious material. Consistent use of personal protective equipment can dramatically reduce the risk of exposure (National Institutes of Health Clinical Center Nursing Department, n.d.). Personal protective equipment includes disposable gloves, protective eyewear (glasses with side shields), masks, laboratory coats, and cover gowns (Seneca, Carroll, & Kuhlow, 1988).

GUIDE TO WEARING GLOVES

G loves should be worn (Lubinski, 1994):

1. When changing a diaper
2. When changing dressing or sanitary napkins
3. When providing mouth, nose, or tracheal care
4. If the caregiver has broken skin on the hands (even around the nails)
5. When cleaning up spills of blood (i.e., nosebleed) or body fluids and wastes and soiled supplies
6. When providing therapy in which you will have contact with an individual's mouth or saliva.

Gloves should be worn when direct care of an individual may involve contact with blood or body fluids. It is recommended that gloves be worn as well for urine, feces, and respiratory secretions. Gloves that are torn or defective in any way need to be thrown away and not used. Gloves should be discarded after each use and never reused. Hands should be washed whenever gloves are taken off. Gloves are the most common protection used by an SLPA, even in a school setting. Sometimes more protection such as gowns and protective eyewear may be needed, especially if splattering of body fluids is possible. If you are doing therapy with an individual who is an inpatient with an infectious disease, you may have to wear a gown, gloves, and a mask. These specifications will be posted on the patient's door.

If you are confronted with a blood spill when you are unprepared, like a fall on a playground or a nosebleed, and gloves or other personal protective equipment are not readily available, use a barrier. A barrier can be anything from a diaper, towel, or shirt, that you place between your skin and someone else's blood or fluids (Unified Student Services, 1999). Some places prepare little kits that contain gloves and gauze in a sandwich bag that are available to take on outings or on the playground. Remember that hands need to be washed immediately when they come in contact with blood.

SIDELIGHT: *Quick Thinking in an Emergency*

Jackie worked as an SLPA at Fireside Elementary and part of her duties included bus duty before school a few days a week. She was helping children off the bus on a snowy day when a little girl fell on the ice and cut her cheek, next to her eye. This type of injury tends to bleed a lot, and this time was no exception. Jackie remembered that she had a handkerchief in her pocket that she could use to help stop the bleeding and serve as a barrier. She quickly pulled it out and started applying pressure to the wound. She brought the girl to the nurses' office where a nurse starting cleaning and taking care of the cut. Jackie quickly went into the faculty restroom and washed her hands.

Needles or Sharps

You may work in an environment that uses disposable needles and syringes called **sharps**. These items can contain and transmit infected fluids and a great deal of precaution is needed when working with them. Needles always need to be placed in a puncture-resistant container. Never try to recap, bend, or manipulate used needles because you may get stuck. Never reuse a needle.

Cleanup

Most facilities that employ SLPAs have specific policies on how spills should be cleaned up. These policies will usually be shared with you during an orientation meeting; if not, contact your SLP supervisor and find out the correct procedures for your work environment. General guidelines for the cleanup process include wearing gloves; mopping up the spill with paper towels or other absorbent material; using a solution of 1 part household bleach in 10 parts of water (wash the area well); and disposing of gloves, soiled towels, and other waste in sealed double plastic bags in the garbage (Mohawk College of Applied Arts and Technology, 1997).

FIRST AID AND CPR

The following information provides a general overview of first aid and **cardiopulmonary resuscitation** (**CPR**)— before attempting either, be sure you have received proper hands-on training. The information included in this chapter is a general overview. You may be required to take a first aid and CPR class for your job, especially in school and health care settings.

First Aid

First aid is the help that is provided after an accident, illness, or injury has occurred. Many guidelines have been developed to deal with the major emergencies that may be encountered, such as allergic reactions, breathing problems, drowning, injuries, poison, and shock, to name a few. The main ones that will be addressed in this text include breathing problems, seizures, shock, stroke, and wounds. These are the most common ailments you may come across as an SLPA.

Breathing Problems

Breathing is essential to life. As you inhale, your chest expands and you take in air through your nose, mouth, and windpipe to your lungs. The oxygen then gets into the bloodstream and is pumped throughout the body by your heart. Breathing problems may occur at any stage of this process. Injury, sudden illness, or ongoing medical problems (such as heart disease, emphysema, chronic bronchitis, or asthma) can also cause breathing difficulties (American Red Cross & Handel, 1992). Shortness of breath can also occur at high altitudes.

SIGNS OF BREATHING DIFFICULTIES

Signs and symptoms of breathing difficulty include (American Medical Association, 2000):

- ■ Shortness of breath
- ■ Cough
- ■ Gurgling, wheezing, or whistling sounds
- ■ Labored breathing, tense chest muscles
- ■ Pale or bluish lips and fingernails

Asthma is a breathing difficulty that affects many children and adults. It is a condition caused by the slow or sudden narrowing of the passageways to and within the lungs. Breathing may be difficult on exhalation. Sometimes the individual is exposed to something he is allergic to, which causes the linings in the lungs to become inflamed and start to narrow. Emotional factors can also bring about breathing difficulties for those with asthma. When an individual with asthma is having difficulty breathing it is common to hear wheezing when he exhales. This is caused by the narrowing passages (American Red Cross & Handel, 1992).

Seizures

A seizure or convulsion is a result of an upset in the electrical activity in the brain. It leads to a series of uncontrollable movements that can occur with partial or complete unconsciousness. Most seizures last 1 to 2 minutes. "Seizures can occur with a head injury, brain tumor, poisoning, electric shock, withdrawal from drugs, heatstroke, scorpion bites, poisonous snakebites, hyperventilation, or high fever. Seizures also occur in people who have epilepsy, a disorder that results when brain cells temporarily become overactive and release too much electrical energy". (American Medical Association, 2000, p. 237). Despite what you may have heard, a person having a seizure is not in danger of biting off or swallowing his tongue. Do not put any objects into the victim's mouth. Injuries may occur while the individual is having the series of uncontrollable movements; you can remove obstacles or potential injury-causing items from the individual's way and decrease the chances of injury. When you see someone having a seizure, call 911 if the person is not known to have epilepsy or if the seizure lasts more than 5 minutes (American Red Cross & Handel, 1992). Keep the individual safe by removing furniture or moving the individual away from stairs or glass doors, and catch him if he falls. Stay with the individual until he recovers, and check for injuries.

SIGNS OF SEIZURE

Seizures may involve any or all of the following symptoms (American Medical Association, 2000):

- A short scream or cry
- Rigid muscles followed by jerky, twitching movements
- Breathing temporarily stops
- Face and lips turn blue
- Eyes roll upward
- Rapid heart rate
- Loss of bladder and bowel control
- Drooling or foaming at the mouth
- Unresponsiveness
- Sleepiness and confusion after the seizure is over

Stroke

A **stroke** occurs when there is an interruption in the blood flow to all or part of the brain. A clot inside an artery supplying blood to the brain may cause the interruption in blood flow. The sooner the individual who has had a stroke receives medical attention, the more successful the treatment may be and the better the chances are of limiting the amount of brain damage. If you think an individual is having a stroke, call 911 for medical help. You can keep the individual comfortable until help arrives.

SIGNS OF STROKE

The symptoms of stroke may include any or all of the following (American Medical Association, 2000):

- Sudden headache
- Sudden paralysis, weakness, or numbness on one side of the body; the corner of the mouth may droop
- Loss or slurring of speech
- Possible unconsciousness or mental confusion
- Sudden fall
- Impaired vision or double vision
- Pupils of different size
- Incoordination
- Difficulty breathing, chewing, talking, or swallowing
- Loss of bladder or bowel control
- Strong, slow pulse

Wounds and Cuts

An open wound is an injury with broken skin. Remember to use personal protective equipment or a barrier if you are trying to stop a bleeding wound. The injured individual is at risk for both becoming infected and infecting you and others. The American Red Cross and Kathleen A. Handel. (1992) give the procedure for dealing with cuts and wounds. Use direct pressure if the bleeding is severe. If it is not, wash your hands with soap and water, put on gloves, and then apply direct pressure to stop the bleeding. When bleeding has stopped, wash the cut or wound with soap and water. Gentle scrubbing may be necessary to remove any dirt or foreign objects in the cut. If a foreign object is implanted deep into the skin, do not attempt to remove. Pat the wound dry and cover with a sterile dressing (Band-Aid). Seek medical attention if the wound is deep, if the bleeding does not stop, if the wound was caused by a dirty object, a human or animal bite, or if you see signs of infection (fever, redness, swelling, increased tenderness at the site of the wound, pus, or red streaks from the wound toward the body). Cuts to the scalp may be accompanied by heavy bleeding even if it is a minor wound. See Jackie's story earlier in the chapter.

OPEN WOUNDS

The objectives in treating an open wound include:

1. Stopping the bleeding

2. Preventing contamination and infection

3. Preventing shock

4. Seeking medical attention if the wound is severe or if the victim has not had a tetanus shot within 5 years

Puncture wounds are small but deep holes from a pin, nail, staple, fang, bullet, ice pick, sticks, or any other penetrating object. The depth of these types of wounds may be difficult to determine and they tend not to bleed. Puncture wounds are very susceptible to infection, and tetanus is a danger with these types of wounds (American Medical Association, 2000). All puncture wounds need to be seen by a doctor.

CPR and Upper Airway Obstructions

CPR stands for cardiopulmonary resuscitation (cardio refers to the heart, pulmonary refers to the lungs, and resuscitation means to revive from a condition resembling death). CPR is performed when an individual is not breathing or you are not able to find that individual's pulse (Trefz, 1988). CPR is performed to provide oxygen to the brain, heart, and other organs until medical professionals restore normal breathing and heart actions. Speed is critical and prompt action by trained individuals can save lives (American Medical Association, 2000).

You will be required to have the official CPR training to be certified in CPR. The certification lasts 1 year so the training is required annually. The training is required so you can practice these techniques under the supervision of a certified CPR trainer.

Upper Airway Obstructions

If an individual's airway is blocked, thus cutting off the flow of oxygen, the result can be fatal. "The term 'café coronary' has been used to describe a choking incident in a restaurant, when upper airway obstruction has been mistaken for a heart attack" (Trefz, 1988, p. 39). Without oxygen, brain damage will start within 4 to 6 minutes. Rapid first aid for a choking victim can save a life.

SIDELIGHT: *Taking the Initiative*

John had been working at Peaceful Valley Nursing home for almost 5 years and kept his first aid certification current. Today he was assigned to work with Ralph on his communication skills during his lunchtime. Ralph sat at a table with two other gentlemen, Henry and Richard. John and Ralph were working away when Henry made a quick movement and held his hands to his throat, indicating he was choking. John quickly got up from his seat and performed the Heimlich maneuver while Henry was seated. The piece of food was quickly dislodged and Henry appeared to be doing better. As a precaution, John found the registered nurse on duty and told her what had happened so Henry could be examined for injuries done during the Heimlich maneuver. Henry had no injuries and cautiously finished his meal.

As an SLPA, you can be aware of choking hazards and address them before they become a problem. If you work with children under the age of 3, put away toys that can fit in a film canister. According to the American Medical Association (2000) there are three types of airway blockages.

The first is partial airway obstruction with good airflow. With good air exchange, the victim will cough forcefully and wheeze between coughs. The second is partial airway obstruction with poor air exchange. Poor air exchange can be recognized if the person coughs weakly, strains to breathe, makes high-pitched, crowing sounds, and possibly shows blueness of the lips and fingernails. The third type is a complete airway obstruction that completely blocks all airflow. The universal sign for choking is putting two hands around the neck. An individual with a complete obstruction cannot talk or breathe, and may stagger around with his neck straining using the universal choking sign to communicate the severity of the situation. If an individual has an airway obstruction, you may use the Heimlich maneuver to help him dislodge it. Another tool to remember when you are giving emergency care is AID. A - Ask for help, I - Intervene, and D - Do no further harm (American Red Cross & Handel, 1992).

AVOIDING UPPER AIRWAY OBSTRUCTIONS

People can avoid upper airway obstructions by (American Red Cross & Handel, 1992):

- Cutting their food into small, easily chewed pieces
- Limiting alcohol intake
- Avoiding laughing and talking while eating
- Making sure dentures fit snugly
- Keeping small objects away from infants and small children
- Not allowing children to walk or run with food in their mouth

OTHER MEDICAL ISSUES

With more medically challenged individuals in schools as a result of disability legislation as well as medically fragile in hospitals and nursing homes, you may be exposed to latex allergies, physical transfers, tube feedings, respiratory care, and oxygen use. An SLPA may be asked to assist in some of these areas, but the ultimate responsibility is on the medical staff. In the Nurse Practice Act of 2001, Section 12-38-132 details that a nurse is able to delegate nursing tasks, but the responsibility and liability stay with the nurse. So in a school setting, a nurse may train a teacher or a paraprofessional to give G-tube feedings, but ultimately the G-tube feedings are the nurse's responsibility (Colorado Nursing Board, 2001). If you are in a setting that wants you to be trained in medical procedures usually carried out by a registered nurse and you do not feel comfortable performing the medical procedures, you may refuse to do those procedures, according to the Nurse Practice Act of 2001.

Latex Allergies

Latex is a combination of tree sap and chemicals, which make it durable, strong, and elastic. Latex is found in many medical products. Items that may contain latex include gloves, catheters, tape or elastic bandages, wheelchair cushions or tires, crutch pads, balloons, rubber balls or toys, baby bottles or pacifiers, art supplies, and diapers or elastic clothing. A growing number of individuals are demonstrating an allergic reaction to latex. A significant number of individuals with chronic conditions such as spina bifida, and urological anomalies have also been identified to have latex allergies. Health care workers and children with histories of multiple surgical procedures or many allergies may also be at risk. You need to be aware of this condition when you are working with individuals.

SIDELIGHT: *Josie's Latex Allergy*

Josie, a 6-year-old girl, had a shunt put in when she was 6 months old owing to pressure from extra fluids in her brain. As she grew, she had undergone several surgeries to make adjustments to the shunt. Through the process of these surgeries and having a latex shunt, Josie had developed an allergy to latex. After several months struggling with wheezing in her lungs and constant watery eyes, it was determined that the latex allergy was the cause of her symptoms. She was scheduled for surgery next week to remove the current shunt and put in a latex-free shunt. The surgery was scheduled to be performed in a special latex-free operating room so Josie would not be exposed to any latex and stir up her allergies.

An allergic reaction to latex may include watery eyes, wheezing, rash, hives, swelling, and in severe cases, anaphylactic shock. Manufacturers of health care products are now making alternative nonlatex products to help individuals with latex allergies. The alternative products may be made of vinyl, silicone, or plastic.

Transfers

A common activity you may be asked to participate is in transferring an individual from one place to another. This may be moving a person from a wheelchair to a bed, or a from a school chair to the floor. The elements of safe **transfers** are a combination of physical capabilities of the one doing the transfer, proper equipment, and techniques that are best for the patient's abilities. "Firm, stable surfaces for the patient to move to and from are required for all transfers" (Ellwood, 1971, p. 429). Hydraulic or mechanical lifts are commercially available for individuals who require extensive assistance. A small person can use these devices very safely if properly trained. Some individuals can help with the transfer, whereas others cannot. In hospital settings, physical therapists train individuals after surgery, strokes, or other medical procedures to make safe transfers. After time, hopefully the individuals will become more independent and can do transfers by themselves. An SLPA may be asked to assist in transfers or perform them with the individual he is working with during therapy sessions.

SIDELIGHT: *A Successful Transfer*

Ramona works in a nursing home and when she arrives Mildred is usually in her wheelchair ready to go to therapy. Ramona was surprised to find Mildred still in bed when she arrived today. Mildred said she felt fine and was ready to work with Ramona. The nurse on duty told Ramona they were short handed today and were not able to get Mildred in her wheelchair for her. The nurse instructed an aide to help Ramona transfer Mildred into her wheelchair so she could go to therapy. Ramona had received excellent training on how to do transfers when she started working at the nursing home so she felt comfortable helping with the transfer.

Two Person Transfers

If an individual is over a certain number of pounds or is very fragile medically, he may require two people to lift him from one place to another. Usually one person lifts the upper body (head and chest) and the other person lifts the lower body (legs). Two-person lifts are indicated in an individual's medical plan. If you are concerned about not being able to make a transfer by yourself, it is a good practice to ask someone to help (Parlay International, 1990).

Lifting Basics

Whenever dealing with transfers or lifting, three basic lifting fundamentals need to be remembered: bend your knees, "hug" the load, and avoid twisting (Parlay International, 1990). Other helpful hints include wearing shoes or boots that will not slip, making sure the path is clear, knowing where you are putting the load before you lift, never hurrying, and checking the condition of mechanical aids before loading (Plainsense, n.d.).

Bend Your Knees. Bend your knees, not your waist. This helps your leg muscles do the work instead of your back. It also helps you keep your center of balance. When your knees are bent, your legs and back can work together to carry the weight.

"Hug" the Load. Remember to keep the load as close to your body as possible. That is why it is called "hugging" the load. When making any kind of person transfer, the individual you are transferring needs to be as close to you as possible (i.e., chest to chest). This helps decrease the chances for injury. Then gradually straighten your legs to a standing position so you can walk with the load.

Avoid Twisting. Twisting while you carry a load increases the pressure on your spine and can lead to serious injury. To avoid twisting, keep your knees and body moving in the same direction when lifting. If you are lifting something to put on a stack, bend your knees and grab the load close to your

body, straighten up slowly, and then turn your body so you are facing the place where you want to put the load. These extra steps can mean a great deal to the health of your back.

Tube Feeding

Some children and adults are unable to take in nutrients through their mouth. They may have difficulty swallowing, and to prevent food and liquids from going into their lungs and causing pneumonia, a gastrostomy tube (**G-tube**) may be surgically inserted to feed them. Food and liquids are fed directly into their stomach. Other reasons for using a G-tube include having an obstruction in the esophagus and having difficulty taking in enough food orally (through their mouth) to sustain nutritional needs.

Individuals with G-tubes can be fed on a continuous drip type system or given "food" every 2 to 3 hours. A G-tube may go under clothing and does not restrict a person's daily living activities. In a school setting, the school nurse is responsible for G-tube feedings. You will probably not be required to be involved in this process, but you need to be aware of the procedure.

G-Tube Procedures

The person doing the procedure needs to wash his hands, assemble materials, and put on gloves. The cap to the G-tube is removed, and the tubing is attached to the G-tube. Several things are done before feeding, such as checking for residuals and removing bubbles from the tubing. Then the liquid feeding solution is poured into a syringe and gravity is used to get the contents into the stomach. (Another method includes a pump wherein the liquid feeding solution is pumped on a regular basis into a person's stomach.) Then water is used to flush the tubing. Everything is disconnected and the G-tube is closed. All equipment must be washed after every use. Finally this person needs to take off the gloves, dispose of them in an appropriate container, and wash his hands. All of the amounts and specific procedures for each individual will be prescribed by a doctor or written in a plan by a school nurse.

Respiratory Care

Many of us have seen individuals carrying around oxygen tanks with a tube placed under that person's nose. If a person is unable to get enough oxygen from the air around him, he may need additional oxygen to stay healthy. An individual could have problems along any part of the respiratory system. To get oxygen to our body we inhale through our mouths. The air travels through the larynx and trachea (or the windpipe) to the bronchi, which are in the lungs. It then goes into alveoli and into the bloodstream, where the oxygen is taken to every cell in our body. Our brain tells our body to breathe on a regular basis. It happens hundreds of thousands of times throughout our day and we tend to be unaware it is even happening. Some people have problems with the muscles in the respiratory system, whereas others may have had brain damage that affected the brain's ability to tell the body to breathe. Others may have problems in the breathing structures of the windpipe or lungs. These problems may make it necessary for a person to need intermittent or continual oxygen use.

Oxygen Use

You may be exposed to oxygen use and other types of respiratory care on your job. Several safety precautions need to be observed when around oxygen and may be found in Figure 9-3. Oxygen is usually in gas form contained in a tank. The tank is turned on and off with a wrench. Oxygen is carried from the tank through tubes and then either through a nasal cannula or oxygen mask. A nasal cannula is a piece of tubing that goes under the nose with two small parts (prongs) that fit into the nostrils. The tube is then threaded around a person's ears to help hold the cannula in place. The oxygen mask is a plastic mask that fits over an individual's nose and mouth and held on the face by a piece of elastic that goes around the head. The other major part of an oxygen system is a flowmeter. It tells how much oxygen is going through the tank to the individual. A physician prescribes the amount of oxygen an individual should receive. Oxygen is measured in liters per minute, and a common range of oxygen is 1 to 5 liters per minute. Babies and small children may take less than 1 liter a minute, and their flowmeter may be set at $1/4$, $1/3$, $1/2$, etc.

To set up the system, first you need to wash your hands. Then you connect the tubes to the flowmeter and turn on the regulator to the prescribed amount of oxygen. Always check that the oxygen flow is coming out of the cannula or mask. If you hold it up to your ear you can hear it or feel it against your hand. Then place the nasal cannula or oxygen mask on the individual. Wash your hands again. You will probably not set up an oxygen system, but you may need to

---

Oxygen Safety Precautions

1.
Do not smoke or allow open flames near oxygen. Store oxygen away from heaters and the hot sun.

2.
Never put anything over an oxygen gas tank.

3.
Have spare equipment available: oxygen gas tank, tubing, and tank equipment (wrenches).

4.
Be careful that the oxygen tubing does not become kinked, blocked, punctured, or disconnected.

5.
Notify the fire department that oxygen is in use in a school.

6.
Know the name of the home oxygen supply company and return defective equipment to the company for replacement.

7.
Use plugs, caps, and plastic bags to protect "off-duty" equipment from dust and dirt.

8.
Do not allow oxygen equipment to get near any oil or grease.

Figure 9-3 Safety around oxygen use. *Note.* From *Oxygen Equipment Safety Information*, by Allied Healthcare Products, Inc., n.d. Retrieved July 26, 2002, from http://www.life-assist.com/recallinfo.html. Reprinted with permission.

troubleshoot a system if it does not appear to be working (i.e., a tube gets disconnected or the cannula comes out of the client's nose). SLPAs may work with individuals on oxygen and therefore need to be aware of the signs of when these individuals may not be getting enough oxygen.

SIGNS OF DIFFICULTY WITH OXYGEN USE

The following is a list of observations you may see when an individual on oxygen is having difficulty breathing and needs immediate attention:

1. Shortness of breath or a rapid breathing rate

2. Agitation

3. Blueness or pallor of the lips, nails, or earlobes

4. Pulling in the muscles at the neck or chest

Nebulizer Treatments

Nebulizer treatments deliver medication in a mist directly to the lungs. They are usually given to children and adults with asthma. They may also be used to deliver antibiotics or other medications. An air compressor is hooked up to some tubing and a medicine cup. When the air in the compressor reaches the medicine cup, it breaks it up into a mist where it is breathed directly into the lungs. A nurse usually administers a nebulizer treatment under orders from a physician.

Ventilators

A mechanical ventilator is used to breathe for a person who is unable to breathe sufficiently on his own because of a stroke, head injury, coma, or paralysis. It may also be used to assist a person who needs help breathing, such as an individual with emphysema who has a cold. A mechanical ventilator is usually attached to a person through an incision in the neck called a stoma. The actual mechanical part of the ventilator may be mounted on a wheelchair. An individual with a ventilator usually has people around who are trained

specifically in this type of specialized care. With more medically fragile people out in the community, you may be exposed to an individual on a ventilator in your setting.

CONCLUSION

Health and safety are an important part of the training for an SLPA, especially if employment is in a field that primarily helps people in medical settings. Many of you choose to work in schools, hospitals, clinics, or home health care, which will have their own health and safety training programs you will be required to take. The principles of infection control are universal precautions that help protect you and others from spreading infection and diseases. First aid is the procedures and knowledge you use to treat injuries in an emergency. CPR is the way to keep someone breathing and the heart beating until medical assistance arrives or until the individual starts breathing or until the heart starts beating on its own. All of these are principles you can use both in your private and professional life.

This chapter has reviewed several methods to prevent the transmission of infections. Your personal health and safety regimen, however, should always begin with hand washing. Hand washing is the key component of infection control. This helps stop the transmission of infections that are spread by touching them and then touching your mouth, eyes, or nose. It also is an extra precaution before and after working with individuals so you do not spread germs from one individual to another or to yourself. The second way of stopping the spread of bloodborne infections is the use of universal precautions. The four components of the universal precautions include wearing gloves when in contact with bodily fluids, using a new clean pair of gloves with each individual, washing your hands after throwing the gloves away, and properly disposing of all blood-contaminated materials.

Other issues that the SLPA will need to be familiar with include latex allergies, how to perform safe patient transfers, tube feedings, oxygen use, nebulizer treatments, and ventilators. These medical procedures have become more common in the school setting with the integration of children with

significant medical issues. As an SLPA, you will not be responsible for this level of care of an individual. However, you need to be aware of these medical procedures because you may be asked to assist your supervising SLP or another professional in the care of patients with these unique needs. With the proper training in health and safety, you will be ready to handle all types of health care issues and emergencies.

DISCUSSION QUESTIONS

1. Describe the need for hand washing. When should it occur and how often should it happen? What are the proper steps to hand washing?

2. What are the universal precautions? What specific area do they apply to?

3. Describe the process of how infection is spread. Include information about bloodborne pathogens and airborne pathogens.

4. How is HIV transmitted? Can you get it from shaking someone's hand or being in the same room?

5. What precautions need to be taken when working with an individual who is using oxygen to breathe?

SUGGESTED ACTIVITIES

1. Contact a local hospital and talk to someone about the hospital's disease prevention policies. Do they include hand washing and universal precautions? What other training do they offer that was not included in this chapter? Is disease prevention training required for employment?

2. Take a CPR and first aid course if you have not already done so within the last year.

3. Interview an individual who has a dependence on a ventilator or has a tracheostomy. How has this affected his life? What activities is he able to do, and what activities is he not allowed to do? Is he more suscepti-

ble to colds, the flu, and other infections? Does he have to be careful about the amount of time that he is out in public?

REFERENCES

American Journal of Infection Control, & Larson, E. L. (1995). APIC guideline for hand washing and hand antisepsis in health care settings. *American Journal of Infection Control, 23,* 251–269.

American Medical Association. (2000). *Handbook of first aid and emergency care.* J. B. Leikin, & B. J. Feldman (Eds). New York: Random House.

American Red Cross (1993). *Preventing disease transmission.* Baltimore: Author.

American Red Cross, & Handel, A. (1992). *First aid & safety handbook.* Boston: Little, Brown.

Centers for Disease Control and Prevention. (1987). Recommendations for prevention of HIV transmission in health care settings. *Morbidity and Mortality Weekly Report, 36*(Suppl.), 3S–18S.

Centers for Disease Control and Prevention. (1988). Universal precautions for prevention of transmission of human immunodeficiency virus, hepatitis B virus, and other bloodborne pathogens in health care settings. *Mobidity and Mortality Weekly Report Supplement (MMWR), 37,* 377–382.

Centers for Disease Control (1988, June 24). *Guideline for handwashing and hospital environmental control, 1985.* Retrieved February 4, 2002, from http://www.cdc.gov/ncidod/hip/guide/handwash.htm#handwashing

Colorado Department of Human Services: Division of Child Care. (2001, November). *Rules and regulating child care centers.* Denver, CO:Author.

Colorado Nursing Board. (2001). *Nurse Practice Act of 2001.* Retrieved March 13, 2001, from http://www.dora.state.co.us/nursing/statuesandrules/npa.htm

Ellwood, P. M., Jr. (1971). Chapter 17: Transfers—Method, Equipment and Preparation. In F. H. Krusen, F. J. Kottke, & P. M. Ellwood (Eds.). *Handbook of physical medicine and rehabilitation* (2nd ed.) Philadelphia: W.B. Saunders Company..

Hospitals Infections Program: Centers for Disease Control and Prevention. (n.d.). *Universal precautions for prevention of transmission of HIV and other bloodborne infections.* Retrieved August 19, 2001, from http://www.cdc.gov/ncidod/hip/blood/universa.htm

Kemp, R. J., Roeser, R. J., Pearson, D. W., & Ballachanda, B. B. (1996). *Infection control for the professions of audiology and speech-language pathology.* Chesterfield, MO: Oaktree Products.

Lubinski, R. (1994). Chapter 21: Infection Prevention. In R. Lubinski, & C. Frattali (Eds.). *Professional issues in speech-language patholo-*

gy and audiology: A textbook (pp. 269–281). San Diego, CA: Singular.

Mohawk College of Applied Arts and Technology. (1997). *Material handling*. Retrieved August 12, 2001, from http://www.mohawkc. on.ca/dept/ohas/loadSafety.html

National Institutes of Health Clinical Center Nursing Department. (n.d.). *Institution of universal precautions*. Retrieved May 15, 2001, from http://www.cc.nih.gov/nursing/univer.html

National Pediatric and Family HIV Resource Center (NPHRC). (n.d). *Universal precautions*. Retrieved May 15, 2001, from http://www.thebody,com/nphrc/universal.html

Occupational exposure to bloodborne pathogens: Final rule, 29 C.F.R. § 1910.1030 (1991). *Federal Register* 56(235): 64004-64182, December 6, 1991.

Parlay International. (1990). *Lifting basics: Techniques for safe lifting*. Retrieved August 12, 2001, from http://www.inform.umd.edu/ CampusInfo/Departments/Envirosafety/ os/erg/lift.html

Plainsense. (n.d.) *Protect your back when lifting*. Retrieved August 12, 2001, from http://www.plainsense.com/health/general/lift_it.htm

Rosenfeld-Johnson, S. (2002, January). *Oral-motor exercises for speech clarity. Proceedings from Keynote Presentation*, 16th Annual Colorado Public School Speech/Language Symposium, Denver, CO.

Rustein, R., Conlon, C., & Batshaw, M. (1997). Chapter 9: HIV and AIDS. In M. Batshaw (Ed.), *Children with disabilities* (163–182). Baltimore: Paul H. Brookes.

Seneca, C., Carroll, M. A., & Kuhlow, N. (1988). *About universal precautions*. (1988-612-742/80034). Washington, DC: U.S. Government Printing Office.

Trefz, B. W. (1988). S*ave life: The ABC's of CPR*. Park Ridge, IL: American Academy of Orthopedic Surgeons.

Unified Student Services. (1999, September). *Health #5: Universal precautions for school settings*. Retrieved May 15, 2001, from http://boston.k12.ma.us/dept/uss_health5.htm

U.S. Department of Health and Human Services, Public Health Service. (1988). *Update: Universal precautions for prevention of transmission of human immunodeficiency virus, hepatitis B virus, and other bloodborne pathogens in health-care settings*. Rockville, MD: Author.

CHAPTER **10**

Observation

Key Concepts

Observation is a skill that takes time to develop.

People observe for many different reasons.

Observation is an effective tool for learning about the individuals you serve.

Objectivity and accuracy are cornerstones of observation.

Seven documentation methods are available for observation.

Overview

Why Is Observation Important?

Ways to Observe

General Guidelines for Observing—
How to Observe

Factors That Influence Observation

Process of Observation

Methods of Documentation—How to
Write It Down

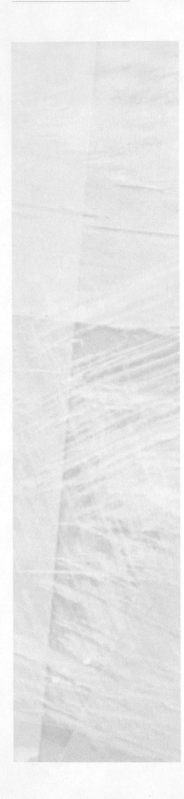

INTRODUCTION

Have you ever gone to a mall to "watch people" or find your-self watching people in a restaurant, airport, or another public location? We use **observation** skills everyday during interactions with people and of our environment. We must recognize that observation and looking are not synonymous. We look and listen to the events that take place before us and absorb what is happening, and that is observation. We are aware of people's verbal and nonverbal communication. We use that information to determine if people understand what we say, if they are happy or angry, and how the interaction is progressing. Usually people do not observe objectively what is taking place around them. Colker (1995) believes that how we react to what we observe is based on our needs, the situation, and other factors such as personal interests, temperament, and cultural background. According to Richarz (1980), observation is one of the oldest and most basic forms of research. Observation also makes us slow down and get to know those around us better (Jablon, Dombro, & Dichtelmiller, 1999). In a way, we all are observers.

In this chapter we will discuss ways and types of observation as well as ways to document what you have observed. A skilled observer needs to be trained what to look for. It takes time and practice to fine-tune your observation skills to use them effectively as an SLPA.

The scene is a preschool classroom, and you have come to visit and watch. You notice a small girl sitting at a table playing by herself with a piece of clay. You step closer to see what she is doing. The girl (we will call her Rosa) smiles as you approach, and asks if you want to play with her. You say "yes," and she gives you her clay. Rosa watches very carefully as you roll the clay into a large ball and then very carefully divide it into two equal parts. You hand her one portion of the clay and tell her, "Now we both have just as much to play with." Rosa nods and smiles again, takes her ball of clay and rolls it around on the surface of the table. You take your part and flatten the piece into a pancake. Rosa notices and shouts, "Hey, your piece is bigger, I want that one!" You do not want to get in an argument with this child so you trade your piece for hers. She smiles and goes back to playing.

You have just observed a child's behavior in a particular situation. You have taken information in through your eyes and ears. What has happened? What have you seen? What could you say about the process you just observed? What could you say about Rosa?

It greatly depends on the perspective you are coming from when you observe (Curtis & Carter, 2000). For example, if you were an early childhood education teacher, you could say which developmental stage the child is in. A parent might notice that the child plays in such a way that is consistent with her play at home. An SLPA may notice that the child's speech is easy to understand and that she talks in complete sentences. A social worker might notice that the child yells when she wants something or when she perceives something is wrong or unfair.

One may think that observation is an easy task, but it involves many intricate parts that fit together to make an observation. You may think that we just use our eyes and ears to take in information about a given situation or person, but we use all of our senses as well as our experiences and background. One major difficulty is that humans are not tape recorders or video cameras and cannot record everything they see in a given situation. The other difficulty that arises is we are individuals with an extensive background of experiences and we tend to "filter" what we see through our belief system and the experiences we have had. What we perceive from a given situation can vary from person to person. Take as an example a car accident scene. Several people might have seen the accident but may highlight different parts or relay the events differently. Police have known for some time that eyewitness accounts of the same accident may vary greatly. If you listen to the TV when they give descriptions of suspects in a crime, the descriptions tend to be general with some variation: "It is a white male approximately 5'9" to 6'0" in his late 20s to early 30s." To be a keen observer, you must learn the parts of observation and then practice to improve your ability to see and hear clearly.

WHY IS OBSERVATION IMPORTANT?

Goodwin and Driscoll (1982) say that observation allows measuring many behaviors of individuals that may otherwise be unmeasureable. Watching people in their daily activities gives us information about who they are, what they like and do not like, their level of skill in communication, fine and gross motor skills, and their social interaction abilities. Giving a formalized test also gives us information about how an individual behaves in a particular area, such as expressive language skills. Observation gives us a broader base of information in everyday life unlike a formalized test looking at specific areas of an individual's abilities in that testing situation (Borich, 1994).

Using more "authentic" means for assessing an individual, professionals realize that observation is one of the most authentic means of learning about an individual and what they know and are able to do, especially when it occurs in their natural environments. "Observation is perhaps the most objective method of assessment" (Taylor, 2000, p. 65). However, different people may see the same event and notice different details about that event.

REASONS FOR OBSERVING

The following is a list of reasons adapted from Martin (1994), in no specific order, why people observe

■ To ensure safety

■ To determine if someone is healthy

■ To pick up on changes in behavior

■ To see what someone eats

■ To learn about what interests a person

■ To see how long a child can focus on an activity

■ To notice what someone's fine and gross motor skills are

■ To learn about a person's social interaction skills

■ To determine if a program is effective

- To see how someone is feeling
- To watch a child's play behaviors
- To learn about an individual's problem-solving skills
- To look at how space is being used and whether more is needed
- To determine if routines are going smoothly
- To watch how someone handles transitions
- To document development
- To report information to parents or other professionals
- To see how a child's language facilitates learning in a classroom
- To determine if someone has difficulty with swallowing
- To obtain documentation for legal purposes
- To gain information for a report card
- To listen to a professional's voice quality
- To see how a person uses nonverbal communication
- To determine a person's learning style
- To learn more about how a person uses his or her eyes
- To watch a communication interaction
- To help build skill in observation
- To appreciate people's differences
- To see what situations a person experiences disfluencies
- To determine how a child's speech is developing
- To see how someone reacts to a new situation
- To learn more about an individual's personality
- To determine a person's conversational skills
- To watch a child's play in order to determine its complexity

Observation as a Method of Gathering Information

Professionals and providers use effective observation as one of their assessment tools. In the past, formal standardized tests were often the focus during assessments, and individuals were asked to sit at a table to complete a wide variety of tasks. We are learning that watching a child or adult in her natural environment is just as valid an assessment as the standardized tests and may reveal more information and is more representative of the individual's abilities. In more recent years, tools have been developed that use observation as the primary method of gaining information. For children, the observation tools may be used as well as parent interviews. Parents and family members are the experts on their child or family member and as professionals we need to tap into that valuable resource. Parents observe their children all the time and see things and understand how their children function like no one else does.

Young children use play as a tool to learn about their world. Watching what they do during their play gives us information about their cognition, language, speech, motor skills, and social interaction skills. Because play is what children do, it is developmentally appropriate to use observation as an assessment tool to evaluate their play. "This is one of the primary tools of many clinicians and researchers who are involved in assessing the behavioral, social, and emotional problems of children and adolescents, and it holds a prominent position as one of the most empirically sound assessment techniques" (Merrell, 1999, p. 48). Observation also has value for SLPAs in working with adults. Observation is widely used as an assessment tool along with standardized tests. This tends to give a more accurate representation of an adult's abilities. How an adult interacts and communicates with others can provide important information regarding current functioning levels.

SIDELIGHT: *Observing Kiki*

Joani was asked to observe Kiki in her preschool class for 20 minutes. Joani took her notebook and sat in a corner, where she could watch Kiki without being a disruption to the classroom. The preschool was having free choice time so the children were able to choose from playing make-believe at the house, putting together puzzles, playing on the computers, pushing cars around on a road carpet, and coloring. Kiki chose to play in the house with her friend Kate. Joani observed their interaction and wrote down what both girls said and what they were doing every few minutes. She followed Kiki when the preschooler decided to play with the puzzles, where she sat down with David and Fredrick. It was challenging to write down what the boys said and did, but Joani was able to keep up. With this information and some formalized tests, Joani's supervising SLP would determine if Kiki qualified to receive speech-language services.

WAYS TO OBSERVE

Merrell (1999) describes three ways to observe: naturalistic observation, analogue observation, and self-monitoring. This section highlights the main characteristics of each method.

Naturalistic Observation

Naturalistic observation is when you observe an individual in her natural environment. For children the observation could be at home with their family, at school with their friends, or in a classroom with their teacher. For a teenager it may be where they work or hanging out with their friends at a mall. For an adult in may be at work, at home, or at a social gathering with peers. This type of observation differs from the other two methods because it uses observing people in their typical, day-to-day situations and these environments that can produce very accurate observational information on everyday functioning. The main emphasis of this method is to observe in a way that does not bring attention to the observer and change the behavior of those being observed.

Analogue Observation

Analogue observation is designed to simulate the conditions of the natural environment. It is to provide a highly structured and controlled setting where behaviors of interest are likely to be observed (Merrell, 1999). Analogue observations may take place in a clinic or laboratory where a natural type of environment is set up. A clinic could have a room for children with toys that are set up in an inviting way for them to play. Specific toys may be chosen to look at different behaviors. For example, if you are looking at how a child produces the "s" sound, you may choose toys that begin with the letter "s": sand, sack, saddle, salad, salt, sandwich, seed, seesaw, seven, sink, sister, six, soap, soccer, soda, soft, soil, song, sound, sugar, or sun. Or you may want to watch how teenagers interact socially so you set up a living room situation in a school to complete the observation. You may want to observe communicative interactions among adults during a conversation group. Analogue observation takes more

inference about behaviors than naturalistic observation. This type of observation has its advantages because then you can control the environment to get at certain behaviors. The environment needs to resemble the natural setting in which the individual is having difficulty as close as possible. This way the observation information is close to what you might obtain in a natural setting.

Self-Monitoring

The third method of observing is self-monitoring, which means an observer is trained in observing and recording her own behavior. This type of observation is efficient and has a very low cost. Self-monitoring can be used with behaviors that are difficult for an outside observer to gain adequate amounts of information like eating habits or sleep patterns. Doctors may use this method when they are determining what foods a person may be allergic to. The doctor may have the patient document what food is eaten throughout the day and what, if any, allergic reactions occur. The patient may observe that she had peanuts for a snack, and that night she developed watery, itchy eyes, hives around the mouth, stomach cramps, and a runny nose. One drawback of self-monitoring is the reliability of the observations. It may be difficult to train an individual who is experiencing the event to be objective.

As an SLPA, you may use all three methods of observation, but the analogue observation is used most frequently.

GENERAL GUIDELINES FOR OBSERVING—HOW TO OBSERVE

The following guidelines give you a framework to work from in preparation, actual observation, and documentation of the observation. Three informal observation procedures are available for use. The first is observed in a natural environment, with the observer being someone in her natural environment (parent, teacher, or a day care provider). The next is when an outside observer watches in a natural setting, and the third method is when the observer is not present in the

natural environment but is watching through a one-way mirror or videotape (Bentzen, 1997).

Preparation

To get ready for an observation, several factors must be considered as well as the preparations that must be made. The first part of preparation is to define your purpose for observing. Your purpose for observing defines everything else you do during your preparations. For example, your SLP may request that you observe a particular student in a classroom to document carryover of specific articulation goals worked on in therapy. Objectives need to be defined precisely enough so that the observational task is broken down into a manageable size.

The second factor to consider is where you are planning on doing the observation. This may be derived easily from your purpose. For example, if you are planning on watching geriatric patients' social interactions, then a nursing home or senior center may be the best place to set up your observation. If the choice of settings is limited, for example, you live in a small town with one hospital, clinic, and nursing home, that will restrict your choice of where you will observe. The purpose of your observation may change a little if this limitation exists.

The third factor is determining what you are allowed to do in the setting. Some settings may give you considerable leeway to do what is necessary to accomplish your objectives, whereas others may be more formal and not allow certain things. Some places may require you to interact with the individuals you are observing and not allow you to take notes unless you are outside the room. In this situation you will have to rely on your memory until you are able to write down your observations. The setting may also dictate what type of recording technique you use, for example, a tape or video recorder or paper and pen. A checklist would allow you more flexibility to be involved if necessary, whereas an elaborate **narrative description** would not allow you to be able to interact with the students at the classroom at all. Some settings may require you to sign a permission slip before the observation, which lists their guidelines for observation. If a particular setting has limitations that affect your purpose in observing, you may need to pick another setting that will accommodate your needs.

SIDELIGHT: *Tape Recording Observations*

Kristen was taking a class in her SLPA program on communication skills of adults and she was interested in individuals who had sustained a head injury. For an assignment, she needed to be able to record with a portable audiotape recorder the interactions she was observing so she could transcribe the interaction at a later date. The first rehabilitation center she called would allow her to do on-line transcription, but she could not bring a tape recorder into the therapy session she was observing. Because the taping was part of her assignment, she called another rehabilitation center. The SLP agreed to let Kristen audiotape the session if the individual with the brain injury agreed and was willing to sign a release form.

Inconspicuous Observation

"There is a principle that says that observing a phenomenon changes it. Observing people can change their behavior, although we may not know how much their behavior changes. Their awareness of the observer's presence can distract them or motivate them to behave in ways they believe will please the observer" (Bentzen, 1997, p. 41). The more inconspicuous you are in an observation setting, the more natural the behavior will tend to be. The *American Heritage Dictionary* (2000) defines inconspicuous as "not readily noticeable" (p. 888). This phenomenon of changing behavior when an observer is present concerns many researchers. We are all researchers in one way or another if we are looking at behavior and then along the process that behavior is analyzed and interpreted in certain ways. The observer needs to be as invisible as possible to gain the most information from the observation.

One way to help minimize changes in behavior is through participant observation. This means that the observer becomes part of the group and participates in as many activities as they can for a given situation. Teachers are natural participant observers and they can observe without adversely affecting those being observed. This can be very different for an unfamiliar person coming into a setting to observe. Eventually researchers feel that the novelty of the unfamiliar person wears off and the behavior of those being observed is not affected. Some feel like the individuals who are being observed will always perform for the observer to some degree (Kozloff, 1994).

SIDELIGHT: *Participant Observation*

Richard had been working on listening skills with Jimmy for 3 months in his classroom, especially with teacher directions. Today his supervising SLP wanted Richard to observe Jimmy to get some information about how he was doing. Because Richard was expected to participate in the classroom, he needed to do his observation as a participant observer. The teacher was explaining an activity in which the students would break into small groups and make a teepee. Richard watched Jimmy as the directions were given and he appeared to be using the strategies that he had been taught. He got to his small group and was able to participate with the group, with minimal cues from Richard. Richard carried a clipboard and wrote down his observations as Jimmy participated in the group. See Figure 10-1.

According to Thorndike and Hagan (1977), young children have not developed the covers and camouflages to conceal themselves from being observed as well as older siblings. Therefore, the effects of an unfamiliar observer may be minimal with younger children. Inconspicuous observation tries to prevent or minimize unwanted influence on the behavior being observed.

Difficulties of Remaining Inconspicuous

Being inconspicuous is not always easy. A new person to a situation is likely to get at least some attention of those being observed until the novelty has worn off. In some places there may be observation booths that can be used to observe without being seen. See Figure 10-2 to see an observer in an observation room. A one-way window is placed between the main room and the observation room so the individual in the observation room may watch without being seen by those in

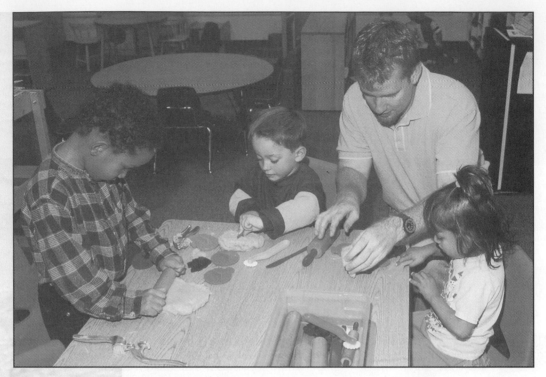

Figure 10-1 An observer is engaging in participant observation. By becoming part of the group he has become inconspicuous as an observer.

TIPS FOR SUCCESSFUL OBSERVATION

The following list contains some tips to help ensure inconspicuous observation:

- Avoid eye contact and facial expressions that initiate communication.
- Wear comfortable but plain clothes. Watch out for fancy belts and jewelry that may especially attract a child's attention.
- Try to avoid obvious staring. This makes people feel uncomfortable.
- Distance yourself so you can hear what is going on but not in the individual's personal space.
- If an individual gets you into a conversation, simply state what you are doing and end the conversation. Make sure if you promise to do something later that you follow up on that commitment.

the main room. From the main room, it looks like there is a mirror on a wall, and the participants most likely will have no idea that anyone is on the other side. This type of observation definitely interferes less with normal behavior.

During most observations, you will need to document or write down what you are seeing, which may be distracting especially because children may be curious about what is being done and what is being written. If a child asks you what you are doing, you can tell her that you are working, or you can give some other brief explanation that is true. Try not to tell those being observed that you are watching them and writing down everything they are doing. That will definitely affect their behavior and make those being observed nervous, self-conscious, or uncomfortable.

Language is difficult to observe from a distance because the observer must be able to hear what is being said. Usually getting that close to someone with a notebook or even a tape recorder can bring attention to the observer.

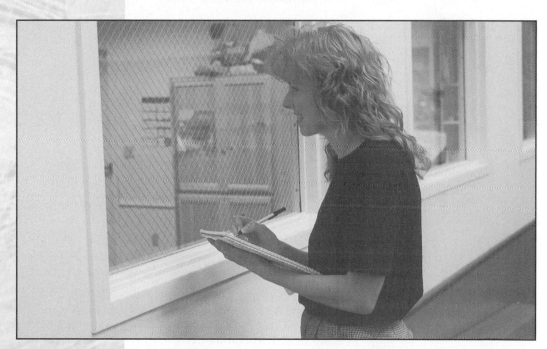

Figure 10-2 Some schools and clinics have observation rooms with one-way windows and counter desk tops.

When you are observing, there will be little reason to interfere with what is going on in the situation you are observing. If you are a participant observer you will be very involved in what the people you are observing are doing.

Even with the difficulties explained above, it is possible to observe without interfering in such a way as to change behavior within the requirements of the observation and the place you are observing. When you are observing it is important to be as detached as much as possible, which means watching for spontaneous behavior, not behavior that is prompted or instructed to happen without becoming a part of the behavior being observed. Observing in a natural environment is different from observing during a testing situation. In the testing situation, the tester is requesting that the individual perform a certain way.

Professional Ethics and Confidentiality

As described in Chapter 7, ethics plays a critical role in all professional activities, and that includes observation. In most places where you observe, you are a guest and a representative of the institution you are from (college). Your behavior therefore reflects not only on yourself, but also on the school you represent. You may also have obligations to those who come behind you, because your behavior may affect whether others will be allowed to come and observe at a later time.

Research using human subjects is closely monitored. A researcher is under some very specific guidelines on what she can do with human subjects. The rights, safety (physical and psychological), and privacy of the individual must be held in the uttermost importance. In a way, your observations are a form of research so these principles must be observed. During an observation you are watching behaviors, documenting those behaviors, sometimes making interpretations, and watching changes over time. Dealing with people and gaining information about them must be done with care and sensitivity. Objectivity is one of the best ways to be sensitive and demonstrate caring. Objectivity in an observation is describing behavior just as it occurs—what happened, what was said, and what actions were made. This does not

include making judgments or "value" of the behavior. Remember that even objective documentation may reveal information that may be embarrassing or could be misused to make someone look bad. To help this situation from occurring, it is helpful not to use names in your documentation. This helps keep the information confidential.

Another practice that facilitates confidentiality includes not talking to others about those individuals you have observed unless you have specific permission from the one being observed. That means do not talk to your parents or friends about what you observed. This practice is easily violated; therefore, you must take extra care not to breech confidentiality. If you do discuss the individual(s) you have observed with the appropriate people, make sure that the individual(s) in question do not overhear your discussion. You need to take extra measures especially with children to make sure they are not close by and can overhear what you are saying. Children are very sensitive to information being shared about them. This practice does not rule out discussing an individual privately with an instructor or in a formal classroom setting. In these situations the purpose is to help in your understanding of the observation process or to solve difficulties you experience when you observe. These discussions may be done without violating the individual's rights to privacy and confidentiality especially when names are not used. Remember that when dealing with children, parents' rights are not violated. If a parent does not want her child to be observed and information about this child documented, you are obliged not to do the observation.

When you do an observation, you must have permission to do so. Permission must be granted before making the observation. In places such as clubs, Sunday schools, Girl Scouts or Boy Scouts, or similar organizations where the roles of adults are much less defined, it is recommended that you obtain written permission from parents before the observation. Permission is not required in public areas such as a shopping mall, swimming pool, or playground, but you still need to be unobtrusive. With public settings, it is wise to just observe and not try to interact with those you are observing in any way. When observing children, you especially want to just watch, because interacting with a child may be taken in

the wrong way. Remember that stranger training when you were growing up. If you are documenting behaviors in a public setting, it would be polite to explain to the individual or her parent(s) what you are doing and receive verbal permission. "Asking is a gesture of courtesy, and it may help avoid suspicion" (Bentzen, 1997, p. 46).

When you are carrying out your role as an SLPA, you need to follow professional ethics and behave in a professional manner. This requires that at times you set aside your own wants and needs. This professional behavior must occur when doing a variety of SLPA tasks, but especially when you are doing observations.

FACTORS THAT INFLUENCE OBSERVATION

Making accurate and clear observations can be a challenging task. The following are several factors that may influence your observation. You need to consider these when planning, doing, or recording an observation.

Sensitivity and Awareness

Sensitivity or acuity to observe specific behaviors is a skill that comes with time. As you perform an increasing number of observations and if you concentrate on improving these skills, they will get better over time. You will be able to notice subtle behaviors as well as intricacies of interactions. As you learn about specific speech and language behaviors, they will be easier to notice in a natural environment.

Tiredness, Illness, Discomfort

Tiredness, illness, discomforts, and "things on your mind" can easily influence your ability to make accurate observations. "Things on your mind" may be personal problems, anxiety, fear, or just trying to do too much at once. You need to make a conscious effort to leave those things behind and focus on what you are doing, an observation. One way to offset the effects of these things is to avoid them altogether. You may need to postpone an observation if you are tired, sick, or physically uncomfortable. You may also want to break an observation into several parts to help alleviate tiredness or distraction during a long observation.

Environment

Sometimes things within the environment will distract you from your observation. For example, the room may be too hot or too cold, your chair may be uncomfortable, or there may be poor lighting. The physical setup of the space you are observing in may be confined and it may be difficult to remain inconspicuous. The equipment and materials available to the individuals you are observing may influence the behaviors you see and therefore affect your observation also. Awareness of these factors helps decrease the effect the environmental distractions may have on your observation.

SIDELIGHT: *Darwin's Story*

Darwin had difficulty sleeping last night. When he got to work, he needed to observe a high school student's social skills in a history class. His supervising SLP had provided Darwin with a social skills checklist to use during the observation. As the students worked in small groups planning a trip to California in a covered wagon, Darwin found a location in the room where he was not noticed—but it also happened to be next to a heating vent. He quickly noticed that the warm temperature and his lack of sleep the night before made it difficult to keep focused. He found himself yawning and found that several minutes had gone by and he had not written a language sample. Knowing that incomplete data might negatively affect the SLP's assessment of the student, Darwin shifted his position and tried to wake himself up. He was able to rouse himself enough to finish the observation. He hoped to sleep better tonight.

Your Personality and Biases

It may be challenging to sort out who you are from what you are viewing. You come to any situation with your own unique set of past experiences, attitudes, needs, fears, and desires. These tend to become filters for whatever you hear and see.

An observer may project how she is feeling onto the individual she is observing. For example, the observer may feel that a child who is playing by herself must be lonely, or when watching an interaction between two adults and one of them raises her voice, the observer thinks she must be mad. These biases can affect what you look at as how much you focus on certain behaviors. This can especially be true when the behaviors are not liked by the observer or even consider unacceptable. There is a tendency to make judgments in your observation instead of just reporting the facts. We all have biases and we need to learn to control them so they do not interfere with the observation process. The main goal of observation is to be as objective as possible.

Look at the pictures in Figures 10-3 and 10-4 and list 10 observations. Figure 10-3 is a picture taken at a sporting event in a high school football/track field.

The following are 10 objective observations of the scene. Compare them to your observations.

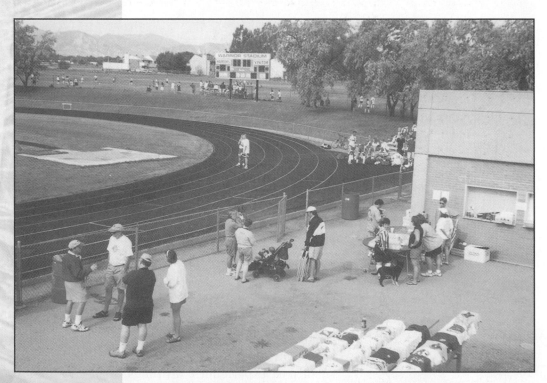

Figure 10-3 Provide some observations about this event at a high school track and field competition.

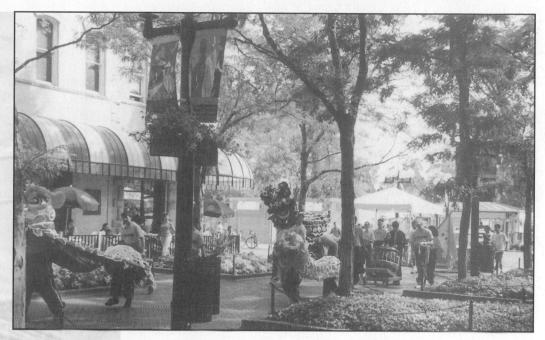

Figure 10-4 Provide some observations about this Chinese New Year parade.

1. Parents and family are standing around talking. A group of four and another group of four standing around a stroller are standing behind a chain-link fence talking.

2. Shirts are laid out neatly on the bleachers.

3. A table has food and drink items on it.

4. Two adults are standing next to the table talking.

5. One adult is leaning over the table.

6. A child with a dog is standing next to the table.

7. One adult is turning away from the table with a cup in his hand.

8. Two teenagers in blue shorts and white shirts are standing on the track talking and looking at something on the football field.

9. A group of teenagers are congregated around a set of bleachers.

10. On a field next to the track, kids in uniforms are running around kicking a ball while others are standing or sitting next to the field.

Try making 10 observational statements while looking at Figure 10-4 where a Chinese New Year parade is occurring on an outside mall.

Here are 10 sample observation statements of Figure 10-4.

1. Three oriental dragons are in a parade.

2. Three people are walking next to the dragons.

3. One person in a black oriental outfit is playing a large black drum in the middle of a group of seven people.

4. People next to the man playing the large black drum are playing other instruments.

5. A person is walking behind the people playing instruments carrying a blue flag.

6. The parade is in front of a sidewalk café.

7. People are eating at the outside café.

8. Behind the group of people walking are two large canopies and two smaller canopies.

9. Bikes are parked next to the café.

10. A man is sitting on a bench.

Did your observations match the ones that are given? Did it contain subjective statements like "The people were not watching the parade because they did not like it"? Did you include lots of details or were your statements general?

Objectivity

Objectivity is the cornerstone of observation. This happens when you report exactly what you see and then document it in some form (this will be covered under Methods of Documentation). Here are two statements of the same situation. Decide which one is more objective.

1. The child was tired and did not participate in the activity the other children were doing, coloring an activity sheet.

2. The child yawned and put her head on the table. She set her crayon down and watched the other children color their activity sheets.

The second is much more objective than the first. It describes exactly what happened instead of making judgments about the actions as seen in the first statement. Try it again.

1. A girl about 20 years old picked up a pack of cigarettes and put them in her pocket. She then walked out of the store. No one noticed.

2. A 20-year-old girl stole a pack of cigarettes from the store and walked out unnoticed.

The first statement is the more objective one and gives much more information than the second. In your observation of the mall scene, were your statements objective or do they reflect how you view the world and include judgments?

Objectivity is defined in the *American Heritage Dictionary* (2000) as "have or having to do with a material object, having actual existence or reality, uninfluenced by emotions or personal prejudices or fair" (p. 1212). According to this definition be careful about making things up that did not actually happen and just state the facts of what you saw. Remember that completely objective observation is not possible just because we are human, but we can try to make it as objective as possible. Objective descriptions may be very useful to your supervising SLP, who needs information on how a student is performing in a classroom, or how an elderly patient in a nursing home tells the nursing staff her needs. This information is then used to make or change current treatment plans for those individuals. One way to determine if you are really objective is to ask yourself if you are describing things in such a way that anyone viewing the same scene would describe it in the exact same way (Colker, 1995, p. 7).

Interpretation

Instead of being objective in an observation, you may be tempted to interpret what you are seeing. Avoid that tempta-

tion. When you interpret what you see, it defeats the purpose of the observation and eliminates your objectivity. Remember that the purpose of the observation is to give an accurate picture of the individual or group you are observing or how the program is working. Interpretations are your opinions and they may be true, but they may not be supported by what is observed. Colker (1995) describes the following things that cannot be observed, including intelligence (how smart a person it), feelings (such as frustration or happiness), reasons for doing things (she was unhappy), or self-concept (that person suffers from a low self-esteem). These are all subjective judgments rather than objective observations.

Accuracy

Accuracy emphasizes that you are both factual and exact in your description. This will be most helpful to your supervising SLP. Record exactly what you see and as completely as you can. Be as specific as you can in reporting your observations. For example, in an early childhood setting, report what takes place, how children use materials, and how they relate to each other. The more information you write down, the better sense of the activity you are observing will be, and it will be less likely to be misinterpreted later. Ambiguous words like *crowded*, *too many*, *wild*, *roughhousing*, and *messy* are relative terms with no transferable meaning. To accurately describe a setting, count the number of people, give comparative measures, and describe the arrangement of the area and materials. "For example, rather than saying that the water props are inconvenient for the children to get on their own, you might note that the water props are stored on the top ledge of the area divider and that the child who went to use them had to stand on her tiptoes and stretch her outreached fingers to get them off the shelf" (Colker, 1995, p. 7). The more exact description, the better your observation results will be and the more helpful you will be to your SLP. The purpose of your observation will also dictate how much information you need for your observation as well as the method you use to document the information (see Methods of Documentation).

PROCESS OF OBSERVATION

As an SLPA, you will be a part of the first step of observation. The three stages of observation are objective description, interpretation, and evaluation. The first is the key part of the observation because everything else depends on it. Objective description consists of recording what you see very precisely and with the amount of information that will make it complete according to your objectives. The second and third steps are reserved for your supervising SLP. The second step is interpretation, which is giving meaning to what was seen. For example, if you saw a little girl fall off the slide and start crying, that is an objective description. If you added, "because she was hurt," that would be an interpretation. Someone else may say that the girl cried because of fear and frustration instead of being hurt. Those are two different interpretations of the same event. An individual is trying to identify the cause of the behavior of crying and it assigns motives to that individual's actions. The third step is evaluation. At this point an individual's values and opinions come into play concerning the observed behavior and maybe the individual's character and personality.

Groups or Individuals

As you determine the purpose for your observation, you will need to decide if group or individual observation will most effectively meet your purpose. It also determines how the information may be used at a later time.

Groups

Group observation looks at how the group functions during an activity. A group is defined as a collection of individuals who are assembled in a particular place and may be as unstructured as those who are at the grocery store or as structured as a football team where everyone has a designed role. You may want to look at how a class of fourth graders moves through the school—to the lunchroom, outside for recess, or you may want to see how a group of people interact while riding an elevator. When you are observing a group, you are looking at the whole. It is impossible to gain specific information about a specific individual while watching a group. You may watch how individuals function within a group, but not specific information about an individual. One other drawback around observing groups is that it is difficult to listen to every conversation and see what every person is doing at the same time. With the help of videotaping technology, this has become more possible, especially when viewed repeatedly.

SIDELIGHT: *Observing a Conversation Group*

Jennifer was going to be working with a group of adults who had aphasia in a conversation group. She expressed her desire to observe the group before she started with her SLP. Her main goal in observation was to see how the group was run and how the individuals interacted in a group setting. She was introduced to the group and took a chair outside the circle so she could observe without becoming part of the group. She gained many ideas about running the group and wrote them down in her notebook.

Individuals

An individual is one person who may be in a group with other individuals or may be by herself. When watching an individual, you have much more freedom to look at how she behaves in different environments. Observing individuals does not have the limitations of watching groups because the observation is specifically one on one. One person watches another person. As an SLPA, you will be observing an individual's speech or language skills rather than observing groups.

METHODS OF DOCUMENTATION—HOW TO WRITE IT DOWN

Seven different ways of recording an observation are discussed in this section: narrative description, sampling, anec-

dotal records, diary record, frequency counts, and checklists. To make recording easier, use a pencil, paper, wristwatch, and maybe a golf counter. Using audio and videorecordings also makes recording easier, especially when you are learning to observe. With a permanent record of what happened, you can go back as many times as necessary to get the information you are looking for. You will notice over time that you will not need to rely on the audio and video as much. Documentation is a vital part of an observation so you have a record.

Narrative Descriptions/ Running Record

A **narrative description**, sometimes called a running record, basically is when everything an individual does is recorded as it happens in as much detail as possible. The individual may be with other people or may be by herself. The main goal of narrative description is to get a detailed, objective account of an individual's behavior. An observer can use this method with little observation experience, but a more experienced observer will be able to record more detail, describe more accurately, and avoid personal bias. It is important in a narrative description to record the context the behavior is in as well as what those who interact with the individual are doing and saying. A good description is found when the reader of the description can close his eyes and get a good mental picture of what is happening. The goal would be to record much like a video camera. The limitation of a narrative description is the short amount of time you are able to observe because of physical and mental fatigue that may happen during this type of recording. You may not want to do this type of recording for more than an hour.

The main advantage to this method is how complete the record is of an individual's behavior stream. It also includes context as well as behavior that gives a great amount of information for the SLP to interpret. The narrative description also is very helpful if it is done several times over a period of time; then the sequential records may be compared and analyzed. The main disadvantage is that it can cost a lot of time and energy to acquire a narrative description. It also takes a great amount of skill to be able to observe as well as write on a continuous basis. The narrative description shown in Figure 10-5 gives a complete record of an observation.

Sampling

Sampling is a method that looks at smaller pieces of the whole instead of the whole. If you are sampling a box of 50

Observer's Name   Alice Thompson (Teacher)

Child/Children Observed   Melissa L.

Child's/Children's Age(s)   4 years, 3 months   Child's/Children's Sex   Female

Observation Context (home, child care center, preschool, school)   Children's Delight Preschool

Date of Observation January 10, 1999   Time Begun 9:20 A.M.   Time Ended 9:30 A.M.

Brief Description of Physical and Social Characteristics of Observation Setting

Children are busily engaged in various free play activities. The overall mood seems upbeat. Of the usual 15 children who are enrolled, only 12 are here today—3 are ill, according to the parents' telephone communications with the director this morning. Although the children's moods seem good, they are more quiet than usual—not as much loud talking as sometimes takes place.

Objective Behavioral Descriptions (OBD) and Interpretations:
Narrative Description

OBD 1: [Time Begun 9:20 A.M.   Time Ended 9:22 A.M.]
Melissa (M) arrives about 35 minutes after the other children have arrived and started their activities. She puts her coat in her cubby and then stands in the doorway of the main classroom and looks around; she remains motionless for about 1/2 minute, moving only her eyes as she glances at other children and their activities.

Interpretation 1:
Melissa seems shy, almost withdrawn. From moment of arrival, she seemed reluctant to enter into things. May be because she didn't want to come in first place; her reluctance was mentioned by her mother several days ago. No specific reason was offered.

OBD 2: [Time Begun 9:22 A.M.   Time Ended 9:24 A.M.]
M. walks toward reading area on far side of the room from the cubbies. As she walks, she scrapes the toe of her right foot at each step, doing this for about 5 feet. She passes by the puzzle table where two children are seated; no communication is exchanged. She walks to a table with some books lying on it. Tina, José, and Miguel are seated at the table; José and Miguel are sharing a book, Tina (T) is watching them "read." Melissa says nothing to the three children as she sits down.

Figure 10-5 Narrative description—school setting (continues)

Interpretation 2:
Melissa still seems uncertain; even her motor behaviors seem restricted; she walks slowly, shuffling, as though unsure of herself and of her relationship with the other children or her environment. Seems to have trouble deciding what to do. Not at all communicative; makes no overtures to any of the children who were "available" for such.

OBD 3: [Time Begun 9:24 A.M.   Time Ended 9:29 A.M.]
José and Miguel don't look up or acknowledge Melissa in any way. Tina says "Hi, Melissa, wanna read a book with me?" M. cocks her head to one side and says, "I don't know how to read." T. replies "We can look at the pictures." M. looks over toward the big block area and without looking at T., says, "OK." Tina smiles and goes to a shelf containing a number of books. M. picks up one of the books already on the table and flips through the pages. T. returns with a book and says, "I like this one, let's look at this one." M. merely nods; T. sits down close to M., but M. moves slightly, keeping a distance of about 6–8 inches between her and Tina.

Interpretation 3:
Tina seems outgoing and friendly as Melissa approaches; M. is still uncommunicative; still seems shy and uncertain; speaks softly as though afraid of being heard. Tina persists in spite of M.'s apparent lack of enthusiasm. M. also seems distractable or inattentive. She shies away from T.'s efforts to get close physically. Tina moves at a quick pace—much more energetic than M.

OBD 4: [Time Begun 9:29 A.M.   Time Ended 9:30 A.M.]
José looks up and says, "Hey, you two, wha'cha doin'?" Tina tilts her head upward, thrusts out her chin slightly and says, "Never mind, we're busy." Melissa says nothing, but gets up from the table and walks toward big block area. Miguel still reads.

Interpretation 4:
Tina is much more outgoing and sure of herself than M. T. didn't interact too much w/ José and Miguel; may have felt left out of their activity. T. definitely seemed pleased to see M.; displayed no unfavorable response to M.'s "unsocial" behavior. T.'s response to José was quite assertive, but in a friendly way; almost like she claimed Melissa as her playmate, maybe in retaliation for the two boys ignoring her earlier. M. still seems uninterested, even uncertain of what to do.

Figure 10-5 (continued)

pieces of chocolate, you only have to taste one or two to determine the status of that chocolate. You do not need to eat all 50 pieces to determine if the chocolate is good or not. Another example of sampling is when samples of sale or new items they want people to purchase are handed out at the grocery store. People are given a small amount to let them determine if they want more. Sampling is also used in looking at behavior. If you do not want the entire time documented, you may want parts of it that may represent the whole. Two major types of sampling exist: time sampling and event sampling.

Time Sampling

Time sampling is taking small chunks of time out of a specified time you are observing. It may be broken down into 3-minute segments taken every 10 minutes over an hour. You therefore end up with 15 minutes of observed time of one individual over the total time of 1 hour. To make the observation more effective you may want to watch three different individuals each for 3 minutes over an hour time period. Or you can break it down and watch 25 students in the classroom 1 minute. When you do time sampling, you may look for a specific behavior during each of the sampling times. You may be looking at sharing behavior in preschoolers, watching each child for 1 minute and making a mark if you see sharing during that 1 minute you observe with each child. For example, if you move from Sara to Betsy and Sara shares with Betsy, you may not mark that down because now you are watching Betsy for sharing behavior. Coding methods are usually used with time sampling because you do not have much time to write detailed descriptions. A check mark may be all you have time to do during your time sampling. When designing your coding methods, make sure that each possible category is separate from the others. Say you are looking at articulation difficulties in several children and you design your categories as follows:

1. Substitution: d for g
2. Substitution: t for k
3. Omission of g or k
4. Misarticulate g
5. Distortion of k

In these categories a child could produce a d for g and two categories would need to be marked: Substitution of d for g and Misarticulate g. If a child produced a k for g, then you would check the Misarticulate g category.

Time sampling, as seen in Figure 10-6, is mainly used when looking at how often behaviors occur. The main disadvantage of time sampling is that if coding methods are being used, it misses the details of the context, the behaviors and how the situation turns out, and how the behaviors change

Observer's Name   Carmen Gonzalez

Child/Children Observed   Melissa (Tina, Miguel, and José are also involved, but only data on Melissa are included in this example)

Child's/Children's Age(s)   4 years, 3 months   Child's/Children's Sex   Female

Observation Context (home, child care center, preschool, school)   Mother's Love Child Care Center

Date of Observation   February 12, 1999   Time Begun   9:30 A.M.   Time Ended   9:45 A.M.

Brief Description of Characteristics of Physical and Social Environment:
Children seem in a good mood; some are physically active, others are engaging in sedentary activities. All 15 children are present today. Some children are playing with children with whom they do not ordinarily play.

Recording Intervals

Behavior Category	1	2	3	4	5	6	7	8	9	10
General Response to Setting										
1. Enters setting willingly (specify which areas are involved—big block area [BBA], reading area [RA], Snack Area [SA], Free Play [FP], Art Area [AA], Main Classroom [MC], etc.)		②	③	④						
2. Enters setting reluctantly	①2									
3. Refuses to enter setting										
General Response to Environment										
4. Uses equipment/materials freely										
5. Limited or sporadic use of equipment/materials					①5					
6. No use of equipment/materials										
General Response to Others										
7. Seeks or is in contact with peer(s)										
8. Seeks or is in contact with adult										
9. Avoids or breaks contact with peer(s)										
10. Avoids or breaks contact with adult										
11. Reluctant contact with peer(s); contact lacks motivation or concentration on part of child					①11					
12. Reluctant contact with adult; contact lacks motivation or concentration on part of child										
	1	2	3	4	5	6	7	8	9	10

Children Observed

1. Melissa   3. José
2. Tina   4. Miguel

Figure 10-6 Time sampling description of one child

over time or in different contexts. For example, you are watching for aggressive behaviors in 5-second intervals for each child in the classroom. While you are watching Jean she yells, " Get out of here you mean boy." You determine that that is an example of aggressive behavior so you check it off. What you did not see is that Jean was pretending to be a mommy in the playhouse and was pretending to be aggressive. Time sampling does not treat behavior as it occurs naturally. A behavior may begin or end before or after the specified time has occurred. The advantages of time sampling include there are no restrictions of the kinds of behaviors that can be studied, it is economical on time and energy, it is efficient when used with coding methods, and the data are reliable (Bentzen, 1997).

Event Sampling

Event sampling uses the same sampling technique as time sampling except that sampling is done on an event basis. Our lives are one continuous event after another. You pick one specific event and then watch for it to happen. The event may be anything from quarrels, social interactions, or dependency behavior (Bentzen, 1997). When the event occurs you record what happens. You may use coding methods, narrative description, or a combination of both. In event sampling you only take one sample from the individual's behavior stream, unlike time sampling in which you take several. Event sampling closely resembles narrative description although it defines what will be observed.

Event sampling has several advantages. If narrative description is the method of documentation, it may provide a detailed account of an event. It is also practical to use especially with behaviors that do not occur frequently. Another advantage is that coding and narrative description may be combined to give more information about a particular event. The disadvantage of event sampling is that it only looks at one specific event in the flow of many. See Figure 10-7 for an example of event sampling. Event sampling examines one event in a series of events.

Observer's Name   Ursula Ostertag

Child/Children Observed   Melissa

Child's/Children's Age(s)   4 years   Child's/Children's Sex   Female

Observation Context (home, child care center, preschool, school)   Preschool (FunTime Care Center)

Date of Observation October 13, 1999   Time Begun 9:20 A.M.   Time Ended 9:35 A.M.

Brief Description of Characteristics of Physical and Social Environment

The children are fairly active today—seem to be in a good mood. The teachers and aides also share the children's mood. The activity areas are in a bit of disorder—equipment and materials are strewn about, which might reflect the general emotional mood of the class. The general demeanor is in somewhat sharp contrast with yesterday's emotional climate.

Objective Behavioral Descriptions (OBD) and Interpretations: *Event Sampling*

OBD 1: [Time Begun 9:24 A.M.   Time Ended 9:29 A.M.]
Melissa approaches the reading table where Tina, José, and Miguel are seated. M. sits down, but says nothing to the others. Tina responds immediately to M.'s presence; greets her with "Hi, wanna read a book with me?" M. replies that she (M.) can't read. T. replies that they can look at the pictures. M. agrees with a soft spoken, "OK." Tina smiles and goes for a book. M. does not look at or speak to José and Miguel, nor they to her. T. comes back and tries to sit close to M., who responds by moving away slightly, keeping about 6–8 inches between them. José speaks to the two girls, asking them what they're doing. T. responds, "Never mind, we're busy." M. says nothing but gets up from the table and moves toward the cubby area.

Interpretation 1:
Melissa seems shy, withdrawn, apathetic. She doesn't respond to Tina's greeting, barely even looks at her; seems not even to notice José and Miguel, who also ignore her. M. avoids close contact with Tina; seems to reject physical or psychological proximity. M. is easily distracted, does not focus well socially, as evidenced by her lack of eye contact with Tina and by her looking around the room as T. tries to engage her in a social exchange. M.'s actions don't appear to stem from any dislike of Tina; no evidence of hostility— indeed, M. is emotionally bland. Appears to have no interest in the company of others.

OBD 2: [Time Begun 9:29 A.M.   Time Ended 9:30 A.M.]
M. breaks contact with Tina and José and walks toward the big block area.

Interpretation 2:
Melissa still seems withdrawn and uninterested; she makes no response to José's friendly overture,

Figure 10-7 Event sampling of social behavior

Anecdotal Records

Anecdotal records are a written description of a particular event that has occurred and tend to be used by teachers. A good example of this is a parent recording in a baby book such events as when the baby rolled over, when the first tooth came in, or when the first steps were taken. These types of records may follow a child through her school years. According to Goodwin and Discoll (1982) anecdotal records have five characteristics. First, the record must be from a direct observation of the child. Second, the record must be a prompt, accurate, and a specific description of the event. Third, the record must contain the context in which the event occurred. The fourth characteristic is that any inter-pretation of the event is kept separate from the objective description. The last component is that it is recorded whether the behavior being described is typical or not for that particular child. These guidelines help keep rumors and other descriptions of a child out of her record.

The main advantage is that an anecdotal record gives a continuous record of a child's behavior within specified set-tings. It also may be used as a comparison of a child's behav-ior and therefore may be a good indicator of change. It is easy to use because it has no specific guidelines for how it is recorded. The disadvantage of using an anecdotal record is that bias can easily creep into the description of an event. Then these records may be passed on to others who may make their own judgments of the child's behavior. See Figure 10-8 for an anecdotal record.

> Jimmy came to school today with his pet goldfish. He was so excited when all the students gathered around him and asked him questions. He was smiling and answering everyone's questions. When it was time for class to start, he appeared sad when he was asked to put his goldfish on the back counter until sharing time. He walked slowly to the counter, set the fish down and dragged his feet as he walked to his desk pouting. He grumbled something about wanting to keep the fish on his desk.

Figure 10-8 Anecdotal record

Diary Records

A **diary** is something that is written in on a daily basis summarizing the events of an individual's day and is the same for documenting diary records. This method is great for looking at change over a long period of time. Diary records tend to focus on new behaviors as they occur in an individual's life. This method is wonderful for looking at a child's growth and development. Diary records require continuous contact between the individual and the observer and usually a parent, guardian, caregiver, or teacher can only achieve this. See Figure 10-9 for an example of diary records.

The main advantage to this type of observation recording is that it tends to provide a detailed account over a long period of time. It is a very helpful way to look at changes over time. Diary records tend to be permanent records and can then be compared with other forms of observational data, for example, developmental norms. The main disadvantage is that it tends not to be useful way to document most observations. The continuous contact needed makes it useful for a small number of observers.

Frequency Counts

Frequency counts are a record of how often a particular behavior has occurred. Usually the observer just makes a mark on an observation sheet every time a behavior occurs. These records are useful for baseline measurements or to see a change in a behavior. It is very easy to use and gives immediate data after it has been counted. The information can then easily be put into graphic form for ease of reading the data. The frequency count gives limited information about the behavior, just that it has occurred.

An example of frequency counts could be the number of times George initiated conversations with peers with his AAC device in the classroom and during recess: 11111 / 11111 / 11111 / 11 = 17.

Monday, 12/1 - Sophia recognized 2 letters in isolation, s and a.

Tuesday, 12/2 - Sophia said a 4 word sentence, "I want go home". Played with Teren in the water table for 5 minutes.

Wednesday 12/3 - Sophia was in a good mood, greeted teachers at the door with a big "hello".

Thursday 12/4 - Sophia was a chatterbox today. She used 2-4 word sentences.

Friday 12/5 - Mom said Sophia had difficulty sleeping last night. Sophia was a little grumpy and not willing to try new things.

Monday 12/8 - Played in the motor room today catching a ball.

Tuesday 12/9 - Sophia interacted with Margarita in the pretend house making soup.

Wednesday 12/10 - Sophia tripped on the playground and bumped her knee - skin was not broken. Needed a hug before she would go back to playing.

Thursday 12/11 - Sophia sang "Twinkle Twinkle Little Star" in a group with the hand motions. Seemed to like the song.

Friday 12/12 - Sophia was full of energy, going from activity to activity. She engaged John in a short conversation about his painting at the art table.

Figure 10-9 Diary record of observations of a preschool child

Checklists

Checklists are a list of items that you look for during an observation and check off when they are seen. They are very easy to use and have many uses. A to-do list or a class attendance record are examples of checklists we use everyday. You can use published checklists or create your own. See Figure 10-10 for an example of a checklist that follows developmental norms. If you are going to watch how a stroke patient performs daily living skills such as eating, walking, dressing, and so on, you need to make sure you include all the behaviors you think you want recorded. By including everything you want to observe, your efficiency will improve during the observation. Brandt (1972) says that checklists "are especially appropriate when the behavior alternative with respect to a given problem are somewhat limited, mutually exclusive, and readily discernible to observers" (p. 8).

One example of a published checklist is the *Denver Developmental Screening Test II* (Frankenburg & Dodds, 1990). The *Denver II* provides norms for behaviors in four developmental areas: gross motor, language, fine motor-adaptive, and personal-social. The examiner is provided with questions she can ask the child for certain behaviors and see if the child could demonstrate those behaviors. If the child can, the examiner then checks the item. The child's performance is then compared to the norms for her age. Another published checklist is the *Bzoch-League Receptive-Expressive Emergent Language Scale Second Edition (REEL-2)*. This checklist for children birth through 3 years of age is used either when observing a child or during a parent interview. It has three questions under each age range for both expressive language and receptive language skills. An examiner may mark it with a "+" or a "-" depending if the behavior is observed or if the parent reports having observed it. Then the number of "+"s are added up and you receive a standardized score for the child. Another checklist is a phoneme awareness checklist to determine a child's ability to hear sounds in words and in isolation and manipulate them by putting or taking them out of words.

Checklists are efficient, easy to use, and usable in many different situations. Checklists can put relatively complex behavior patterns into a form that can be easily observed.

Child's Name _____ Date of Birth _____

Date _____ Teacher's Name _____

Directions: Check only those statements which you feel are really true of the child. Do not guess if you are not certain.

		Yes	No
1.	Puts together 3-piece puzzle	☐ Yes	☐ No
2.	Snips with scissors	☐ Yes	☐ No
3.	Picks up pins or buttons with each eye separately covered	☐ Yes	☐ No
4.	Paints strokes, dots, or circular shapes on easel	☐ Yes	☐ No
5.	Can roll, pound, squeeze, and pull clay	☐ Yes	☐ No
6.	Holds crayons with fingers, not with fist	☐ Yes	☐ No
7.	Puts togehter 8-piece (or more) puzzle	☐ Yes	☐ No
8.	Makes clay shapes with 2 or 3 parts	☐ Yes	☐ No
9.	Using scissors, cuts on curve	☐ Yes	☐ No
10.	Screws together a threaded object	☐ Yes	☐ No
11.	Cuts out and pastes simple shapes	☐ Yes	☐ No
12.	Draws a simple house	☐ Yes	☐ No
13.	Imitates folding and creasing paper 3 times	☐ Yes	☐ No
14.	Prints a few capital letters	☐ Yes	☐ No
15.	Copies a square	☐ Yes	☐ No
16.	Draws a simple recognizable picture (e.g., house, dog, tree)	☐ Yes	☐ No
17.	Can lace shoes	☐ Yes	☐ No
18.	Prints capital letters (large, single, anywhere on paper)	☐ Yes	☐ No
19.	Can copy small letters	☐ Yes	☐ No
20.	Cuts pictures from magazines without being more than 1/4 inch from edge of pictures	☐ Yes	☐ No
21.	Uses a pencil sharpener	☐ Yes	☐ No
22.	Folds paper square 2 times on diagonal, in imitation	☐ Yes	☐ No
23.	Prints name on paper	☐ Yes	☐ No
24.	Kicks large ball when rolled to him	☐ Yes	☐ No
25.	Runs 10 steps with coordinated, alternating arm movement	☐ Yes	☐ No
26.	Pedals tricycle 5 feet	☐ Yes	☐ No
27.	Swings on swing when set in motion	☐ Yes	☐ No
28.	Climbs up and slides down 4 to 6 foot slide	☐ Yes	☐ No
29.	Somersaults forward	☐ Yes	☐ No
30.	Walks upstairs, alternating feet	☐ Yes	☐ No
31.	Catches ball with 2 hands when thrown from 5 feet	☐ Yes	☐ No
32.	Jumps from bottom step	☐ Yes	☐ No
33.	Climbs ladder	☐ Yes	☐ No
34.	Skips on alternate feet	☐ Yes	☐ No
35.	Walks balance beam forward without falling	☐ Yes	☐ No
36.	Runs, changing direction	☐ Yes	☐ No
37.	Jumps forward 10 times without falling	☐ Yes	☐ No
38.	Jumps backward 6 times without falling	☐ Yes	☐ No
39.	Bounces and catches large ball	☐ Yes	☐ No

Figure 10-10 Checklist for preschool development

They are good tools to establish baselines. For example, a teacher might administer a checklist to her students at the beginning of the school year to establish a place where each student skills start. Then the teacher may use the same checklist at the middle or the end of the year to determine how much the students have grown over the school year. A checklist may also be a starting place when observing certain behaviors in an individual. If those behaviors are present, another more detailed observation may look more closely at those behaviors. The main disadvantage is that the checklist does not record the context. Checklists are an excellent method of documenting an observation.

CONCLUSION

Observation is a skill that is developed with practice and fine-tuning and may be performed for many different reasons. It is an effective tool to get a true picture of an individual and her abilities. When an observation is done, one needs to prepare, work on being inconspicuous, and remember issues in professional ethics and confidentiality. Several factors may influence an observation such as physical factors, environmental factors, and personality and personal bias factors. When you observe, you usually will be watching one child or adult unless you are looking at how a specific program is run or how effective it is. Objectivity and accuracy are the cornerstones of an effective observation. Seven methods of documenting observations are commonly used for observations and each one is very useful for different types of observation goals. The choice of a specific system needs to be guided by the characteristics of the behavior under observation. You will find that observation can be an effective tool you can use to assist your SLP in planning and implementing interventions and charting progress.

DISCUSSION QUESTIONS

1. Describe the seven methods of documenting an observation. Which one would you use for watching an

individual at a nursing home during a meal and why? Which one would you use for a 2-year-old child playing at the park and why? Which one would you use to observe a eighth grade classroom and why?

2. Compare and contrast group observation and individual observation.

3. List the qualities that improve an observation and then list qualities that take away from an observation. Describe which of these qualities would be a strength for you and which one would be a weakness.

4. Why do people do observations? Why would your supervising SLP ask you to do an observation?

5. Define objectivity. Are you an objective observer? Do you notice details when you observe? Do you analyze what you see before you document it?

SUGGESTED ACTIVITIES

1. Take out a blank piece of paper and draw a picture of the Touch-Tone phone pad then think about the following questions: How often have you observed a phone pad in your life? How well did your memory serve you in this exercise? Were you able to draw a close approximation? Did you remember to include the "start" and "pound" keys in your drawing? Did you include the letters of the alphabet? Did you include items in your drawing specific to a particular phone pad (redial button or hold)?

2. Go to the closest mall. Sit and watch a crowded area for about 15 minutes. What did you see? How many people? How many children? Were children with families? Was the group made up of teenagers or adults? Did you see senior citizens? Were they wearing coats or shorts? What was the outside temperature? What were they doing? Eating? Walking? Running? Pushing? Carrying? How did you document your observation?

3. Set up an observation with a practicing SLP in the area of your interest. Watch the way the SLP interacts

with the individuals, how they respond, and how the room is set up. Write down your observations. Get together with a peer and discuss your observation with them. What things did you notice that they did not and vice versa? Discuss ways to improve your observation skills.

REFERENCES

American Heritage Dictionary of the English Language (4th ed.) (2000). Boston, MA: Houghton Mifflin Company.

Bentzen, W. R. (2000). *Seeing young children: A guide to observing and recording behavior* (4th ed.) Albany, NY: Delmar Publishers.

Borich, G. D. (1994). *Observation skills for effective teaching.* New York: Maxwell Macmillan.

Brandt, R. M. (1972). *Studying behavior in natural settings.* New York: Holt, Rinehart and Winston.

Bzoch, K. & League, R. (1991). *The Bzoch-League Receptive-Expressive Emergent Language Scale Second Edition: Profile/Test Form.* Austin, TX: PRO-ED.

Cohen, D. H., Stern, V., & Balaban, N. (1983). *Observing and recording the behavior of young children* (3rd ed.) New York: Teachers College Press.

Colker, L. J. (1995). *Observing young children: Learning to look, looking to learn* (videotape and book). Washington, DC: Teaching Strategies.

Curtis, D., & Carter, M. (2000). *The art of awareness: How observation can transform your teaching.* St. Paul, MN: Redleaf Press.

Frankenburg, W. K., & Dodds J. B. (1990). *Denver Developmental Screening Test (Denver II) II.* Denver, CO: Denver Developmental Material, Inc.

Goodwin, W. R., & Discoll L. A., (1982). *Handbook for measurement and evaluation in early childhood education.* San Francisco: Jossey-Bass.

Jablon, J. R., Dombro, A. L., & Dichterlmiller, M. L. (1999). *The power of observation.* Washington, DC: Teaching Strategies.

Kozloff, M. A. (1994). Chapter 10: Direct Observation. In *Improving educational outcomes for children with disabilities: Principles for assessment, program planning, and evaluation.* Baltimore: Paul H. Brookes.

Martin, S. (1994). *Take a look: Observation and portfolio assessment in early childhood.* Don Mills, Ontario, Canada: Addison-Wesley.

Merrell, K. W. (1999). Chapter 3: Direct Behavioral Observation. In *Behavioral, social, and emotional assessment of children and adolescents* (pp. 48–71) Mahwah, NJ: Lawrence Erlbaim.

Richarz, A. S. (1980). *Understanding children through observation.* St. Paul, MN: West.

Taylor, R. L. (2000). *Assessment of exceptional students: Educational and psychological procedures* (5th ed.) Boston, MA: Allyn and Bacon.

Thorndike, R. L., & Hagan, E. P. (1977). *Measurement and evaluation in psychology and education* (4th ed.) New York: Wiley.

CHAPTER 11

Documentation and Record Keeping

Key Concepts

■

Record keeping and organization are an important part of an SLPA's responsibilities.

■

A record of each therapy session must be written, and documentation must be kept current.

■

A computer can be a valuable tool for record keeping and documentation.

■

Recording accurate data is essential to the measurement of an individual's progress as well as documentation of ongoing assessment information.

■

Language sampling is an excellent tool for determining an individual's language abilities.

■

Several analyses help document language abilities.

■

Portfolios are another method of documenting how language abilities change over time.

Overview

■

Record Keeping

■

Language Samples

■

Portfolios

INTRODUCTION

Documentation and record keeping are vital parts of an SLPA's role. Keeping records is all part of a day's work. Other than seeing individuals for therapy, your duties may include filing, materials management, ordering supplies, telephone use, computer use, Internet use, taking attendance, following lesson plans, taking data, writing progress notes, scheduling, laminating, faxing, photocopying, organizing client files, billing, or preparing insurance claims. The paper trail can seem endless at times, but if you have skills in organization, this part of your job will come naturally. Record keeping is a natural part of any job, especially when working with people. Records must be kept to keep track of an individual's progress in therapy, as well as how to contact him or the professionals in his life. One needs to know how often an individual attends therapy, when an assessment was performed, and when the individual was discharged from therapy. Records must be kept for accountability purposes and sometimes for legal purposes.

Taking a **language sample** and analyzing the different aspects of **language** is one part of assessing an individual's language as well as documenting changes. Computers are valuable tools to keep track of client records as well as analyzing language samples and scoring standardized tests. Portfolios are another way of documenting changes in language. You may participate in collecting observations as well as putting all the collected information into a photo album or scrapbook. Record keeping and documentation have many facets.

RECORD KEEPING

One of your important jobs as an SLPA includes helping the SLP maintain quality and up-to-date records and to organize the paper trail. This may include documenting phone conversations, taking data in a therapy session, compiling or writing progress notes, putting client files together in an organized fashion, organizing and maintaining therapy materials, ordering new protocols, keeping track of your work

hours, and maintaining other records required by your supervising SLP. Paperwork and record keeping are a vital part of every professional's life. Learning organization skills will make your job run much smoother.

Let us review the process of working with a new client and discuss the areas that will require different types of record keeping. Depending on the setting, the individual contacts the SLP through a referral to a clinic, doctor's orders, referral from a classroom teacher, or from a parent or family member. Sometimes a general screening is performed and those who do not pass the screening are then referred for an assessment. For example, in some school districts, the kindergarten students are screened for speech-language difficulties. During the first contact with an individual desiring speech-language services, it is critical to get the vital information from him, including his name, address, phone number, E-mail address, referral source, insurance information, description of the difficulty, and so. Many settings have a protocol for the initial contact. For example, a hospital may require the individual to register through a main registration line to get all the pertinent information before continuing on in the process and scheduling an initial meeting with the SLP.

The next step is setting up and performing an assessment. Once the assessment is scheduled, a release of information needs to be signed so information from a doctor, school, or others may be obtained to help acquire information needed for planning an assessment. Sometimes forms may be sent to the individual to fill out before the assessment. A map or directions may be included in this information along with a general welcome letter. Then the specific assessment tools are chosen and materials are prepared. The SLP performs the assessment. The information gathered from the assessment must be scored and analyzed before the SLP interprets and shares the results. A report is then written and sent to the individual and to anyone else specified by the individual. If the individual qualifies for **therapy**, then one will need to be contacted to schedule therapy. The SLP will write a treatment plan with long-term goals and short-term objectives. From this guide the SLP will make a session plan and you will need to collect the materials and organize data collection tools to use during the therapy time. After the therapy session, you will need to write some type of note describing what happened during the session and reporting the data that were collected. Sometimes this is called a progress note or SOAP note. All along this process paperwork is being completed and materials are being used. Developing a system to help you manage these tasks will help you stay organized and able to find information when it is needed.

In its accreditation standards ASHA's Professional Services Board (1994) requires that "accurate and complete records shall be prepared and maintained for each client. Records shall be accessible to appropriate personnel and systematically organized to facilitate storage and retrieval" (p. 12). PBS requires specific information in a client's record (see the following sidelight), but does not specify a certain format for those records. Client reports are a vital record-keeping method and as an SLPA, you will be involved in organizing and keeping this record current. Client records must also be "protected with respect to confidentiality, destruction, and loss" (Professional Service Board, 1994, p. 13). See Chapter 7 on Ethics to review issues around confidentiality.

REQUIRED INFORMATION FOR CLIENT RECORDS

The following list contains information that must appear in client records (Hegde & Davis, 1999):

1. Client identification data: telephone number, address, file number, and so on

2. Referral source: name of the individual or agency that referred the client

3. Pertinent information about the client: client history, including related information from other agencies (medical reports, individualized education plans [IEPs], psychological assessments, etc.)

4. Name of SLP responsible for client care and SLPA providing services

5. Assessment reports, treatment plans, treatment reports, and prognostic statements as well as notations regarding conferences held with family or other professionals

6. Chronological log of all services

7. Dated and signed information release forms

8. Daily progress notes reflecting current status of treatment objectives

In the health care setting you will hear and see medical terms that reflect a medical model of diagnosis and intervention. Two basic forms of records are used. The first and most common is the **unit record**. "It is a compilation of all the care provided to a single patient in a health facility. Unit records may be sectioned according to health specialty, or progress/patient-care notes may be integrated among all health-care providers. Information is presented in chronological order, and all illnesses, disorders, or problems are discussed concurrently" (Cornett & Chabon, 1988, p. 93). According to Flower (1984), five sections must be included in the unit record:

1. Application data, including patient information and payment information

2. Initial assessment, chief complaint, history, provisional diagnosis

3. Progress notes

4. Special assessments and treatment records

5. Authorizations and correspondence

The second is the **problem-oriented record** (POR). It is organized according to the patient's problems such as speech or language difficulties (Cornett & Chabon, 1988). Each section may be a different diagnosis or components of a diagnosis. These types of records were initially designed to be used in acute-care hospitals and are now used in many settings, such as hospital outpatient clinics, private clinics, rehabilitation centers, and university clinics. For clients who are hospital inpatients, the medical records are kept close to the patient or on the hospital computer system and are a key in communication between professionals (Bray, Ross, & Todd, 1999). They facilitate the coordination of information from a multidisciplinary team about contacts, assessment findings, diagnosis, intervention, progress, and recommendations. Entries in these records are required and need to be very clear and concise as well as relevant. Individuals in this health care setting may not have time to read more than the bare essentials. You may have other avenues for communication besides the client file, such as hospital rounds, case conferences, and meetings with specific professionals (Bray,

Ross, & Todd, 1999). An example of an entry into an adult client file is "Drowsy and confused, language comprehension moderately impaired; speech output restricted to unintelligible jargon; motor skills unaffected in feeding and speech (SLP signature and date)." Records may be kept in a unit record or a problem-oriented record style.

Coding systems are used in hospital or clinic settings to help provide common terminology for patient diagnoses. These codes are used for administration, reimbursement, educational, and research purposes. Codes are recorded in the patient records and on billing forms to help identify the patient's problem and the specific assessment or treatment services provided. The most widely used coding systems used in the United States are the ICD-9, CPT-4, and DSM-III. Your setting will inform you of the coding system to use. Manuals will be provided so you can look up specific information you need (Cornett & Chabon, 1988).

In contrast, the terminology used in schools reflects an educational orientation or model for documentation. Schools use the IEP for documentation. For more information on the IEP, refer to Chapter 8, Legislation. Public Law 94-142 established the requirements for ensuring that children with disabilities receive a "free, appropriate education in the least restrictive environment." The IEP is the written document that ensures the law is being fulfilled for each child. The IEP documents all the programs, services, methods, equipment, and materials that are needed to provide an appropriate education for a student with disabilities. An IEP is developed by the parents, teachers, and professionals in the school in a team effort to determine the best way of providing the specific child an education (Cornett & Chabon, 1988; Roth & Worthington, 1996). The terminology and methods for documentation are reflective of the school setting.

Progress Notes

The most common format for **progress notes** in a health care or medical setting is identified by the acronym **SOAP**. Each letter stands for one aspect of the note according to Cornett & Chabon (1988) and Hegde and Davis (1999). **S** represents subjective data that include the concerns of the

individual or family member and subjective observations by the clinician. For example: The client appeared very alert and cooperative. He said, "I work hard." The **O** represents objective data and encompasses specific clinical findings, test results, and a summary of the data collected during the therapy session. For example: The individual produced "s" in initial position of words with 80% accuracy in 40 out of 50 trials. **A** stands for assessment and compares the subjective and objective sections as well as compares the individual's performance across sessions. For example: Production of four-syllable phrases increased from 65% accuracy last session to 78% accuracy during today's session. The **P** represents plan and states a course of action to be followed. The plan must demonstrate the pursuit of the treatment plan or may indicate modification or reorientation of that plan. For example: Continue current treatment activities. See Figure 11-1 for a sample of SOAP form of progress notes. In a school-based setting, SLPs maintain records of student progress in working files or notes that then inform updates on the IEP/IFSP on a regular basis.

Forms of Communication in Health Care Setting

Written communication is key to keeping records as well as interacting with the client and other professionals. Several forms of communication are used by the SLP and the SLPA, including assessment reports, clinical reports, letters, treatment plans, session plans, progress notes, discharge summaries, and referrals. Assessment or assessment reports are the beginning of communication. These reports give background information, a description of tests and procedures done during the assessment, summary of results, diagnosis, and recommendations. Clinical reports may be written on a regular basis (may be every 6 months to a year) and give a summary of treatment and progress. They may also include reasons why therapy needs to be continued. Letters are correspondence with other professionals that are written for a specific purpose. Treatment plans identify the goals and objectives for therapy as well as provide a summary of background information, including previous assessments and

---

Sample SOAP notes

Example 1:

S: Gary was in a good mood and was very responsive to therapy. He greeted the clinician with his augmentative communication device.

O: He was able to locate 15 out of 20 vocabulary items in the social category. He needed minimal cues to locate the correct category and activate the appropriate vocabulary.

A: During role playing, Gary accessed the vocabulary and kept the conversation moving. He is starting to take ownership of the augmentative communication device and making it his voice.

P: Review vocabulary in the social category and start working on the daily living vocabulary on the augmentative communication device.

Example 2:

S: There was little change in the production of final consonants in Sara's conversational speech.

O: Acceptable final consonant productions achieved by imitation of words ending with /k/, /g/, /d/, and /t/, 19 or 20 out of 20 for each sound. Inconsistent acceptable productions of imitation words ending in /p/ and /b/, 5 out of 20. Accurate productions of final consonants in spontaneous naming of 12 of 20 pictures of words.

A: Although some progress is apparent in structured speech activities, no carryover as yet has been achieved.

P: Continue with current therapy plan.

Figure 11-1 Sample progress notes in the medical SOAP note form

therapy. Session plans specify what is going to happen during a therapy session, the rationale for each activity, and how data will be collected. Progress notes summarize what happened during a therapy session and the data that were collected. Specific to hospital programs, discharge summaries

are written when an individual has met the goals and objectives have been set for them and therapy is ending. A discharge report is a summary of background information, met goals and objectives, summary of therapy, and recommendations. There may be times when an individual may need to see another professional for services. The SLP may write out a referral suggesting several individuals in the particular specialty area for an individual to see. You may have a part in some of this communication as an SLPA, but primarily you will be writing only progress notes on therapy sessions. The SLP may have you make copies, look up addresses, or mail out reports or referrals. In contrast, the IEP/IFSP provide a formalized process for updating information and documenting changes according to the student's goals in the public school setting.

Recording Session Data

Your SLP will write goals and objectives to meet the individual's needs. From these measurable goals and objectives, he will determine lesson plans for you to follow as an SLPA. A crucial part of those lesson plans is in defining how to record the responses of the child or adult receiving services. The data you gather during a therapy session give the SLP critical information to modify the plans if they are not meeting the written objectives, or they can help indicate when an individual needs a change or needs to be discharged (Pietranton, 1995).

Data must also be collected during group sessions. Although it may be possible to record all responses produced by a child or adult on every objective during the individual therapy time, it is not possible when you are treating more than one individual at a time. The sampling method is a feasible alternative. If you have two 7-year-olds in a language group, you may want to take data on one student for 5 minutes and then switch to the other student for 5 minutes. You could also pick one objective that all individuals share and take data just on that one objective. Let us say a group is working on listening to two-step directions. As a student gets the direction correctly, a tally mark is put under her name. A total number of directions are given to all the members in

RECORDING SESSION DATA GUIDELINES

The following guidelines include information critical to recording session data from Roth and Worthington (1996).

1. Specific recording sheets must be designed before the therapy session. These sheets will usually be provided for you by the SLP, but if they are not, you may need to design one yourself.

2. The notation system or the way the information is documented needs to provide the type of information that is most relevant to the specific individual's goals and objectives. You can use 1 = correct and 0 = incorrect or a scale 1 to 5 to indicate responses. Another method for phonologic therapy may include a "+" if the child makes the correct production on the first trial, a "-" if the child produces it correctly with a visual cue (pointing to a particular area of the mouth or throat), or a check mark if the child produces it correctly with a model.

3. The data collection system needs to be flexible enough so the clinician can see clearly when a response is imitative, cued or prompted, self-corrected, or spontaneous.

4. Reinforcement tokens or stimulus items can be used as an alternative to paper-pencil on-line recording of client responses. One approach has the stimuli or token in groups of 10 (often called the base 10 approach). You then can count the remaining tokens to determine a number of incorrect responses or a percentage. If you have three tokens remaining, that means that the individual had seven answers correct. That easily translates into 70% correct. If you use stimuli cards, you can place the correct identification of those cards in one pile while the incorrect go into another pile. Then you can count the number in each pile to determine the correct and incorrect numbers.

5. Record every stimulus response. The absence of a response may yield very important information and may be recorded with an NR, indicating no response.

6. When therapy tasks reach the conversational level, it may be difficult to collect data on every correct or incorrect response. You may need to take data in a timed way. For example, you may take data for a minute and then repeat the 1 minute of data collection every 5 minutes.

the group and then a percentage correct can be figured for each person. Another example is an adult aphasic group working on conversation skills. You could keep track of the amount of time it takes for each person to respond or make a comment. You have to be careful when taking data in groups to make sure you are taking data on all of the objectives for all the individuals in the group over a period of time. If each individual has two objectives and you meet with them twice a week, you could take data on the first objective during one session a week and the second objective during the other session that week.

SIDELIGHT: *Enrique's Story*

Enrique, a bilingual, developmentally delayed adult, was coming to see Mary Lou for speech intervention. Mary Lou's supervising SLP had performed the assessment and written a comprehensive treatment plan. Enrique's speech was intelligible to the unfamiliar listener 50% of the time and it was determined that his misarticulation of /s/ was influencing his intelligibility. Mary Lou prepared for her therapy session and collected some picture cards that started with the /s/ sound to use in conversation. As Enrique produced the initial /s/ words, she would place the card in one pile if he produced it correctly the first time, a second pile if he produced it correctly on the second trial with a cue, and a third pile if he was unable to produce it correctly. She had chosen 20 cards so it would be easy to calculate percentages from the three piles of cards.

Young active children pose a challenge for data collection. During these sessions, you may be interacting with the child and using many materials to keep the child's interest. Remember to follow the child's lead during these sessions. Because this requires you to move around the room with the child and frequently be on the floor, you will need to figure out a way to carry a paper with you to take data. Some clinicians find it useful to hang a small spiral notebook around their neck for easy access or you could tape a recording form to the wall in different areas of the room so one is accessible for the different activities. You could also put masking tape on your leg or place a piece of self-sticking paper on your nondominant arm. Depending on the child's needs, you may need to be creative in your method of data collection. Counters are often successful tools to help you collect data.

Ways to Record

Many ways to record responses are available. The way you record may vary greatly on the individual's objectives and

needs during therapy. Susan Meyer (1998) describes a horizontal versus a vertical system of data collection. The horizontal method records responses from left to right on a line, whereas the vertical method records responses from top to bottom. The horizontal method is easy but may not collect the type or amount of data needed. This system only records the first response. For example: NNNYYNYNYY. Keeping 10 responses together can help in calculating percentages quickly. The horizontal recording method may be modified to include every response an individual gives, but some type of notation must be made in between the stimulus items. For example, NNNY / NNY / Y / Y / Y / NNY / Y / NY / Y / Y / NY.

If the slash marks had not been made, someone looking at the data would assume that 20 stimulus items had been presented instead of the 10. This gives much more information than just a straight horizontal notation system. In the given example, the individual was able several times to come to the correct response after the second or third attempt. This type of notation does not include whether the individual received a cue, just that the individual obtained the correct response within a certain number of trials.

The vertical system records responses from top to the bottom of the page. The vertical system looks more like a chart and makes it easy to record multiple trials on a single stimulus.

1. NNY
2. NY
3. Y
4. Y
5. NY

From these data you could quickly determine that the individual got 40% correct and corrected the errors on the second try twice. The vertical method is much easier to scan quickly and obtain the results, but it does take up more space on a page unless you use columns.

Accountability

Accurate records are extremely important for effective therapy. In most settings, the SLP is held accountable for the

therapy decisions that are made and you as the SLPA are held accountable for the actions you take in serving an individual. Keeping accurate records meets the professional standards and demonstrates that you have acted responsibly. Records are used for many purposes and are vital to providing the best services. If for some reason litigation occurs with one of the individuals you have worked with, those records may be used to defend what was done with that individual. Our clinical records are the primary way we communicate to other SLPs or SLPAs, health and education professionals and administrators, government agencies, and third-party payers.

Computers

Computers are an invaluable tool for the SLPA. Many aspects of record keeping and documentation can now be done on the computer. Some settings may require you to use the computer for specific aspects of charting in client's records, scheduling, writing correspondence, and keeping vital information on clients. Computers are also being used during therapy as well as scoring standardized tests and analyzing language samples. You may be asked to input data into programs designed to score standardized tests and provide detailed analysis of the data. Databases are great for keeping track of client's basic information, attendance, and progress notes. You will also need to be familiar with a word processing program. Understanding of a drawing program or a picture-based program like Boardmaker will help you design creative therapy materials. You may need to use the Internet during therapy to research a particular topic or disorder, or to look up information needed by the SLP. Computers have become part of our everyday lives and are an essential part of the SLPA's job.

Scheduling

One of the duties of SLPAs may be to schedule their own clients. In hospitals and clinic settings, a secretary may be responsible for scheduling your clients, but in the schools,

you may be responsible for your own schedule. Initially, you need to block out times that you are not able to see students such as required meetings, lunchtime, conference or planning time, clerical duties and paperwork, and assessment assistance. Then you need to block out times for seeing clients, patients, or students. Flexibility is key to scheduling especially to meet the needs of the individuals. You may group some students together because some may not be able to come at the scheduled time. You may need to change your schedule throughout the year as students' needs and schedules change. "Master schedules can change, new classrooms can be added, existing classrooms can be divided into other classes, classroom schedules can change, new students can arrive, current students can move away, programming for any child can change in a number of ways" (Thomas & Webster, 1999, p. 55). Some parents want their children to stay in their regular classrooms as much as possible, so you may be providing speech-language services within the classroom. This service model requires collaboration with the classroom teacher.

You may experience similar challenges with scheduling hospital- or agency-based patients or clients. Remember to keep lines of communication open and problem-solve challenging scheduling issues with your SLP.

Part of record keeping is keeping track of who attends therapy and the reasons for missed therapy. You can make an attendance book and make notations whether an individual is present or not. You could design a code for certain types of cancellations. For example, I = illness, V = vacation, L = late, etc.

LANGUAGE SAMPLES

A language sample is a way of writing down what a child says, and it is an excellent way to measure a child or adult's expressive language skills. It also can be an effective tool to document changes over time and the effectiveness of language intervention. The desire is that a language sample is representative of the child's overall productive language. A written record of what has been said is called a transcript. "The transcript should reflect the way the child usually talks

SCHEDULING IN SCHOOL-BASED PROGRAMS

According to Thomas and Webster (1999), the following items need to be considered when scheduling in school-based programs:

1. Each teacher needs to be contacted and asked when he prefers his students to be pulled out of their classroom. Direct academic instruction in reading, writing, and math should not be disrupted by speech-language therapy. Children also do not like to miss specials, such as physical education, art, music, computer class, recess, or lunch.

2. Group therapy is most productive when the group's goals are the same. Similar difficulties and similar ages can be grouped together.

3. Try to keep groups made up of students from the same grade level. Groups work well with three to four students.

4. When scheduling, you must keep in mind that other programs may also pull the child out and you will need to coordinate with those teachers also. For example, a child may receive special education, occupational therapy, and speech-language therapy. One option if scheduling conflicts occur is to provide therapy together if both can reach their goals during the same time. Otherwise, one of you will need to find another time to see the child.

5. It needs to be communicated with the teacher that the student is not responsible for the academic material covered when he is with you in speech-language therapy. Be conscious of what the child is missing. You may even bring in some of the work the child is missing as part of your therapy session if you can meet the goal objectives set out by the SLP.

6. Middle and high schools may have strict policies about when students can be pulled out. Consider study hall or advisory and activity times. Some campuses may use a rotating schedule so students will not miss the same class consistently.

and what he or she talks about" (Miller, 1981, p. 9). Language samples are often used to assess a child's language and are an extremely valuable tool to get a "read" for a child's speech. The SLP will be able to use the information from a language sample to determine the child's developmental language skills and in what specific areas an individual needs help. The information from a language sample may also be used to write long-term goals and short-term objectives. How to collect and record a language sample, procedures for analyzing free-speech samples, and how to elicit an expressive

language sample are discussed next. Edwards and Knott (1994) discuss assessing spontaneous language abilities of aphasic speakers. Language sampling will be an important tool in the SLPA's bag of tricks.

Collecting

The first step in using a language sample is to obtain a language sample. Individuals talk to make requests, demands, tell stories, play, share information, or comment to other people about the things they want or things that interest them. Individuals respond to the requests, questions, or demands of those around them. It is the job of the SLPA to elicit language in some type of interaction or to observe the individual with others in an interaction to obtain a language sample. "The primary goal in collecting a free-speech sample is to record what is representative of the child's usual productive language. The term *representative* implies both reliability and validity" (Miller, 1981, p. 10). According to Miller (1981), five factors affect whether a language sample is representative of a child's spontaneous language: nature of the interaction, setting, materials, **sample size**, and context. These factors are discussed in the context of collecting samples from children, but the concepts are generalizable to collecting narratives or discourse samples from adults.

Nature of Interaction

You can take a language sample of an interaction between you and child, the child and its mother, two or more children, or the child and a teacher. When a child is between the ages of 9 and 30 months, he may have difficulty separating from his parent or caregiver. Some children have difficulty talking with strangers and may refuse to talk. It is beneficial in these situations to have the child's significant individual, such as a parent, be the partner in the interaction. You may instruct the parent that you want to see how the child talks when he is at home. Other interactions may be child to child or child to sibling. If you are in an educational setting, you may want to obtain a language sample between the teacher and the child.

The SLPA will need to monitor the interaction to make sure that it is spontaneous and maintains the child's interest and whether the interaction is between the parent and the child, the SLPA and the child, a sibling and the child, the teacher and the child, or a peer and the child. Interaction styles were discussed in Chapter 4 and may be reviewed if questions arise. The main thing to remember when participating in an interaction is to limit the questions you ask. Research demonstrates that asking questions limits a natural interaction and the child's language output. Asking questions encourages sentence fragments that cannot be analyzed with many systems of analysis like computer programs. You can ask open-ended questions ("Tell me more," "What happened?" or "What's next?"), but primarily make comments on what the child is doing ("You are coloring with the yellow crayon"), or respond to what the child has said (child: "I will cook and you set the table"; adult: "I will put on the plates and silverware"). When a child has poor intelligibility, it may be helpful to repeat what he says. Repeating what the child says will help with the **transcription** of the interaction. If you are in the interaction, you will need to record the interaction in some way such as audio or video, so you can transcribe or write down exactly what the child says at a later time.

Children need to feel comfortable with the clinician before they will start talking. The clinician needs to be warm, friendly, and interested as well as being sensitive to the child's level of development. If a child is talking at the one- or two-word level, it is does not facilitate language production if the clinician is speaking in phrases that are six to seven words long. In some ways it helps to "match" the child's level, especially expressively. It also helps if you give some pause time between when the child says something and when you respond. This way you are allowing the child to be ready when you talk and can listen and respond. A rule of thumb is to count to 3 and then say something. Allowing some time for the child to warm up will also increase the quality and quantity of the language sample.

SIDELIGHT: *Jimmy's Story*

Jimmy is a very shy kindergartner and the SLP had talked with his teacher about his concerns regarding Jimmy's language skills. The supervising SLP asked the SLPA to take a language sample and because Jimmy is shy, she recommended watching him in the classroom first and then working with him in a play situation to do a language sample. The SLP and SLPA decided this was the best way to proceed so Jimmy could become familiar to her before she took him out of the classroom. After watching him in the classroom and recording his language, the SLPA brought Jimmy to the office the next day to play. The previous day the SLPA called Jimmy's mother and found out that Jimmy loved to play with dinosaurs, so dinosaurs were spread out on a table for him to play with. The SLPA played quietly beside Jimmy and after about 10 minutes, Jimmy started talking and interacting with the SLPA. She had a tape recorder running next to the table to record the language sample so she could transcribe it at a later time.

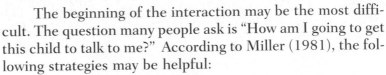

The beginning of the interaction may be the most difficult. The question many people ask is "How am I going to get this child to talk to me?" According to Miller (1981), the following strategies may be helpful:

1. Saying nothing beyond the initial friendly greetings for the first 5 minutes. This one is especially beneficial with children who are hesitant to talk or shy.

2. Play next to the child doing something similar to what he is doing (playdough, building blocks, pretending to cook, etc.). You may want to talk to toys instead of directly to the child. This strategy works well for children functioning below the 30-month level.

3. Interactive play with little talking during the first few minutes. You can share toys by just stating, "I'm going to play with the blue ball. You can play with the green ball." If you ask the child to play, he is likely to say no. This strategy is good for children with cognition in the 3- to 5-year-old range.

4. Interactive play without introductions. The clinician and child can work together.

These strategies correspond with general development to meet the child's perceptual, visual, auditory, and motor capabilities. The nature of the interaction will determine how the SLPA needs to respond to obtain a language sample.

Setting

Language samples may be obtained in four major settings: home, school, residential facility, and clinic or hospital (Kemp & Klee, 1997). A representative sample may be collected almost anywhere as long as the constraints are recognized and monitored. For example, some settings may allow for only certain kinds of speech to be used, depending on the activity. If a fourth grade class is reading a social studies text on Christopher Columbus and the teacher is lecturing and asking the students questions, the language sample of one particular child may be very limited or restricted, whereas if the students are given free time to make something with clay, the language sample may be more representative of a student's spontaneous language. Each situation must be evaluated to determine if an appropriate language sample can be collected. If you are collecting language samples from several children, collect the language samples under the same conditions. If a child comes to a clinic or hospital setting, the environment may be set up to elicit certain types of interactions. The setting will determine the type of language sample that will be collected.

Materials

The materials used in obtaining a language sample need to focus on facilitating language production. They are tools, not an end in themselves. The materials need to be at the cognitive, interest, auditory, visual, and motor levels of the child. Pretend play items tend to be the best at facilitating spontaneous language for younger children up through early elementary age. These toys may include eating utensils, stove, refrigerator, dolls, barns and animals, gas station with cars, people, school bus and school, or blocks or Lego. They are familiar items that a child sees in his everyday life; therefore,

the child can interact and talk during his play with the familiar toys. New toys can also promote spontaneous language. Materials around a routine may not produce spontaneous language. One example may be games where individuals may say, "It's your turn," repeatedly. Another example may be familiar storybooks that tend to produce language such as "Once upon a time. ..." It would be beneficial to discuss with the parents the specific toys a child likes before the session. This can facilitate your choice of appropriate materials.

Toys can be presented one at a time or left out in an inviting way for the child to find. The first option is helpful to control the presentation and order of materials. This can be helpful if you are going to get language samples from more than one individual and you desire to compare them. The second option maximizes the child's interest because they get to choose what toys they want to use. The second option tends to be the best for children up to the ages of 7 and 8. Older elementary students through high school may be given pictures to discuss or make up a story about instead of setting out toys for them to play. The older students may not need the props that younger children need to produce spontaneous language. Your supervising SLP will be able to help you determine the appropriate materials if you are unsure. When the interaction is very structured, the less varied the language sample may be and could affect measures like **mean length of utterance (MLU)** (Leadholm & Miller, 1992).

When you are interacting with children, you will want to keep a few things in mind. The first thing to remember is to be a good listener. If you listen carefully to what the child means, then you can give a thoughtful response to show that you are on the same topic or focus. The next key to keep in mind is to be patient. Be careful about overpowering the child with requests or actions. Give the child space and time to do what needs to be done. Do not be afraid of long pauses. The next is to follow the child's lead, which will help keep his interest and focus. After the child has chosen what to do and talk about, keeping his attention on the interaction will be easy. A part of following the child's lead is keeping the same pace as the child and trying not to rush on to the next activity. Recognizing the child's comments as important and worth your undivided attention will show the child that you value him. Children respond to warmth and friendliness in a

positive way. Be careful not to play the fool by not asking questions that the child knows you know the answer to. Learn how to think like a child and gain his perspective at different levels of development. These interaction keys will help you when you work with children and will help you in obtaining a complete language sample. The choice of materials will facilitate a productive language sample. It is critical that transcriptions reflect not only what the child says, but what the adult/caregiver/peers say as well. This is a way to assess whether the sample is biased.

Recording

Three methods are available for recording what children say: audiotaping, videotaping, and writing down the interaction as it occurs. The main goal for recording is to get the most accurate and representative recording of exactly what the individual says. If you are the one interacting with the individual, you may want to use the audio and videotape recording methods so you may concentrate on the interaction instead of documentation.

A good quality cassette tape recorder and microphone are essential for an accurate **transcription** of the dyadic interaction. The microphone inside the tape recorder may give you a sufficient sound, especially in a quiet environment. If it does not, a multidirectional microphone placed close to the child is preferred. Cordless microphones may also work well and will not limit movement. A child may be distracted by the tape recorder at first, but after about 5 minutes the novelty will wear off. You may need to show the child the tape recorder before he is ready to play with the toys you have set out. You could also start the tape recorder before the child's arrival and put it close to the area in which he will be working. The child may not even notice it. With a tape recorder, you do not have the benefit of seeing what is taking place during the interaction. You may want to make brief inconspicuous notes of the child's activities to help with the transcription. Remember that you will not be able to remember as much as you think you will, so writing down notes during or just after the session will greatly increase the quality of your transcription.

Videotaping gives the most information of an interaction. It provides visual as well as auditory information to help with the transcription. With the advent of home video cameras, children and adults are used to video cameras but may be distracted initially. The main drawback to videotaping is the quality of the audio signal. Depending on quality of the audio signal of your camera, you may need to repeat some of what the individual says so you will be able to understand it when you transcribe the tape.

Both audio and videotaping require transcribing the interaction at a later time. The final way to record the language sample is to do an on-line transcription. You can only do this if you are not the one interacting with the child. You may also want to do on-line transcriptions when you need immediate results. Two things must be considered when deciding what type of on-line transcription to do. The first is how much the child talks. It is not possible to write down everything a child says when he is very vocal and you are recording over a long period of time. The second aspect is what aspects of language are the focus of the language sample and what will be analyzed at a later time. Language components include **phonology**, syntax, semantics, or pragmatics as well as turn taking and intelligibility. Phonology analysis needs phonetic transcription, whereas syntax and semantic analysis needs the child's utterances as well as the context. Looking at a child's pragmatics needs the transcription of both the child's utterances as well as the utterances of the interaction partner. So determining the purpose of the transcription will aid in deciding the type of transcription method to use.

Two general approaches are used for on-line transcription (Hadley, 1998). The first is just writing down everything the child says and the second is time sampling, which is writing down everything at regular intervals of time. The first approach is good for young children who have limited verbal production and may need phonetic transcription for articulation errors. The second approach works well for a child who is very vocal. The observer records what the child says for a limited time through the observation period. You would transcribe for 1 minute and then rest for 4 minutes and repeat for the entire observation time. Time samples will cover a variety of contexts and give a more reliable transcript

than one made in a single 5- to 10-minute on-line recording session. For more information on time sampling, see Chapter 10, Observation.

On-line transcription gets easier with practice. According to Miller (1981), on-line transcriptions are very reliable compared to transcriptions done from an audio or videotape for experienced clinicians. Also remember to set up the way you are doing your transcription before you start to improve your accuracy of transcription.

Sample Size

Sample size is the number of utterances you want to collect for your language sample. Some language sample analysis tools specify a number of utterances you need to perform the analysis. This could be 50, 100, or 200 utterances. The method of analysis may require a certain number of utterances (Systemic Analysis of Language Transcripts [SALT] = 100 utterances, developmental sentence scoring [DSS] = 50 utterances). These numbers may sound high, but for a verbal child it may not take much time to accumulate 200 utterances. The other way to determine the sample size is by specific period of time. This approach tends to be much more flexible and you may only have a specific amount of time to interact with a child. Remember that young children can tire quickly. Typically, a 30-minute interaction can produce 100 to 200 utterances based on the age of the child (Retherford, 1993). For children under the age of 2, you can expect fewer utterances (30 to 60 utterances in 30 minutes). For very young children (under 12 months), you may need to supplement your language sample with information or logs kept by parents or a caregiver to give you an accurate representation of the child's language skills.

If you are doing 30-minute sessions, you may want to divide it up into two 15-minute play sessions. The first 15 minutes could be with the mother or caregiver and the second 15 minutes with you, another clinician, or another child. Transcribe every utterance for the 30-minute period, including both the interaction partner and the child. This gives the SLP more information when performing the interpretation of the language sample. Always remember if you

are going to take the time to transcribe the child's speech to do it right. The analysis is only as good as the transcript.

Context

Context can play a vital role in the language sample. Objects and events that happen around an individual's speech is defined as context. You will put much thought and effort into setting up an environment that is inviting and interesting to the child. Language is difficult to separate from the environment, especially in play situations so it will be important to make contextual notes telling exactly what the child is doing at particular times during the interaction. Recording the context is vital to the interpretation of the child's and adult's language samples (Retherford, 1993).

Context includes not only the materials and what the individual is doing, but also the verbalizations of the interaction partner. The individual may have responded to what was said and that information needs to be documented to see a complete picture of the individual's language. This tends to be even more critical when a child is under the age of 3 or an adult who has had a stroke when his spoken output is under three to five words at a time. For example, if a child says, "Mommy ball," this could mean mommy has a ball, mommy play ball with me, mommy get the ball, look mommy there is a ball, or it could mean mommy's ball. If an aphasic adult says "wife drive," it could mean my wife drove me today, I do not like when my wife drives, or tell my wife to drive me home. You need the context to determine the correct meaning.

Several methods are available to record the context along with the actual words the individual says. First, you could make a separate column next to the transcription and put important contextual cues next to the words when they occur. Another way to record is to include it with the exact words spoken with parentheses. For example, "She has it": She [Mommy] has [is holding] it [the doll]. This may be done as you are transcribing on-line, transcribing from a tape, or at a later time. Try to write down the context as soon as you can if you are transcribing on-line because your memory will quickly fade after the event.

Knowing the analysis that will done on the transcription will determine if you need to write down contextual cues. If you are just doing an MLU, no contextual cues are needed. The shorter the individual's utterances, the more context you will need. Longer utterances do not need as much context because those utterances will probably include context. As you practice doing language samples, you will learn what contextual cues need to be written as well as when they are needed. Your supervising SLP may request a specific transcription method. When learning, you will want to write more contextual cues so when you are finished you have enough for the SLP to do her analysis. A good guide is whether someone who was not present during the language sample can get a good visual picture from your transcription. If he cannot, you need more contextual cues.

Cultural Diversity

Language sample analysis is recognized as a valuable assessment procedure for a linguistically diverse population because it is culturally sensitive, flexible, and accessible (Stockman, 1996). Language should be judged as delayed only when it deviates from the range of normal in the native linguistic community. Language samples provide a flexible method to assess an individual's language and compare it to a linguistic community from which it originates. Standardized tests do not demonstrate this same flexibility. Language sample analysis does not provide a comparison of behaviors across children at comparable developmental stages to determine if the language sample represents a delay or not. Stockman suggests that language sample analysis may provide a valuable screening tool for linguistic minority preschool children. Language samples provide an excellent representation of culturally and linguistically diverse individuals.

Transcription

How do you do an actual transcription? A sample transcription is shown in Figure 11-2. Most of the analyses available only require a transcription in Standard English. Phonetic transcription may be needed for an individual who has

Language Sample

Name: John Smith
Age: 2-7
Date: April 26, 2001

Source: Videotape
Setting: Home
Time of Day: 10:00 A.M.

1. J: me eat cracker
2. M: you're eating a cracker
3. J: this fit in there
4. M: this one too?
5. J: yea
6. M: that fits
7. J: the bike no go in there
8. M: ok, the bike stays out here
9. J: me up here
10. M: you're up there
11. J: I sit down
12. M: I'll sit down too
13. J: this is a cowboy
14. J: this my cowboy
15. J: this my horse
16. J: this my horse
17. J: no fit in there
18. M: no, he doesn't fit
19. J: right here
20. M: hey, I want a ride
21. J: ok
22. M: thank you
23. J: ride horsies
24. M: you ride
25. J: walking home
26. J: horsie go home
27. M: walking home
28. J: this horsie go home
29. M: bye horsie
30. J: bye

Figure 11-2 Language sample transcription

speech difficulties. Your supervising SLP will make it clear what type of transcription is needed for his goals. Make sure you include unintelligible utterances down to the syllable if possible, because most utterances that are not intelligible still have the intonation of a typical sentence or question. Usually you will be able to tell when there is a break between unintelligible utterances. The unintelligible utterances can give important information to the SLP in planning his treatment plan or writing his assessment report. Phonetic transcriptions are needed when looking at an individual's speech production but not when looking at language.

Analysis

Many different analyses are available to help examine all the aspects of a language sample. Language can be analyzed with phonetics, semantics, syntax, and pragmatics. An SLPA may have the opportunity to help with these analyses and then the SLP can interpret the results.

Phonetics

One method of documentation is phonetic transcription. **Phonetics** is the study of the perception and production of speech sounds. When an individual has speech difficulties and a speech analysis needs to be performed, phonetic transcription is the best method of documenting his specific speech difficulties. You have had or will have a complete course on phonetics and how to do phonetic transcription. The following description is just a summary of phonetics. The English language has 42 to 44 **phonemes**; the range is based on different phoneticians counting the phonemes. The sounds are broken down into vowels and consonants. The consonants are divided into seven basic categories based on the place of articulation within the mouth, and six are based on the manner of articulation. The vowel category also includes dipthongs and is divided into placement subcategories. The vowels are divided by where they are produced in the mouth: front category / i, ɪ, e, ɛ , æ, a/, the central category / ɝ, ɜ, ɚ , ʌ, ə / and the back series / u, ʊ , o, ɔ, ɑ /. The six categories based on the place of articulation include stops, nasals, fricatives, liquids, glides, and affricates. The seven categories based on place of articulation are bilabials / b, p, m, w, ʍ /, labiodentals / f, v /, interdentals / θ, ð /, alveolars / t, d, s, z, l, n /, palatals / ʃ, ʒ, tʃ, dʒ, j, r /, velars / k, g, ŋ, w, ʍ / and glottals / h, ʔ /. (Bernthal & Bankson, 1998; Shriberg & Kent, 1982). A sample transcript can be found in Figure 11-3.

One of the major issues in phonetic transcription is accuracy. The SLP or SLPA must have an accurate phonetic transcription of an individual's speech skills to perform a valid analysis. Another key to phonetic transcription is that one must practice his phonetic transcription skills on a reg-

Phonetic Transcription

1. moon	/ mun /	11. palms	/ pɑmz /
2. creed	/ krid /	12. would	/ wʊd /
3. long	/ lɔŋŋ /	13. daylight	/ dēɪlāɪt /
4. range	/ rēɪndʒ /	14. slurred	/ slɝd /
5. clue	/ klu /	15. cousin	/ kʌzn /
6. grew	/ gru /	16. sirloin	/ sɝlɔ̄ɪn /
7. bleed	/ blɪd /	17. mercy	/ mɝsi /
8. teamed	/ timd /	18. ruined	/ rund /
9. bald	/ bɔld /	19. wrong	/ rɔŋ /
10. through	/ θru /	20. gems	/ dʒɛmz /

Figure 11-3 Phonetic transcription

ular basis because they are easily lost (Louko & Edwards, 2001). Some clinicians may not use diacritical marks or phonetic symbols and stay with a broad transcription. Diacritical marks and phonetic symbols provide necessary information as well as many advantages in their use. Phonetic transcription is an essential tool for working with phonologically impaired individuals as well as non-native speakers (Louko & Edwards, 2001). When an individual's speech contains just a few errors, the phonetic transcription can be done on line. For an individual with multiple articulation errors, the transcription may need to be done on line and then backed up with an audio or videotape. Your expectation of what you are going to hear can affect the outcome of a transcription. Knowing what the speaker is trying to say can help or hinder a transcription (Oller & Eilers, 1975). You may fill in gaps for the speaker and not notice certain articulation errors, or knowing what they are saying may help you focus on specific aspects of speech production.

According to Carol Stoel-Gammon (2001), when you are taking a speech sample of very young children (under the age of 3), you may need to transcribe both the intelligible and unintelligible utterances to get an accurate speech sam-

ple. These children may be too young for a typical articulation test and may need to be "tested" through a spontaneous speech sample. It is difficult with this age group to distinguish between an unintelligible utterance, an attempt at meaningful speech, and babbling, nonmeaningful vocalizations. The context of the interaction may prove to be extremely useful when analyzing the speech sample. One may need to audio or videotape the interaction to make sure that the transcription is complete. The transcription may need to be done in stages: transcribe segments first using standard symbols from the International Phoenetic Alphabet (IPA), add stress markers on multisyllabic productions, add diacritical marks as needed, and add comments: utterance was whispered, very high pitch, produced more quickly than other utterances (Stoel-Gammon, 2001). An example of an IPA transcription is included in Figure 11-3.

Semantic Analysis

Semantics is the study of language content made up of word meanings and the principles of expression. This is one level of analysis that can be performed on a language sample to gain more information on an individual's language abilities. For children, Bloom (1973) and Nelson (1973) designed categorization procedures to analyze one-word utterances. Bloom divides words into three categories: substantive, naming, and function. A substantive word refers to an object or event (ball, cookie, or chair). Naming is a word that is used to label objects or events (mom, kitty, or brother). Function words refers to words that refer to more than one object (up, broke, or more). Nelson's categorization was developed to describe the first 50-word vocabularies of children around 18 months of age. Nelson uses five categories to describe words: nominals, action words, modifiers, personal-social, and function words. Nominals can be either specific or general and refer to instances of objects, animals, people, letters, and numbers. Action words refer to actions through description (bye-bye or go), expression of attention (look or hi), or demand for attention (up or out). Modifiers are used to describe properties of things, including expressions of recurrence, disappearance, attribution, location, and posses-

sion. Social relationships (please, thank you, yes, or no) and affective states (want, feel) are in the category of personal-social. Function words are used to fulfill grammatical functions (what, where, is, or for). These two analyses are useful in analyzing children's language that is just developing.

Retherford, Schwartz, and Chapman (1981) and Brown (1973) designed an analysis of one- and multiword utterances. The first is a semantic role analysis through categories, whereas the second is a prevalent semantic relation analysis, which incorporates Brown stages of linguistic development. The semantic roles analysis has defined 15 categories for looking at the adult and child's speech: action, locative, agent, object, demonstrative, recurrence, possessor, quantifier, experiencer, recipient, beneficiary, comitative, created object, instrument, and state. Brown stated that the eight prevalent semantic relations he found that occurred frequently later were the foundations for longer utterances. Details for both of these analyses can be found in *Guide to Analysis of Language Transcripts*.

Type Token Ratio (TTR). A vocabulary analysis called **type token ratio (TTR)** was designed by Templin in 1957. This procedure allows you to look at the relationship between the total number of different words used and the total number of words used. Then you compare the information you receive to a chart on ages (Miller, 1981: Retherford, 1993). A sample of 100 utterances is used for this analysis. You count the total number of words in a language sample and the number of different words in a language sample. If the language sample in Figure 11-3 is used, the total number of words used by John was 52. The total number of different words was 29. You divide the total number of different words (29) by the total number of words (52) and come up with a type token ratio of .5576, which rounds up to .56. This is an easy calculation to determine the variety of vocabulary a child uses.

Syntactic Analysis

Syntax is the study of language forms, of how words go together to make phrases and sentences. Several syntactic

analyses are available and they will be described, but only the analysis of mean length of utterance (MLU) and developmental sentence analysis (DSA) will be discussed in depth.

Syntax includes grammatical morphemes, noun phrases, verb phrases, negation, yes/no questions, wh-questions, and complex sentences. Each of these can be analyzed within a language sample of a child who is starting to put two words together up to a child who is putting complex sentences together. Grammatical morphemes include the use of –ing, plural –s, possessive –s, regular past –ed, articles (a, an, or the), among others. As a child develops, he starts using these grammatical morphemes in the correct manner. Using a chart to tally their use can help identify if their use has been mastered. The complexity of noun phrases, verb phrases, negation, yes/no questions, wh-questions, and complex sentences can all be analyzed by using Brown's stages of linguistic development. The complexity of these syntactic parts tends to increase with sentence length. Miller (1981) and Retherford (1993) explain these analyses in detail.

Mean Length of Utterance (MLU). Brown (1973) first designed a procedure to analyze utterance length. The **mean length of utterance (MLU)** is the procedure. The mean length of utterance is a total of words or morphemes in each phrase or sentence of 100 utterances. This number is then divided by 100 and correlates fairly closely to the chronological age of the child. For example a 3-year-old may have an MLU of 3.0 to 3.49, and a 2-year-old may have an MLU of 1.5 to 1.9. Table 11-2 gives MLU ranges and corresponding ages.

An example of counting morphemes is found in Table 11-1. This sample is only a part of a 100-utterance sample but can give you an idea of how to figure out morphemes. It also shows then how to figure out the MLU. If this sample were 100 utterances, then you would divide the total number of morphemes by 100 utterances and reach an MLU. A language sample with corresponding MLU counts are in Table 11-1. If you desire more practice with figuring morphemes, see pages 87–90 in *Guide to Analysis of Language Transcripts*.

Table 11-1: Language Sample with Morpheme and Word Counts

	Morpheme Counts	Word Counts
1. J: me eat cracker	3	3
2. M: you're eating a cracker		
3. J: this fit in there	4	4
4. M: this one too?		
5. J: yea	1	1
6. M: that fits		
7. J: the bike no go in there	6	6
8. M: ok, the bike stays out here		
9. J: me up here	3	3
10. M: you're up there		
11. J: I sit down	3	3
12. M: I'll sit down too		
13. J: this is a cowboy	4	4
14. J: this my cowboy	3	3
15. J: this my horse	3	3
16. J: this my horse	3	3
17. J: no fit in there	4	4
18. M: no, he doesn't fit		
19. J: right here	2	2
20. M: hey, I want a ride		
21. J: ok	1	1
22. M: thank you		
23. J: ride horsies	3	2
24. M: you ride		
25. J: walking home	3	2
26. J: horsie go home	3	3
27. M: walking home		
28. J: this horsie go home	4	4
29. M: bye horsie		
30. J: bye	1	1

= 54 morphemes divided by 18 utterances = 3.0 MLU (morphemes)

= 52 words divided by 18 utterances = 2.88 MLU (words)

GUIDELINES FOR CALCULATING MORPHEMES

The rules for assigning **morphemes** to utterances was originally presented in the literature by Brown (1973), Bloom and Lahey (1978), Miller (1981), Owens (1992) and Retherford (1993). The calculation of morphemes is straightforward. The following guidelines apply:

1. Only assign morphemes to utterances that are completely intelligible.

2. Assign morphemes to 100 consecutive utterances. (You want to stay away from a series of utterances that contain yes/no questions because this can give a lower MLU.)

3. Do not count words that are a result of stuttering, just the main sentence. For example, "I I I wa want to play" is counted "I want to play."

4. Fillers such as um, oh, or well are not assigned morphemes.

5. Compound words are counted as a single word (choo-choo, night-night, quack-quack).

6. Diminutive forms of words are assigned one morpheme (doggie, mommy).

7. Auxiliary verbs are assigned one morpheme. Words like gonna, wanna, and hafta are assigned one morpheme.

8. All inflections, including possessive –s, plural –s and third person, singular –s, regular past –ed, and present progressive –ing are assigned one morpheme.

9. Negative contractions (can't, don't, won't) are assigned two morphemes if the child demonstrates that he uses the full form (cannot, do not, or will not) in other situations.

10. Indefinite pronouns (anybody, anyone, somebody, someone, everybody, and everyone) are assigned one morpheme.

Developmental Sentence Analysis (DSA). Laura Lee (1974) developed the *Developmental Sentence Analysis (DSA)*. This analysis looks at a child's syntax and how it fits into a developmental sequence from an expressive language sample. Normative data help compare the one you are evaluating to other children the same age. This analysis should only be performed on children whose first language is Standard English. The results from bilingual-speaking children or areas where the English is significantly different from Standard English are not reliable and cannot be used. The child's utterances are transcribed disregarding phono-

logical errors and corrections a child makes while talking. For example, a child may say, "Then the… brown dog… uh… sat… I mean laid down on the porch." Taking out the filler and repeated words, the sentence would be, "Then the brown dog laid on the porch." The final sentence would be used in the analyses.

The DSA is made up of two separate procedures. The first is called **developmental sentence types (DST)** and the second is called **developmental sentence scoring (DSS)**. The DST indicates whether grammatical structures are developing in an orderly fashion before the emergence of a basic sentence. DST looks at 100 utterances and those utterances can usually be obtained in a typical 1-hour therapy session. If it cannot, then the DST is not the appropriate analysis for that particular child. Typical transcription for a DST includes primarily one- to three-word phrases (my chair, blue ball, here baby, sit down, look, eat pizza, small brown puppy, etc.). The DST provides a chart broken down into three categories: (1) Single words, (2) Two-word combinations, and (3) Multiword constructions are not complete sentences. Frequency counts in the three areas are tallied and then compared to normative data. Then one can indicate in the multiword constructions, which grammatical stepping-stones are evident. The DST is an excellent analysis for children in the one- to three-word range.

The DSS looks at the developmental sequence of grammar in complete sentences for children 3-0 to 6-11 years old. DSS looks at 50 utterances and the utterance is considered complete if it contains a noun and a verb. For example, doggy bark, baby crying, car go, mommy drink, and so on. Other exceptions to the noun/verb requirement are clearly stated in Chapter 2 of the *DSA* as well as other finer points of transcription. Eight categories of grammatical forms have a developmental progression that is fairly easy to identify:

1. Indefinite pronoun or noun modifier
2. Personal pronoun
3. Main verb
4. Secondary verb
5. Negative
6. Conjunction

7. Interrogative reversal in questions
8. Wh-questions

Each of these categories are scored from 0 to 8 in each sentence (even if it is a zero or an attempt mark). Then the sentence receives a score of 1 if it follows the definition of an adult sentence. These scores are calculated for each sentence and then a total is figured. The number of sentences then divides the total and a DSS score in the range of 1 to 14 is obtained. The final score is then plotted on a chart with the norms, percentiles, and ages. The information from the analysis may be used to design treatment plans, document baseline and final rate information, and document changes over time. A compilation of the developmental sequence for syntactic and semantic development is included in Table 11-2. This is a great resource to help you know what areas may be analyzed in a language sample by your supervising SLP.

Pragmatic Analysis

Pragmatics is the study of how language is used in conversation. Areas of pragmatics that tend to be evaluated include requesting, commenting, referencing presuppositions, turn taking, responding, narratives, and speech adjustments. According to Miller (1981) analysis of pragmatics can be done on four levels: utterance level, discourse level; utterance related, discourse level; speech act related, and social level. Dore (1974), developed two analyses. The first is done with primitive speech acts and conversational acts. The primitive speech acts are categorized into nine areas: labeling, repeating, answering, requesting action, requesting answer, calling, greeting, protesting, and practicing. Once you put each utterance in a category, total them and get a percentage for each area. Coggins and Carpenter (1981) in their *Communicative Intention Inventory* developed a variation on Dore's system. This inventory has eight categories: comment on action, comment on object, request for action, request for object, request for information, answering, acknowledging, and protesting. The *Communicative Intention Inventory* provides percentile ranks to give the user a perspective regarding the frequency of these behaviors in normal 16-month-olds.

Table 11-2: Production Characteristics of Linguistic Development Organized by Brown's Stages

Stage	MLU	Age (months)	Grammatical Morphemes	Negation	Yes/No Questions	Wh-Questions	Noun Phrase Elaboration[d]	Verb Phrase Elaboration[d]	Complex Sentences
Early I	1.01-1.49	19-22[a] 16-26[b]	Occasional use	*no* as single-word utterance (but not as a negative response to a yes/no question)	Marked with rising intonation	*what + this/that*	NP → (M) + N[e] Elaborated NPs occur only alone	**Main Verb:** uninflected; occasional use of *-ing* **Auxiliary:** not used **Copula:** not used	None used
Late I/ Early II	1.50-1.99	23-26 18-31	Occasional use	*no* + noun or verb		*what* + NP or VP		Verb + Particles: occasional use	
II	2.00-2.49	27-30 21-35	1. Present progressive tense of verb *-ing*[c] 2. Regular plural *-s* 3. Preposition *in*	*not* + noun or verb		*where* + NP or VP	NP same as Stage I Object NP elaboration appears: V + NP	**Main Verb:** occasionally marked **Auxiliary:** 1. Semiauxiliary appears 2. Use of present progressive *-ing* without auxiliary **Copula:** appears without tense/number inflection	Semiauxiliary appears: *gonna, gotta, wanna, hafta*

I[d]

II[d]

Note. From *Guide to Analysis of Language Transcripts* (3rd ed., pp. 111–112), by K. Rutherford, 2000, Eau Claire, WI: Thinking Publications. ©2000 Thinking Publications. Reprinted with permission.

Table 11-2 (continued)

Stage	MLU	Age (months)	Grammatical Morphemes	Negation	Yes/No Questions	Wh-Questions	Noun Phrase Elaboration[d]	Verb Phrase Elaboration[d]	Complex Sentences
III	2.50-2.99	31-34 24-41	4. Preposition *on* 5. Possessive *-s*	NP + (negative) + VP			*Wh-* word + sentence *why, who,* and *how* questions appear	NP → {(demonstrative) (article)} + (M) + N Subject NP elaboration appears: NP + V	Main Verb: 1. Obligatory 2. Overgeneralizatin of regular past *-ed* Auxiliary: Present tense forms appear: *can, will, be, do*	Object NP complement; full sentence takes the place of object of the verb
Early IV	3.00-3.49	35-38 28-45		NP + auxiliary + (negative) + VP NP + copula + (negative) + VP	Inversion of auxiliary verb and subject noun	Inconsistent auxiliary inversion *when* questions appear			Simple infinitive phrases appear Simple *wh-* clauses appear Conjoined sentences with conjunction and

III[d]

Table 11-2 (continued)

Stage	MLU	Age (months)	Grammatical Morphemes	Negation	Yes/No Questions	Wh-Questions	Noun Phrase Elaboration[d]	Verb Phrase Elaboration[d]	Complex Sentences
Late IV/ Early V	3.50–3.99	39–42 31–50	No others mastered	No change	No change	No change	NP → {(demonstrative) (article) (M) (possessive)} + (adjective) + N Subject NP obligatory; noun or pronoun always appears in subject position	Main Verb: regular past -ed (double marking of main verb and auxiliary for past in negative sentences) Auxiliary: 1. Past modals appear, including *could, would, must, might* 2. be + present progressive -ing appears Verb Phrase: semi-auxiliary complements take NP	Multiple embeddings Conjoined and embedded clauses in the same sentence
Late V	4.00–4.49	43–46 37–52	6. Regular past tense of verb -ed 7. Irregular past tense of verb 8. Regular third person singular present tense -s 9. Definite and indefinite articles 10. Contractible copula	Past tense modals and *be* in contracted and uncontracted form		See Grammatical Morphemes column (6-14)	NP → same as Stage IV Number agreement between subject and predicate verb phrase continues to be a problem beyond Stage V	See Grammatical Morphemes column (6-10)	Relative clauses appear Infinitive phrases with subjects different from that of main sentence Conjunction *if* used

Table 11-2 (continued)

Stage	MLU	Age (months)	Grammatical Morphemes	Negation	Yes/No Questions	Wh-Questions	Noun Phrase Elaboration[d]	Verb Phrase Elaboration[d]	Complex Sentences
V+	4.50-4.99	47-50 41-59	11. Contractible auxiliary 12. Uncontractible copula 13. Uncontractible auxiliary 14. Irregular third person singular	No data	No data			See Grammatical Morphemes column (11-14) Main Verb/Aux. 1. Past tense *be* appears as main verb and auxiliary 2. Infrequent use of present tense perfect tense with auxiliary marked	Gerund phrases appear *Wh-* infinitive phrases appear Unmarked infinitive phrases appear Conjunction *because* used
V++	5.00-5.99	51-67 43-67	No data	No data	No data	No data			Conjunctions *when* and *so* appear

[a] Predicted age range

[b] Age range within one SD of predicted values

[c] Based on 90% use in obligatory contexts, except stages EI-LI/EII

[d] Stages I, II, and III have been used to describe developments within only noun phrase elaboration and verb phrase elaboration based on sources of these data

[e] The following are definitions of sentence notation:
→ is expanded, or elaborated, as S → NP + VP
(x) the item within the parentheses is optional VP → V + NP
{(x) (y)} either one of the items must occur

Adapted from Assessing Language Production in Children: Experimental Procedures by J. Miller, 1981, Baltimore: University Park Press.

Dore (1978) developed analysis to look at conversational acts. The conversational acts are categorized into eight categories: requests, responses to requests, descriptions, statements, acknowledgments, organizational devices, performatives, and miscellaneous. These are just a sampling of pragmatic analyses that are currently available.

Adult Analysis

Language sample analysis is also used with adults, especially with neurologic impairments. With adults several forms of language samples may be acquired: spoken, written, and reading (Glosser & Deser, 1990). A spontaneous language sample may be used to determine an individual's fluency and content. The Western Aphasia Battery (WAB) (Kertesz, 1982) has a subtest, called Oral Language Subtests, that analyzes spoken language samples. The subtest gives a standardized score in the area of content and fluency. The WAB may be given in the context of the entire test, or it may be used informally as a guide to analyze a language sample. Narrative discourse is another method of language sample analysis. An adult is shown a picture and asked to tell a story about it or describe it. Then the language sample is analyzed. Brownell and Joanette (1993) in their book describe "one particular type of multisentential text, narrative discourse, which refers to the ways in which people link together the bits and pieces of language to create representations of events, objects, beliefs, personalities, and experiences" (p. vii). Other analyses may be of writing or reading samples. Your supervising SLP may have you help in obtaining or transcribing an adult language sample.

Computer-Based Analyses

A variety of computer-based programs are available to analyze language samples. It is important to understand the basis for these analyses to understand the programs and exactly what they do. According to Schwartz (1985), the computer analyses are only as good or accurate as the coded transcription on which they are based. The following com-

puter language sample analysis tools are time saving in the area of frequency-of-use summaries. Computer programs are able to only analyze certain aspects of language, and more complex aspects of language require specialized coding systems for the computer to analyze (Miller, Freiberg, Rolland, & Reeves, 1992). One area programs are not able to analyze are nonverbal components to communication such as eye gaze, gestures, and intonation or the analysis of stylistic variations a speaker may use. One major benefit of computerized language sample analyses is that several databases with developmental norms on language have been developed. One well-known database is called CHILDES (MacWhinney, 1995; MacWhinney & Snow, 1985). Several available computer programs are described here so you can get a sampling of what is available. Your setting may have a specific program they want you to use.

Lingquest 1: Language Sample Analysis. *Lingquest 1: Language Sample Analysis* (Mordecai, Palin, & Palmer, 1982) provides three major types of analyses. The first is a grammatical form analysis looking at frequency of use to opportunities for use comparison of eight categories of grammatical forms (nouns, verbs, modifiers, prepositions, conjunctions, negatives, interjections, and wh-questions words). It identifies analyses of errors and identifies patterns. The second area is a lexical analysis looking at the variety of vocabulary used (TTR). An MLU in words and morphemes will be figured. The third is the structure analysis looking at the variety of phrase, sentence, and question types. You will need to learn how to transcribe using their coding system to help analyze structures. The basic information from each analysis is provided and developmental norms are not included.

Systematic Analysis of Language Transcripts (SALT). *Systematic Analysis of Language Transcripts (SALT)* was written by Miller and Chapman (1983, 1991) and is a very flexible and complicated software program. The SALT performs three types of analysis. The first is a word and morphemic analysis giving you an MLU, TTR, and a summary of omissions. The second is an analysis of language structure consisting of verb, question, and negative form summaries. The third looks at how the phrases before the one being ana-

lyzed and after match. This program has many options that may be selected or created by the user. This program is sophisticated and requires training to use. A tutorial program is provided to help an individual learn the coding system. A reference database has been developed to help compare results with developmental norms but is not included with the program. The developmental norms were taken from 30 children at each of the following ages: 3, 4, 5, 6, 7, 9, 11, and 13 years. Language samples were collected from each of these children in conversation and narration because both are important in an educational setting.

Computerized Language Sample Analysis (CLSA). Weiner (1984) developed the *Computerized Language Sample Analysis (CLSA)*. This program provides the user with summaries of the frequency of occurrence and accuracy of use for 14 grammatical categories. They include nouns, verbs, sentence types, length of utterance, and word usage. More detailed analyses may be chosen. One needs to be familiar with language analysis to be able to interpret the information provided in the summaries. A tutorial is included with the program to facilitate learning the coding system. The updated version of this program is called *Parrot Easy Language Sample Analysis* (Weiner, 1988).

Pye Analysis of Language (PAL). Pye (1987) wrote *Pye Analysis of Language (PAL)* and it performs morphologic, syntactic, and phonologic analysis using procedures by Ingram (1981). By coding the transcript, the user can create other analyses. This program requires the understanding of DOS and its commands for coding and analysis.

Computerized Language Profiling Version 6.1 (CP). Long and Fey (1989) developed The *Computerized Language Profiling Version 6.1*. This program includes many analyses that were formerly done by hand. They include *Language Assessment, Remediation, and Screening Procedure (LARSP)* (Crystal, Fletcher, & Garman, 1991), *PRISM+* (Crystal, 1982), and *DSS* (Lee, 1974). This is the only program that can also perform pragmatic and phonological analyses. Some of the analyses have complex coding systems and may be

time consuming. The *DSS* and *Conversational Acts Profile* have normative data included in the program.

PORTFOLIOS

A new trend is happening in early childhood education and some elementary education programs. **Portfolios** are being used as a way to document changes in a child's language abilities as well as assess a child's language abilities. Standardized tests only tell you how a child performs at a specific point in time in an unnatural setting. According to Kratcoski (1998), portfolios may be used for assessment and assessments as well as measuring learner progress. Portfolios capture what happens throughout the child's day in a natural environment and give a picture of the child over time. With the passage of IDEA, the focus is on functional assessment and portfolios are a wonderful way to achieve this. Teachers and helpers make observations of the children's language in their classroom and write the children's comments on their artwork and take pictures of the children throughout their day. Teachers also take notes from interactions from parents on what the children are doing at home. The information that has been collected is then placed in a photo album, scrapbook or video. Initial referral, language samples, story retell samples, observation notes, work samples, teacher interviews, parent interviews, student interviews, and testing data may also be included in a portfolio (Kratcoski, 1998). The process of making a portfolio creates an ongoing record of the child's language growth and can be used by both the parents and the teachers. According to Gronlund and Engel (2001), "Documentation is evidence of a child's experience and includes photos of the child in action, or work samples, that the child produced. To go along with each photo and work sample, the teacher writes an 'anecdote'—a note describing what was happening with the child at the time the photo was taken or the work sample was made" (p. 2). After all the data are collected, then a narrative statement is written to summarize the information that has been gathered. These summaries can be used in place of formal assessments. Portfolios give wonderful picture of the progress a child has made as well as where they are currently functioning in their language skills. The developmental information is valuable for the teachers and professionals to be able to modify curriculum to meet the needs of each child. You may be a part of taking notes and making observations of a child's language as well as putting together the actual portfolio.

SIX STEPS TO USING PORTFOLIOS IN ASSESSMENT

The California Early Language Development Assessment Process (California Department of Education, Santa Cruz, 1998) six steps to using portfolios in assessment are:

Step 1. Make a Plan: Define clear and realistic goals—identify who, what, when, and how.

Step 2. Collect Information: Observations, prompted responses, product of activities, and information from family members.

Step 3. Create a Portfolio: Includes samples of the child's work and teachers' observations presented in an organized way.

Step 4. Write a Narrative Statement: A summary of child's strengths and needs based on the portfolio.

Step 5. Meet with Family and Staff: Family and staff meet separately to review the portfolio information as well as the narrative statement, discuss instructional strategies and activities that are best for the child.

Step 6. Modify the Curriculum: Information from the above meetings is used to identify and implement curriculum activities to foster the language development of the child as well as the group of children.

Portfolios are great tools for children who are bilingual (California Department of Education, Santa Cruz, 1998). It gives teachers and professionals a way to monitor the development of both languages over time. Portfolios capture language in their natural environment. The California Early Language Development Assessment Process (California Department of Education, Santa Cruz, 1998) contains a circle of six steps that defines how to use portfolios in an

assessment process. The assessment process is considered a circle because it is a continual process going through the six steps many times. Portfolios capture a child's developing language skills with the child's work as well as teacher and parental observations and the written summary may be used instead of a formal assessment. Portfolios free the teacher from the constraints of standardized tests (Grace, n.d.). Portfolios may be an integral part of documenting in your work setting.

CONCLUSION

Record keeping and documentation are an important part of an SLPA's job. Everything from making copies, to documenting phone conversations, to organizing an individual's file is a vital part of the job. Accurate records help keep the SLP and SLPA accountable for what services they provide. Computers can be a very useful tool in keeping track of an individual's attendance, recording SOAP notes, or analyzing a language sample. Computers can make your job easier if used effectively. Progress notes help document what happened during a therapy session as well as record accurate data taken during the therapy session. One method of writing progress notes is called a SOAP note with each letter representing one area of the therapy session. Language can be complex and language samples help give a snapshot of an individual's language abilities. Different strategies are available to help an individual talk during a language sample as well as keep their interest and stay on specific topics. All areas of language (phonetics, semantics, syntax, and pragmatics) can be analyzed from a language sample. This information helps the SLP make critical decisions about placement, intervention, and dismissal. Accurate information is vital. A growing method for helping to document changes in language for preschool children is the use of portfolios. It is a nonbiased way to record and analyze language from culturally diverse bilingual children. Every part of the SLPA's job involves documentation and a general knowledge of keeping accurate and current records.

DISCUSSION QUESTIONS

1. Describe the need for accurate record keeping. Include examples of different types of record keeping you may be required to do for your supervising SLP.

2. Do a self-assessment of your organization and record-keeping skills. Describe three strengths and three weaknesses. Document how you could improve on the areas of weakness. How can your strengths help your areas of weakness? Come up with an action plan to implement over the next 6 months.

3. Describe a portfolio. How is it used and what information goes into a portfolio? Start your own professional portfolio. Include information about the classes you have taken and experiences you have had that will help you when you become an SLPA. Also include any special training or inservices you have attended. What previous experiences will help in your education/training as an SLPA? What are your personal strengths and areas of interest?

4. Compare and contrast phonetic, syntactic, semantic, and pragmatic analyses. Define each of the terms and provide reasons for their differences.

SUGGESTED ACTIVITIES

1. Go out into the community and watch a SLP during a therapy session. Write a progress note to summarize the session. Remember to include all the critical information using the SOAP acronym. Compare it to what the SLP wrote for her progress note.

2. Talk to a school SLP about his method of scheduling. From that information, design your method for scheduling 40 students on a caseload in kindergarten through 5th grade. Each grade level has three classes. How would you start this process? Describe the process you go through to get a schedule that fits with that school.

3. Call an SLPA who is in practice and ask him about

the types of documentation and record-keeping activities he does on the job. Ask what skills he would have liked to develop before becoming an SLPA.

4. Watch a therapy session in the area of your interest. Discuss with the SLP or SLPA before the session what data they will be collecting during the session. Design your own data collection sheet and take data throughout the session. Then compare the information with what the SLP or SLPA took during the session. Were you able to pick up all the desired behaviors? Did you count behaviors or answers that the SLP or SLPA did not? Was it an easy task? How would it be if you were running the session yourself and having to do the same type of data collection?

5. Take a language sample of a child either on-line, videotape, or audio tape. Include 100 utterances. Then do a computerized analysis on the language sample. Learn the coding system for the computer program you chose. What information does your particular program produce in the summary of information?

REFERENCES

American Speech-Language-Hearing Association Professional Services Board. (1984). *Accreditation manual.* Rockville, MD: Author.

Bernthal, J., & Bankson, N. (1998). *Articulation and Phonological Disorders* (4th ed.). Needham Heights, MA: Allyn & Bacon.

Bloom, L. (1973). *One word at a time: The use of single-word utterances before syntax.* The Hague: Mouton.

Bloom, L., & Lahey, M. (1978). *Language development and language disorders.* New York: John Wiley and Sons.

Bray, M., Ross, A., & Todd, C. (1999). *Speech and language clinical process and practice.* Baltimore: Paul H. Brookes.

Brown, R. (1973). *A first language: The early stages.* Cambridge, MA: Harvard University Press.

Brownwell, H. H., & Joanette, Y. (1993). *Narrative discourse in neurologically impaired and normal aging adults.* San Diego, CA: Singular.

California Department of Education, Santa Cruz. (1998). *Assessing and fostering the development of a first and a second language in early childhood: Training manual, resource guide, videotape.* Santa Cruz, CA: Author.

Coggins, T., & Carpenter, R. (1981). The communicative intention inventory: A system for observing and coding children's early intentional communication. *Applied Psycholinguistics, 2*, 235–251.

Cornett, B. S., & Chabon, S. S. (1988). *The clinical practice of speech-language pathology*. New York: Merrill, an imprint of Macmillan.

Crystal, D. (1982). Profile in Semantics (PRISM+). In *Profiling Linguistic Disability* (pp. 139–213). London, England: Edward Arnold.

Crystal, D., Fletcher, P., & Garman, M. (1991). *The grammatical analysis of language disability: A procedure for assessment and remediation*. San Diego, CA: Singular.

Dore, J. (1974). A pragmatic description of early language development. *Journal of Psycholinguistic Research, 4*, 343–350.

Dore, J. (1978). Variation in preschool children's conversational performances. In K. Nelson (Ed.), *Children's language: Vol 1* (pp. 397–444). New York: Gardner Press.

Edwards, S., & Knott, R. (1994). Assessing spontaneous language abilities of aphasic speakers. *Language Testing, 11*(1), 49–64.

Flower, R. M. (1984). *Delivery of speech-language pathology and audiology services*. Baltimore: Williams & Wilkins.

Glosser, G., & Deser, T. (1990). Patterns of discourse production among neurological patients with fluent language disorders. *Brain and Language, 40*, 67–88.

Grace, C. (n.d.). The portfolio and its use: Developmentally appropriate assessment of young children. *ERIC Digest* (ERIC Document Reproduction Service No. EDO-PS-92-11)

Gronlund, G., & Engel, B. (2001). *Focused portfolios*. St. Paul, MN: Redleaf Press.

Hadley, P. A. (1998, July). Language sampling protocols for eliciting text-level discourse. *Language, Speech, and Hearing Services in Schools, 29*, 132–147.

Hegde, M. N., & Davis, D. (1999). *Clinical methods and practicum in speech-language pathology* (2nd ed.). San Diego, CA: Singular.

Ingram, D. (1981). *Assessing communication behavior: Procedures for the phonological analysis of children's language* (Vol. 2). Baltimore: University Park Press.

Kemp, K., & Klee, T. (1997). Clinical language sampling practices: Results of a survey of speech-language pathologists in the United States. *Child Language Teaching and Therapy, 13*(2), 161–176.

Kertesz, A. (1992). *Western Aphasia Battery*. San Antonio, TX: Psychological Corporation.

Kratcoski, A. M. (1998, January). Guidelines for using portfolios in assessment and evaluation. *Language, Speech, and Hearing Services in Schools, 29*, 3–10.

Leadholm, B.J., & Miller, J. (1992, reprinted January 1994). *Language sample analysis: The Wisconsin guide*. Madison: Wisconsin Department of Public Instruction.

Lee, L. L. (1974). *Developmental sentence analysis: A grammatical assessment procedure for speech and language clinicians.* Evanston, IL: Northwestern University Press.

Long, S., & Fey, M. (1989). Computerized Language Profiling (Version 6.1) [Computer software]. Ithaca, NY: Ithaca College.

Louko, L., & Edwards, M. (2001). Issues in collecting and transcribing speech samples. *Topics in Language Disorders, 21*(4), 1–11.

MacWhinney, B. (1995). *The CHILDES project: Tools for analyzing talk* (2nd ed.) Hillsdale, NJ: Erlbaum.

MacWhinney, B., & Snow, C. (1985). The child language data exchange system. *Journal of Child Language, 12,* 271–296.

Meyer, S. M. (1998). *Survival guide for the beginning speech-language clinician.* Gaithersburg, MD: Aspen.

Miller, J. (1981). *Assessing language production in children: Experimental procedures.* Baltimore: University Park Press.

Miller, J., Freiberg, C., Rolland, M., & Reeves, M. A. (1992). Implementing computerized language sample analysis in the public school. *Topics in Language Disorders, 12*(2), 69–82.

Miller J., & Chapman, R. (1983). *Systematic analysis of language transcripts.* Madison: Language Analysis Laboratory, Waisman Center, University of Wisconsin.

Miller, J., & Chapman, R. (1991). SALT: A Computer Program for the Systematic Analysis of Language Transcripts [Computer Software] Madison: Language Analysis Laboratory, Waisman Center, University of Wisconsin.

Mordecai, D., Palin, M., & Palmer, C. (1982). Lingquest 1: Language Sample Analysis [Computer Software]. Napa, CA: Lingquest Software.

Nelson, K. (1973). Structure and strategy in learning to talk. *Monographs of the Society for Research in Child Development, 38* 1–2. (Serial No. 149).

Oller, D., & Eilers, R. (1975). Phonetic expectation and transcription validity. *Phonectica, 31* 288–304.

Owens, R. (1992). *Language development: An introduction.* Columbus, OH: Merrill.

Pietranton, A. A. (1995, November/December). Collecting outcome data: Existing tools, preliminary data, future directions. *ASHA's Managed Care Resource Packet.*

Pye, C. (1987). Pye Analysis of Language [Computer software]. Lawrence: University of Kansas.

Retherford, K. S. (1993). *Guide to analysis of language transcripts* (2nd ed.) Eau Claire, WI: Thinking Publications.

Retherford, K., Schwartz, B., & Chapman, R. (1981). Semantic roles in mother and child speech: Who tunes into whom? *Journal of Child Language, 8,* 583–608.

Roth, F. P., & Worthington, C. K. (1996). *Treatment resource manual for speech-language pathology.* San Diego, CA: Singular.

Shriberg, L. D., & Kent, R. D. (1982). *Clinical phonetics.* New York: Macmillan.

Schwartz, A. (1985). Microcomputer-assisted assessment of linguistic and phonological processes. *Topics in Language Disorders, 6*(1), 26–40.

Stockman, I. J. (1996, October). The promises and pitfalls of language sample analysis as an assessment tool for linguistic minority children. *Language, Speech, and Hearing Services in Schools, 27,* 355–366.

Stoel-Gammon, C. (2001). Transcribing the speech of young children. *Topic in Language Disorders, 21*(4), 12–21.

Templin, M. (1957). *Certain langauge skills in children: Their development and relationships.* Minneapolis: University of Minnesota Press.

Thomas, A. F., & Webster, K. L. (1999). *SLP assistant in the schools.* San Antonio, TX: Communication Skill Builders.

Weiner, F. (1984). Computerized language sample analysis [Computer Software]. State College, PA: Parrot Software.

Weiner, F. (1988). Parrot easy language sample analysis (PELSA) [Computer Software]. State College, PA: Parrot Software.

CHAPTER 12

Screening and Assessment

Key Concepts

Speech-language screening is a quick procedure to detect individuals who may have or be at risk for communication problems. It determines if further in-depth assessment is needed.

Assisting in screening, without interpretation, is within the scope of responsibilities of the SLPA.

Effective screening requires training, familiarity, accuracy, consistency, and flexibility.

The SLPA is allowed to assist the SLP in preparation of materials for an evaluation for eligibility determination or other assessments, but the SLPA cannot administer or interpret standardized assessment tests, formal or informal in nature.

Overview

Screening: What Is It?
Screening Tools
Your Role and Responsibility in Screening

Assessment and Evaluation: What Is It?
Three Purposes of Assessment
Terminology of Assessment
Assessment Methods
Models of Assessment
Your Role and Responsibilities in Assessment

INTRODUCTION

Screening: What Is It and Why Is It Done?

Think back to your elementary school days. Do you remember participating in the annual hearing and vision checks? While you sat in the school nurse's office wearing headphones, you raised your hand when you heard a beep. Then you named alphabet letters on an eye chart. Well, that may have been your first introduction to a **screening**! A screening is done to determine which individuals' behaviors or abilities fall outside a determined range of "normal" behavior. The hearing and vision screenings were done in order to identify whether your hearing and vision abilities fell outside the criteria or specified range. Your performance on these screenings was considered either passing or failing. If you failed the hearing screening, you would have been referred for further audiological assessment.

In the world of speech-language, a screening is a quick procedure for detecting potential communication problems (Feeney, 1996). The **screener** consists of a series of uniform questions or speaking activities that allows a client to show his communication skills to the person who is observing. Shames, Wiig, and Secord write that in screening, "the goal is to decide in a very short time whether there is any evidence that a child might have a disorder and require further testing" (1998, p. 240). Screening can be considered the first step in the process of assessment. However, screening does not always lead to an assessment. If a client were to "pass" a particular screening procedure, then the speech-language pathologist (SLP) would probably not recommend further assessment. Thus, the purpose of screening is simply to identify individuals who need further assessment to determine if they may have a speech and language disorder (Mayer, 1993). In screening, there is no diagnosis made and a client is not identified for ongoing service. Because assisting your SLP supervisor in screening is well within your scope of responsibility as a speech-language pathology assis-

tant (SLPA), you will need a better understanding of what it could look like.

What Is It?

SLPs may be involved in screening procedures and tools that vary, depending on setting and population. Because all states are required to identify children and infants who may be eligible for special services, the systematic process of Child Find Screening is one of the most typical screening processes in existence. Public Law 94-142, or what is now called The Individuals with Disabilities Education ACT (IDEA) (discussed in Chapter 8) covers an age range of 0 to 21 years; however, because most children ages 5 through 21 have typically been identified through a public school screening or referral, Child Find Screenings are usually directed toward children under the age of 5 (Chazdon, 1978). The process of "finding" children can vary from state to state and district to district but usually involves extensive parent and caregiver education in the form of public relations brochures, pamphlets placed in pediatrician's offices, newspaper articles, and free seminars. Activities provide families with information about typical **developmental milestones** such as the ages at which most children begin to walk and talk. The importance of early intervention is consistently emphasized. Those who administrate the Child Find Screening (not to be confused with Child Find multidisciplinary evaluations and assessment processes) can provide their own screening programs but usually work in coordination with school or community programs. Although the components of Child Find can be extensive, the main purpose is to determine whether a child may require a complete assessment of her abilities. Screening across all developmental areas is completed. Thus your SLP supervisor may enlist your assistance in collecting information about the child's speech and language development. The actual screenings can involve groups of children using published screening instruments. Screening could take place in preschools or childcare centers, public schools, or health care settings. Often, paraprofessionals and volunteers are trained and used to help administer the screening tests (Chazdon, 1978). Child Find programs identify, follow, and

bring children to the attention of specific service providers (Nelson, 1993).

Another screening process that is increasingly becoming more prevalent is the Universal Newborn Hearing Screening. Initiated by a panel of the National Institutes of Health (Bureau, 1999) held in 1993, development and research of Newborn Hearing Screening programs in the United States has been significant. A recommendation was made based on research that proves the effectiveness of hearing screenings in detecting hearing loss in newborns as well as the importance of early intervention that significantly supports the development of language and social skills. Specifically, that "all infants should be screened for hearing impairment ... prior to discharge" (Management, 2000). Given the fact that a hearing loss that goes undetected can have significant consequences (Yoshinag-Itano, Sedey, Coulter, & Mehl, 1998), many states have either passed or are considering legislative mandates for Universal Hearing Screening programs (Spivak, 1998). The Walsh Bill, a federal initiative recently passed in Washington, DC, also focuses on national implementation of this procedure. Hospitals that offer these programs are implementing ever-improving technology and are finding more and more evidence for the benefits and cost-efficiency of Newborn Hearing Screenings. As an SLPA you will most likely not be directly involved in this process because Universal Newborn Hearing screening is overseen by an audiologist and often requires specific specialized training of volunteers or other hospital personnel.

Other fairly widespread screening practices are seen in Head Start programs, in which all children are typically screened as part of their enrollment. Many school districts also screen children before starting or at the beginning of kindergarten in an attempt to identify the children who "may not yet be ready to enter the regular school curriculum at the kindergarten level so that assistance may be provided if needed" (Nelson, 1993, p. 328). By screening children before they enter kindergarten, the school may recommend anything from waiting another year to enter kindergarten, further assessment, or placement in some sort of developmental program (Catts, 1997). A team made up of kindergarten teachers, SLPs, special education teachers,

paraprofessionals including SLPAs, and any other individual whom the school appropriately trains, may conduct this type of screening. It is considered a "mass" screening and is usually carried out on days that are specifically set aside for that purpose. Parents bring their preschool children who might move around "stations" at which professionals screen a variety of developmental areas, including motor or physical, thinking skills, and of course, communication (Bruce, DiVenere, & Bergeron, 1998). Sometimes rather than moving from station to station, one trained screener will administer the entire screening test to one student.

Screenings for speech or language difficulties occur in the public schools on an ongoing basis each school year. In some school districts, it is a routine for all kindergartners and third-grade students to be screened. In other districts, instead of grade level screenings, the SLP relies exclusively on teacher referral. When a teacher "refers" a student, it means she asks the SLP to informally listen to a child's speech or expressive language if she has questions or concerns about a particular student. Before actually screening the student, the SLP may have a teacher or parent complete a checklist that lists specific communication behaviors that might be of concern. This assists the SLP in processing more accurate referrals. You may be asked to retrieve a specific referral checklist for the teacher to complete. Then the SLP will screen the child using either an informally or formally published screener in addition to one-on-one observations of a brief communicative interaction. Many districts find a combination of grade level screening and teacher referrals to be an effective approach for identification of students who may require further testing. It is generally the case that once a child has entered the school system, the classroom teacher often becomes the main source of speech-language referrals (Lubinski, 1994). Some school SLPs may screen a handful of students or more each year based on an informal list of "rechecks." This includes the children who were previously screened for whatever reason and were not evaluated but may have demonstrated one or two minor or borderline concerns that the SLP wanted to recheck at a later date.

SIDELIGHT: *Recheck Snapshot*

When she was in second grade, Maya's productions of /r/ were accurate and consistent in spontaneous speech in the initial and medial positions as well as in most blends. However, because some /r/ sounds "sounded distorted" (final /r/ and some /r/ blends were mildly distorted), her teacher had referred her to the SLP. The teacher had no academic concerns. The SLP made a note to check on Maya's /r/ productions at the beginning of third grade to determine whether /r/ had spontaneously self-corrected. Maya was rescreened, or rechecked, at the beginning of third grade and the SLP determined that her /r/ sounds had self-corrected. The SLP checked with the new teacher and through a series of open-ended questioning, confirmed there were no academic or social concerns.

Screenings in the hospital occur in the acute care setting when a patient enters the hospital with a stroke, surgery, or illness, and often in the transitional care setting, when the patient is preparing to leave the hospital (Brookshire, 1997). The physician typically refers the patient to the SLP to determine current status. These screenings are called bedside evaluations and may only be done by an SLP. Other screening tools used in the hospital require specialized training. You will need to check with your supervising SLP in the hospital to determine what your role may be in screening in this setting.

It is probably more common for you to be asked to help with screenings in the transitional care setting. An example of a screening tool that you might use to record observations of behavior is the Mini Mental Status Examination (MMSE) (Cockrell & Folstein, 1988; Crum, Anthony, Bassett, & Folstein, 1993; Folstein, Folstein, & McHugh, 1975), which screens orientation, immediate and recent recall or memory skills, and attention. If the patient is functioning at a higher level, you might be asked to help with the Grigsby Cognitive Screening, which screens the following: attention, working memory, delayed and immediate recall, reasoning processing, and judgment. Some hospitals may design their own screening protocol to screen for a variety of functions that might indicate the need for in-depth evaluation or ongoing assessment by the SLP. Again, the outcome of your screening will help determine if further assessment is needed to inform a diagnosis by the SLP.

A variety of other screening procedures may be used in the hospital, agency, or other settings. However, the important thing to remember is that you will need specific training with tools and protocols used in order to assist the SLPs in this activity. The description for your involvement is clearly outlined in the American Speech-Language-Hearing Association (ASHA), Background Information and Criteria for Registration of Speech-Language Pathology Assistants (April, 2001) (see Appendix A). This stipulates that your job responsibility for this function is to "assist the SLP with speech-language and hearing screenings (without interpretation)" (p. 2). It also stipulates that you "may not screen or diagnose patients/clients for feeding or swallowing disorders and that you may not use a checklist or tabulate results of feeding and swallowing evaluations." (p. 2). These are important considerations, particularly for the SLPA working in a hospital or agency that performs such services. This function demands a level of training beyond the scope of the SLPA.

Screening Tools

Components of Screening Tools

Screening tools vary significantly but most tools designed for screening both speech and language include the following components.

Naming. Screeners often use key words or preselected words that contain a variety of speech sounds. The individual names pictures or real objects, which allows the listener to hear a somewhat larger sample of sound productions than she may have heard in a short conversation or question-answer period alone.

Imitation. Frequently, the screening tool will allow for imitation, which is a direct approach for sampling articulation of speech sounds. For this section, the SLP or SLPA says a word and the client repeats the word. Although this may not be the most natural or typical sample of speech, this technique is often necessary, especially for clients who are reluctant to talk. If using imitation, it is important to make a

notation on the screener form or protocol as to whether the sounds were produced spontaneously (with no model) or in imitation (with model). The SLP will want to know whether an individual could not produce a sound when trying to imitate a model.

Serial Verbalizations. Another typical screening component is serial verbalizations. This simply means reciting of information that is typically stated in some kind of consistent sequence. For example, you may have a client count from 1 to 30, or name the days of the week or the letters of the alphabet. This is another way to gather a short speech sample that most students find both fun and easy, depending on the individual. Many sounds of the English language can be elicited by listing one or more of the above serial verbalizations.

Receptive and Expressive Language Screeners. Screeners may also have sections that address receptive and expressive language. The screener may include items that the individual is required to follow such as single and multi-step oral directions, answer yes/no questions, answer wh-questions, verbalize similarities and differences, describe pictures, complete sentences, provide a word similar in meaning to a target word, or repeat numbers, words, and sentences from memory.

Reporting by Adults or Others. The screening tool you use may have a section for reporting by adults or others. This may be included in the general or additional information section discussed earlier or as a separate space to record objective information from a parent, a teacher, or a patient's spouse. Most often, this information has already been given before the actual screening and may be the reason why the referral was made in the first place. For example, if the teacher had shared her impressions of her student's communication, you may quote comments such as "I can't understand Joey when he gets excited." Or if a parent reported, "Jason is being teased by his older brother because he talks funny," you could quote the parents' concern in this section.

Additional Information. Another screening component is a general section for additional information or notes on any observations that were made during the screening. There

may be a space marked "general information" or "comments" or even a section for descriptions of how a child appears visually, whether you observe any differences in voice production or the fluency of speech. It is here that you may write objective, descriptive statements of what you observe. Use this section to make note of any other additional information that the SLP might consider beyond the performance on screening items.

Criteria for Selecting Screening Tools

Before we consider your role in screening, let us take a look at the criteria the SLP may use for choosing a specific instrument. If you were to ask your SLP supervisor, "Why are we using this particular screening tool?" she will likely have clear reasons for her preference of the screening tools she tends to use. Her preferences may result from her own evaluation of any of the following eight criteria for judging effectiveness and appropriateness of screening tools as suggested by Meisels and Wasik (Meisels, 1990) and Lichtenstein (1984) as cited by Cohen (1994).

1. **Brevity:** The length of time required to administer the screener should be relatively short, given the typically large numbers of patients or students who need to be screened in order to determine whether further assessment is necessary.

2. **Norm Referenced:** The screener compares an individual's performance with the performance of others who have taken the same screener or norm referenced the individual's performance. The normative sample of the screener should include students or patients of similar characteristics and background (age, culture, sex, etc.) to the individual being screened. The standards or norms provide the basis on which we compare a student's performance; therefore, the norms need to be representative of the setting population as a whole (Peterson, 1994). Lack of appropriately normed screening tools has been an ongoing challenge in the field of speech-language pathology, especially due to ever-increasing representa-

tion of "linguistically diverse," minority individuals (Huang, Hopkins, & Nippold, 1997; Jitendra & Rohera-Diaz, 1996; Kayser, 1996; Lidz, 1996; Wyatt, 1997).

3. Inexpensive: What is the cost of the instrument? The answer to this question may factor into the SLP's decision about whether to use the tool. Expense has to do not only with the actual price of the instrument, but how efficient it is in terms of use of time and the ease in which it can be administered. Are there extensive training requirements in terms of money and time? A tool becomes more attractive if a professional or paraprofessional can give it quickly and with a minimum amount of training or budget expense.

4. Standardized Administration: The tool should describe standard and consistent procedures to follow during screening administration. Procedures are clearly stated for instructions, items to be given, and scoring criteria. If the screener were given in the same way, using the same procedures, then a particular client's performance would be the same regardless of who gave the screener.

5. Objective Scoring: Just as the administration of the screener must be consistent between all SLPs and SLPAs who give it, the scoring must be consistent also. If the scoring is done objectively, then personal judgment is not factored into the scores.

6. Broad Focus: Because screening tests are used for the purpose of identifying those who require further evaluation, they should be broadly focused. A screener will be more broadly focused if its items cover different areas of speech or language. If a screener has too narrow a focus, potential communication difficulties could easily be missed.

7. Reliability: Screening tools need to be reliable or repeatable. How consistent are the scores? How

confident are you that the score that Evan got today will be very similar to the score he would get next week?

8. Validity: Validity is the concept that demonstrates that a screener is actually screening for what it claims to be screening (Lewis, 1997). How well does the screener do what it is supposed to do in terms of predicting later performance or tapping the skills it claims to tap? For a screener to be valid, it should minimize both **underreferrals** (screener did not refer the child but the child did need services) and **overreferrals** (screener did refer the child but the child did not need services). Peterson (1994) provides more information on the concepts of reliability and validity.

Now that you have considered the criteria that make a "good" screener, you should recognize that consequences may result from using an instrument that has not been appropriately normed, standardized, or is not sensitive to the population in which it is being used (Stockman, 1996; Wyatt, 1997). If a child needs services and is "missed," his self-esteem as well as his academic and social success could suffer (Cohen, 1983). So too could a child "fail" a screener and be looked on as having potential language "problems" when in fact, the child's language differences according to culture were neither recognized nor respected by the tool or by the examiner. Therefore, it is important for professionals to continue to develop and use instruments that best represent the clients they are screening (Jitendra & Rohen-Diaz, 1996; Kayser, 1996). "Using nationally standardized norms that include children from a range of ethnic and economic backgrounds helps us to guarantee that screening procedures are as fair as we can make them" (Paul, 1995, p. 388).

Sample Screening Tools

Your supervising SLP may train you to use a commercially available screener that has been published with standardized administration and scoring norms. Examples may be found in Figure 12-1.

Examples of Commercially Available Screeners

- Quick Screen of Phonology (Bankson & Bernthal, 1990)
- Receptive-Expressive Emergent Language Scale (Bzoch & League, 1991)
- Screening Test for Auditory Comprehension of Language (Carrow, 1973)
- CELF-3 Screening Test (Clinical Evaluation of Language Fundamentals—Third Edition) (Semel, Wiig, & Secord, 1995)
- Fluharty Preschool Speech and Language Screening Test Second Edition (Fluharty-2) (Fluharty, 2001)
- Joliet 3-Minute Speech and Language Screening Test (Kinzer & Johnson, 1983)
- Kindergarten Language Screening Test (Gauther & Madison, 1983)
- Ages and Stages Questionnaire (ASQ) (Bricker & Squires, 2nd ed., 1999)
- Adolescent Language Screening Test (Morgan & Guilford, 1984)
- Quick Neurological Screening Test (Mutti, Sterling, & Spalding, 1978)
- Screening Test for Auditory Comprehension of Language—Spanish and English (Carrow, 1973)
- Screening Test for Auditory Processing Disorders (Keith, 1986)
- Screening Test for Developmental Apraxia of Speech (Blakely, 1980)
- Screening Test of Spanish Grammar (Toronto, 1973)
- First Step: Screening Test for Evaluating Preschoolers (Miller, 1993)

Figure 12-1 Screening tools that may be used by a SLPA.

For example, the Ages and Stages Questionnaire (1999) has been carefully designed to ensure clarity and ease of implementation and is completed by parents of young children. It is designed to screen children for developmental delays during the first 5 years. It was developed at the Center for Human Development, University of Oregon, using more than 7,700 completed questionnaires with items from a variety of sources, including information about specific developmental milestones such as first words, responds to name, identifies pictures, and so on. The question of whether it assesses what it is supposed to assess is addressed through validity studies that indicate a high percentage of comparative results with other accepted measures. The authors of this screener suggest that this type of questionnaire only takes 10 to 20 minutes for caregivers to complete the items, and the results could easily be tabulated by an SLPA to provide the SLP a basis for interpretation of current functioning levels in speech and language as well as related developmental domains. Questionnaires can be administered at all or some of the following intervals: 4, 6, 8, 10, 12, 14, 16, 18, 20, 22, 24, 27, 30, 33, 36, 42, 48, 54, and 60 months of age. Having parents or caregivers observe and complete the questionnaires is thought to enhance the screening process because of the variety and array of information parents or caregivers have about their children. This approach is consistent with the intent of the Individuals with Disabilities Education Act (IDEA) Amendments of 1997, which call for families to be involved in all phases of their child's assessment. The results, once collected and compiled, provide a basis for determining if further evaluation and assessment is needed to clarify parental concerns and current functioning level of the child.

SIDELIGHT: *Aki's Story*

Aki was preparing materials to send out to a family who had concerns about their 3-year-old son's language skills. Aki's supervising SLP recommended sending out a general information form, a case history form, a release of information, and an Ages and Stages Questionnaire. When Aki received the information back from the family, she scored the Ages and Stages Questionnaire and gave all of the forms to her supervising SLP for interpretation.

In addition to commercially produced screening instruments, your SLP may prefer to use informal tools that have been developed specifically for certain settings or populations. Often, agencies will develop their own screeners to meet the needs of the clients they screen and serve. Frequently, informal screeners are developed by various school districts in order to meet the demands of screening large groups of children in the quickest, most effective way. These informal screeners generally have some predetermined criteria for performances that would be considered passing or failing. This criterion is based on knowledge of developmental norms and the communication behaviors that have been determined as falling within the normal range for the setting and population for which they are being used.

Your Role and Responsibility in Screening

As an SLPA you will have three primary roles and responsibilities in screening the patient/client/student you are working with: supporting the SLP, being accurate and consistent, and remaining objective.

Support the SLP

Your primary role in the activity of screening is to support your supervising SLP. This support may take the form of clerical preparation for individuals or mass screenings such as copying and collating test protocols or entering name, date of birth information, and calculating chronological age. You may gather pictures or objects or help to set up a room that has been designated for a time of screening. In addition, you will be involved in administration of screening tests. You will locate students or patients, administer the screener, take notes and record responses and, finally, score the screener. You may also be responsible for transferring results of screening to specific master lists as indicated by your supervisor.

Accuracy and Consistency

It is your responsibility to follow procedures when you collect information or use a screening tool. Give the screener exactly as suggested by the published manual or by the procedures modeled by your SLP supervisor. Remember that when you stick to the standard and consistent method of giving the test, the scores will be more reliable. If you do not give the tool consistently (in the same manner as another examiner would), the performance you observe will neither be reliable nor valid. Therefore, you must spend a significant amount of time being trained to use a screening instrument. The old saying "practice, practice, practice" can be applied here easily. Practice giving the screener to a friend, roommate, or sibling. It does not matter what the responses are because the experience you gain in giving and scoring the screener as well as in making consistent, clear notations will be time well spent. The more familiar and consistent you are with giving and scoring a screener, the more confident you will be with your results. Your SLP supervisor will also have more confidence in your ability to screen and record responses consistently and efficiently.

It is critical for all of your notations to be accurate (Pellegrini, 1996). If you are the one giving the screener, then your SLP supervisor will not be able to remember the client's responses or behaviors because she was not there! Do not assume that she will know what you mean. In fact, assume just the opposite. Write errors and responses exactly as they occurred, giving the SLP as much information as possible regarding that particular client's performance. The SLP needs to know more than just how many items were right and how many items were missed. She needs to know what the error was. She needs to know how often the errors occurred and in what contexts, if possible. For example, if the student mispronounces the word "stick," then the SLP will want to know more than just the fact that "stick" was not pronounced correctly. Given your training in phonetic transcription, you will transcribe the exact production of the word in error. For example, /tIk/ for "stick." In other words, you must make clear notes of not only *what* was said but also *how* it was said.

In addition to error responses, you may record actions or behaviors that you observe (Pellegrini, 1996). This could include noting significant behaviors that occurred during your interaction with the client. For example, you might note that "Jill was coughing" or "Juan looked away from me. He gave eye contact two times within 5 minutes." Other significant behavior worth noting might include repeating sounds or words; blinking frequently; sounding hoarse or congested; not responding to questions or directions; appearing very tired, ill, extremely nervous; or if many repetitions were needed. Record behaviors such as "the client would not respond or repeat any of the items on the screener." This is all necessary and important information. The SLP takes all of the information that you provide about a student's performance into consideration as she interprets the screening results and makes decisions about the necessity of further testing and assessment. It is the SLP's job to interpret errors in terms of type, frequency, and her knowledge of developmental norms and sound processes. It is *your* job to provide the most accurate and consistent information as is possible.

SCREENING DO'S AND DON'TS FOR SLPAS

Do

- Fill in identifying information on the form or protocol.
- Organize and file screening materials.
- Accurately record responses and related behavior.
- Report objective information to your supervising SLP.

Don't

- Give a screening test that you have not been trained to use.
- Give a screening test that you have not practiced extensively.
- Interpret responses or make recommendations.
- Give a screener if conditions will not allow for the best performance.

Objectivity

Your notes and documentation of responses must be descriptions of only what you observe. When you factor in your own opinions, interpretations, or bias (your own perception, prejudice, or preconceived idea), you are no longer providing objective information. As an SLPA, you may not interpret, categorize, or label any of the client's behavior or responses. (See Chapter 2 for clarification on roles and responsibilities of the SLPA.) For example, you may note that "Hector used word and sound repetitions," but you may not state that he was "stuttering." As an SLPA, you may not diagnose or make recommendations. For example, noting "seemed to need many repetition of screening items" is acceptable but stating "receptive language problem" is not. See Figure 12-2. How would you describe the picture in Figure 12-2? The picture

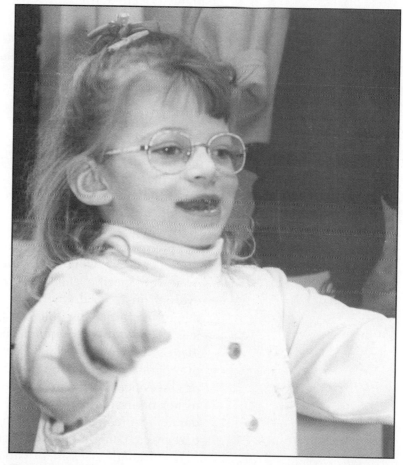

Figure 12-2 A 4-year-old girl eligible for a Child Find screening

was taken at a preschool and the girl is sitting in circle time, singing "The wheels on the bus go round and round." An objective statement describing the picture would be "A young girl with glasses and a pony tail in her hair has her mouth slightly open and her arms extended in front of her." From the picture, one cannot determine if her mouth is open because she is singing, talking, or breathing so that interpretation would need to stay out of an objective description. After giving the screener, you must also score it objectively by avoiding any personal bias or opinion regarding the client's performance as you tally the score. In other words, follow the procedures for getting a score or compiling results. See Figure 12-3 for nine screening habits of the highly effective SLPA.

ASSESSMENT AND EVALUATION

What Is It?

Although these terms are often used interchangeably, you need to understand what assessment and evaluation in the particular setting in which you are working mean. For example, the IDEA, as described in Chapter 8, which mandates certain types of evaluation or assessment be done for children, defines these terms in a specific way. As discussed in Chapter 6, certain predetermined criteria are delineated in the federal law, while state and district level policies determine the specific eligibility criteria to be used. The term **evaluation** is used when the purpose of the process is to determine initial eligibility for particular programs and services. The term **assessment** means an ongoing process to identify the child's unique strengths and needs for purposes of program planning and to measure progress. An evaluation or assessment often includes observing the child or student in her natural environment; reviewing prior medical or academic records; interviewing family members, teachers, or caregivers; completing checklists, or conducting tests.

Although assessment can be accomplished in a variety of ways, Bernstein (1997) discussed three purposes of eval-

Nine Screening Habits of Highly Effective SLPAs

SLPAs who are effective in screening demonstrate the following nine skills or abilities:

1.

Familiarity and training with tool: Has lots of practice with giving, recording, and scoring items on the screener. Knows the tool "backwards and forwards." Knows and follows standard guidelines for appropriate repeating of items, whether prompts are allowed and how to give feedback that will not affect results.

2.

Observation skills: Is consistently objective and can clearly describe communication behaviors. Is able to present screener items, ask questions, record, look, and listen all at the same time!

3.

Clear instructions: Gives instructions that are stated clearly and concisely. Knows how to vary instructions based on the client's age and setting. Recognizes when to clarify or when to repeat (Meyer, 1998).

4.

Accuracy in recording responses: Records all responses and observations with precision. Leaves little room for questions. Knows how to document responses as they occur and provides legible, accurate notes to the SLP (Meyer, 1998).

5.

Warm-up time: If needed, is able to use casual conversation (appropriate to a client's age and abilities) to help the nervous or reluctant person to relax and feel comfortable. Knows how to set a client "at ease" in a natural, appropriate manner and can do so quickly and efficiently.

6.

Questioning techniques: Knows how to use more open-ended questions rather than questions that limit the client to a one-word response. Recognizes that yes-no questions may be needed at first (especially with younger children or very reluctant clients) but then moves toward asking open-ended questions that allow for a variety of lengthier and more elaborate responses. For example, asking "Can you tell me about some of the toys you play with here at school" will likely elicit a longer utterance than to simply hold up a toy and ask, "Is this a truck?"

Figure 12-3 Practices of highly effective screeners (continues)

7.

Pace: Recognizes which clients need a slower or more rapid pace for moving through the screening items. Is able to modify the speed at which they question and the time they allow for responding based on individual needs and comfort level.

8.

Modeling: Has developed skill in providing more than one-word models. Knows that their model of longer sentences will more likely elicit longer utterances from the client. For example, modeling, "My cats are so silly. They chase each other around the house and wrestle. Tell me about your pet and what it does" is more likely to elicit a lengthier response than simply to ask the client if she has any pets.

9.

Flexibility and sensitivity to less-than-ideal screening conditions: Recognizes conditions that are not ideal for best performance from the client. Is sensitive to potential distractions (sound, sight, and physical) and responds with flexibility. For example, if the hallway is noisy, either relocates to another place or closes a door. If the child appears ill or very tired, considers doing the screening at another time. If the game box on the shelf is too distracting to a young child, moves it out of sight.

Figure 12-3 (continued)

uation: identifying individuals with speech or language disorders, developing intervention or therapy programs, and monitoring any changes resulting from invention programs. Some in the field have argued that "traditional" assessment practices (those relying heavily or exclusively on use of standardized test tools) are not able to offer enough direction in terms of planning for intervention such as developing goals

SIDELIGHT: *Marsha's Story*

Marsha's SLP was called by a nursing home to do a functional communication skills screening. Marsha was asked to help with the screening. The SLP administered the screening, and Marsha took a language sample and wrote down the nonverbal cues she noticed. She also took down data while the SLP was giving certain parts of the screener, because it contained information that is difficult to record on-line when giving those sections. The information she collected was very valuable to the SLP.

for the individual family service plan (IFSP) or the individual education plan (IEP) discussed in Chapter 8 (Kratcoski, 1998). As an SLPA, you will not be performing assessments on your own but you will need a basic understanding of the purposes of assessment and how you can assist your SLP in the process.

Three Purposes of Assessment

The three purposes of assessment are as follows.

To Identify Individuals With Speech or Language Disorders

If an individual has been screened or referred for potential speech-language difficulties, an assessment is done to determine whether that person truly exhibits a communication disorder. The assessment process and evaluation allow the SLP to gather information from many sources in her determination of whether a speech-language disorder is present and whether that person meets criteria for eligibility for services. In other words, does this person have a communication disorder and does she qualify (based on standard criteria) for speech or language therapy services? As noted, the criteria for eligibility for certain special education services can vary somewhat from setting to setting but as noted, within the schools, the criteria for determination of a condition and program eligibility are largely governed by IDEA and state and district policies. Sometimes, the SLP is assessing to determine whether a child is showing language differences or a true disorder. It is the role of the SLP to make these determinations. With adults the question may be more straightforward in the sense of "Does this challenge or interfere with daily communication?"

To Develop Intervention or Therapy Programs

The information that is gathered and measured during assessment can also be used to develop an intervention pro-

gram that is appropriate for the individual based on his needs and abilities. In order to design an intervention program that accurately addresses an individual's needs, the SLP will need to gain a better understanding of all components of communication. This means the SLP may assess many different areas, including articulation, phonology, semantics, syntax, and pragmatics as well as reading and writing. In determining intervention, the SLP and the team on with which she works, need to have the best understanding they can of the student or patient who is being assessed. Diagnosis, appropriate intervention, and determination of these least restrictive environment (LRE) are crucial outcomes of assessment (Bernstein, 1997) and are further documented in the IFSP or IEP generated for the child or student. Diagnosis, appropriate intervention, and measurement of benefit from service are critical outcomes when working with adults.

To Monitor Changes Resulting From Intervention

Another purpose for assessment is to determine whether intervention used with an individual has been effective. This type of assessment obviously occurs after such time as a patient has been receiving services. The SLP, the client, and the family want to know whether the program and therapy being used with the client is making a difference. They want to know whether changes need to be made, whether goals have been achieved, and whether the person's communication abilities have improved or become more functional. When the SLP assesses whether intervention has brought about any changes, she is then able to make many decisions as well as document progress and growth for payers of the services such as Medicare and insurance companies. She can decide about program effectiveness, conditions that may be getting in the way of progress, whether a student or individual responds favorably to particular methods, as well as whether the students or individual is applying newly learned behaviors in other communication settings (Bernstein, 1997).

THE THREE PURPOSES OF ASSESSMENT

1. To identify individuals with speech or language disorders
2. To develop intervention or therapy programs
3. To monitor changes resulting from intervention.

Assessment can also be done to effect learning and parent education objectives as parents gain an understanding of their child's abilities, strengths, and needs. In some instances it also serves the purpose of prevention because early identification of challenges in speech, language, and hearing can prevent later delays and disabilities in terms of severity of complications. For example, early identification of deafness can prevent language delays and disorders from developing (Yoshinaga-Itano et al., 1998).

Terminology of Assessment

Once the purpose of assessment has been established, the SLP determines *what* she will assess. Even a summary list of possible areas of communication that can be assessed is seemingly endless:

- Comprehension of language
- Expression of language
- Articulation
- Oral motor functioning
- Phonological processing
- Voice production
- Fluency of speech
- Emerging literacy
- Reading comprehension
- Written language
- Neurologically based disorders
- Dysphagia
- Metalinguistic awareness
- Pragmatic language

- Narrative discourse abilities
- Augmentative or alternative communication

Yes, it can seem overwhelming! You may be feeling grateful at this point that it is the role of the SLP to assess these areas. In any professional arena you enter, you will find it has a "language" of its own. The same is true for the field of speech-language pathology. Let us take a look at a few of the terms associated with assessment so that you will better understand their use as you support the SLP in assessment and evaluation processes.

Case History

Before assessing a client, the SLP or team will gather information related to the individual's difficulties, development, or family history, which is known as her **case history**. Case histories include information that is relevant to understanding, describing, and diagnosing a client's problems. This can be accomplished, in the case of a communicative adult, by simply asking the patient a series of questions surrounding family, school, physiological, speech, and developmental history. In the case of a child or an adult who is unable to respond to this type of information gathering, the SLP may interview the family (Peterson, 1994). Case histories may include reports from other professionals, medical records, hearing screening results, and socioeconomic information. The history information can be gathered as a team, or may involve one professional interviewing the family and then relaying that information to the other members of the team (Bernstein, 1997; Paul, 1995). Despite the fact that a standard case history questionnaire is often used, the interviewing process involves professional interpretation, inference, and skill. Therefore, it is not within the scope of your practice to conduct a client or family interview. You may, however, be asked to gather and complete identifying information (such as name, address, birth date, and phone number) on the questionnaire or to take notes and document responses made by the client or a family member.

Multidisciplinary Team

Multidisciplinary refers to an approach to assessment that involves more than one discipline or area of expertise that will be part of the process. Technically, the term implies that each professional will be responsible only for the areas of assessment (and ultimately, goal setting) that applies to her area. Obviously, if the "experts" are only concerned with their "piece" then the client's needs will not be considered or responded to as a "whole." Members of this team conduct their own assessments, write their reports independently, and typically are little influenced by one another.

Interdisciplinary Team

When a team is an **interdisciplinary team**, it is made up of members from more than one area of expertise; however, their approach to the assessment (and ultimately intervention) is made on the basis of a common goal (Lubinski, 1994). This team is usually coordinated by a **case manager**, who sets up specific methods of sharing information between team members or who facilitates a staffing that will better ensure that each discipline communicates with the others (Nelson, 1993). Interdisciplinary teams involve greater interaction among team members, with each member using information and suggestions from other members in interpreting their data. The report may often be written collaboratively (Westby, Stevens, & Detter, 1996)

Transdisciplinary Team

The term **transdisciplinary** is used to describe the collaborative approach of the team (Nelson, 1993). Multiple disciplines work together in the initial assessment (Westby et al., 1996). Paul (1995) describes it as "one individual may do all or most of the interaction with the child while others observe or make suggestions for the interactor to use during the assessment … team members help each other perform activities traditionally reserved within disciplines." See Chapter 13 for additional information regarding intervention.

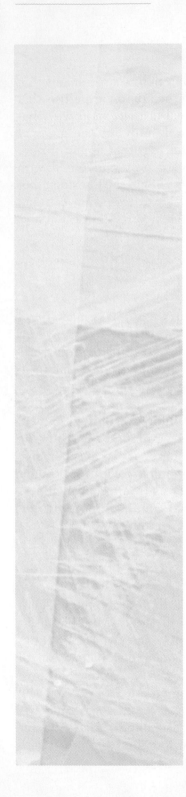

Diagnostic Evaluation or Case Study

When you think of diagnosis, you think of the medical use of the word—as in labeling or categorizing the disease or illness that the patient has. The diagnostic evaluation refers to the process by which the SLP, with a team of other professionals, give input as to their observations and findings regarding the student or client being assessed. The team, represented by a variety of areas of expertise, attempts to develop a whole "picture" of the client's strengths and weaknesses. Ultimately, the team determines a "categorical label used for educational placement or medical treatment" (Paul, 1995, p. 20).

Oral Facial/Peripheral Examination

An oral facial /peripheral examination looks at the structure, strength, coordination, and range of movement of the tongue, lips, teeth, jaw, breathing patterns, and other components involved in producing speech. The tools needed for this examination includes a flashlight, mirror, and latex gloves. The SLP looks at the basic structures of the mouth and then has the individual perform tasks to determine the structure's coordination and movement. One example is having the individual move her tongue from side to side, up and down, and to different areas of her mouth. It is an important part of any assessment of speech and language and may be modified to address the needs of young children as well as adults.

Stimulability

If a person has difficulty producing a particular sound, but can produce it correctly or can approximate the correct production with the help of the SLP providing models or cues, the individual is then considered **stimulable** for that sound.

Intelligibility

The term **intelligibility** relates to the degree an individual's speech is understood by others. It is often described as a percentage that is figured by counting the number of words that have been understood and dividing that by the total number of words spoken.

Assessment Methods

As an assistant to the SLP, you will need a basic understanding of the methods used in assessment. This will not only answer the question "How is assessment done?" but it may also answer the question "What are you doing?" as you observe your supervising SLP administering an assessment. There are four different ways that are often used by an SLP to assess an individual's communication skills: standardized tests, criterion-referenced tools, language and speech samples, and curriculum-based assessment (Maremore, Densmore, & Harman, 2001). Review assessment information from other classes or discuss how you would define and compare each. Even though the SLP will be performing assessments, the SLPA needs to understand the process of an assessment.

FOUR BASIC METHODS OF ASSESSMENT

- ■ Standardized Tests
- ■ Criterion-Referenced Tools
- ■ Language and Speech Samples
- ■ Curriculum-Based Assessment

Models of Assessment

In addition to the different methods of assessment, there are also different models or types of assessment. In Westby et al. (1996), further definitions of the models of assessments may be found. What do the assessments look like and how might you be involved in each of the following models of assessment: family-centered, transdisciplinary play-based, or arena-based assessment; dynamic assessment; and ecological models of assessment.

MODELS OF ASSESSMENT

- ■ Family-Centered Assessment
- ■ Transdisciplinary Play-Based/Arena-Based Assessment
- ■ Dynamic Assessment
- ■ Ecological Models of Assessment

Your Roles and Responsibilities in Assessment

Your role as an SLPA in assessment will vary according to state licensing, employer's guidelines, and your supervising SLP's guidelines, but the general process remains the same and is discussed as follows.

Before Assessment

Before an assessment is performed, you may be asked to:

- ■ Assist in screening
- ■ Prepare or complete a portion of the interview or case history questionnaire
- ■ Collect preassessment information such as hearing and vision results
- ■ Prepare and organize materials as directed by the SLP through verbal or checklist means
- ■ Fill in identifying information on test protocols
- ■ Compute the client's chronological age
- ■ Arrange the testing setting—tables, chairs, and equipment
- ■ Pick up the student or client and accompany her to the SLP's office or room
- ■ Test equipment to ensure proper functioning

During Assessment

During an assessment, you may be asked to:

- ■ Assist with materials, their introduction or removal

- Tally specific behavior
- Take notes from the SLP's dictation
- Elicit and tape record a speech or language sample
- Assist with a patient or student who is difficult to test
- Run a tape or video recorder

After Assessment

After the assessment, you may be asked to:
- Tally or tabulate test responses (no interpretation)
- Determine percentiles or standard scores from test manuals (no interpretation)
- Transfer raw scores to reporting sheets
- Enter data into a computer (software error analysis)
- Refile materials or unused test protocols
- Transcribe a speech or language sample (phonetic or orthographic)
- Tabulate feeding or swallowing results
- Convey brief messages to other team professionals (no interpretation)
- Make copies of the final SLP-written report of finding with recommendations

Supporting Assessment

You may be asked to support your SLP in the assessment processes in many ways. It is important to remember what has been discussed in previous chapters regarding your skill development in observation, your ability to record accurately, and your familiarity with the process of assessment. Knowledge about the types of assessment and your ability to maintain flexibility so that the highest quality of care is provided to the individuals being served is also critical as an SLPA.

CONCLUSION

This chapter has introduced new concepts and reviewed others that were dealt with in previous chapters regarding screening and assessment processes. It is critical that you understand the responsibilities and limitations of your role in screening and assessment activities so that you can provide appropriate assistance to your supervising SLP. This will ensure quality care is provided to those patients/clients/students being served. It is important that you understand the variety of tasks you may be asked to perform and that you seek additional guidance and support from your supervising SLP to fulfill your responsibilities in these areas. As always, your relationship to your supervisor is key with your success in assisting with these very important functions.

DISCUSSION QUESTIONS

1. Explain how observation skills are used in screening and assessment. How is observation different from assessment?

2. Review the following notations made by an SLPA on screening tests that she has given. Give your reasoning as to why the statements are either *within* or *beyond* her scope of practice as an assistant.

   -Shandra is missing top, two central incisors.

   -Evan's speech appears delayed for his age.

   -Jessica gave few responses, answered 2/8 questions.

   -Mrs. Johnson (teacher) said, "Molly isn't very bright."

   -Marco put his head on the table 3x during 10 minutes.

   -Corey stuck his tongue out at me—what a brat!

   -Josh needed frequent prompts to label the pictures.

   -3 misnamings noted: bag/box, fork/spoon, duck/chicken

   -Ladonna needs a full case study.

   -Mrs. Aragon's husband said, "There's nothing wrong with Marta. I want her discharged."

-Kendra is a severe stutterer.

-Mark needs therapy. The first grade articulation group would be perfect.

-2 instances of eye contact in 5 minutes of conversation.

-Vocal nodules if I've ever heard them!

-Be sure to test expressive vocabulary.

-Mrs. White presents with severe dysarthria.

-Mitchell sounded congested.

-There's nothing wrong with this lady's swallowing!

-Colton conversed easily.

3. State the importance of observing and accurately describing behaviors that represent communication delays, disorders, and differences.

4. How can you ensure that the observations you make during screening and assessment support is reliable and valid?

SUGGESTED ACTIVITIES

1. Make arrangements to observe in person or videotape a formal evaluation being conducted by an SLP. As you observe the activity of the SLP, list and describe five ways (within the scope of practice for an assistant) that you could assist the evaluation process.

2. Practice giving a screening tool (tool and number of administrations to be suggested by your instructor).

   Answer the following questions:

   ■ At what time did you begin to feel more at ease with giving the screener?

   ■ What issues arose that required flexibility on your part?

   ■ How consistent were you in your presentation of the items and in scoring performance?

   ■ Describe how results can be unreliable, if you gave or scored the screener inconsistently.

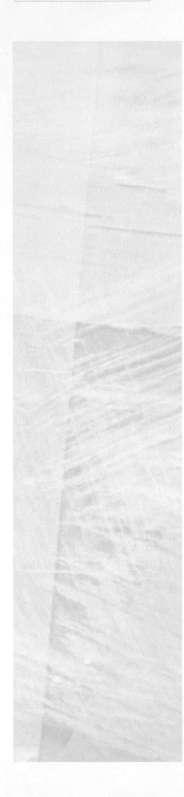

3. Make arrangements to visit a screening program in your area. Describe the qualifications of the individuals who conducted the screening and the population or clients being screened. Describe the instruments and procedures used. Interview one or more of the professionals involved, determining what criteria were considered when selecting their screening instrument.

REFERENCES

Bankson, N. & Bernthal, J. (1990). *Quick screen of phonology*. Chicago: Riverside.

Bernstein, (1997). *Language and communication disorders in children*. Boston: Allyn and Bacon.

Blakely, R. (1980). *Screening test for developmental apraxia of speech*. Tigard, OR: C. C. Publications.

Bricker, D., Squires, J., & Mounts, L. (1999). *Ages and stages questionnaire (ASQ)* (2nd ed.). Baltimore: Paul H. Brookes.

Brookshire, R. H. (1997). Chapter 5: The context for treatment of neurogenic communication disorders. In *Introduction to Neurogenic Communication Disorders*. St. Louis: Mosby.

Bruce, M. C., DiVenere, N., & Bergeron, C. (1998). Preparing students to understand and honor families as partners. *ASHA*, 7(3), 85–94.

Bureau, H. (1999). *Implementing universal newborn hearing screening programs* (p. 36). U.S. Department of Health & Human Services Public Health Service.

Bzoch, K., & League, R. (1991). *The Bzoch-League Receptive-Expressive Emergant Language Scale* (2nd ed.). Austin, TX: Pro-ed.

Carrow, E. (1973). *Screening test for auditory comprehension of language: English/Spanish*. Austin, TX: Learning Concepts.

Catts, H. W. (1997). Clinical exchange: The early identification of language-based reading disabilities. *Language, Speech, and Hearing Services in Schools, 28*(1), 86–89.

Chazdon, C. (1978). *Child Find: A handbook for implementation procedure and recommended guidelines*. Denver, CO: Colorado Department of Education.

Cockrell, J. R. & Folstein, M. F. (1988). Mini Mental State Examination (MMSE), *Psychopharmacology, 24*,689–692.

Cohen, L. (1994). *Assessment of young children*. New York: Longman.

Crum, R. M., Anthony, J. C., Bassett, S. S., & Folstein, M. F. (1993). Population-based norms for the Mini-Mental State Examination by age and educational level. *Journal of the American Medical Associaiton, 18*, 2386–2391.

Feeney, J. B. (1996). The efficiency of the revised Denver Developmental Screening Test as a language screening tool. *Language, Speech, and Hearing Services in Schools, 27*(4), 330–332.

Fluharty, N. (2001). *Fluharty Preschool Speech and Language Screening Test (Fluharty-2)*. Austin, TX: Pro-ed.

Folstein, M. F., Folstein, S. E., & McHugh, P. R. (1975). Mini-Mental State:A practical method for grading the state of patients for the clinician. *Journal of Psychiatric Research, 12*, 189–198.

Hadley, P. A. (1998). Language sampling protocols for eliciting text-level discourse. *Language, Speech, and Hearing Services in Schools, 29*, 132–147.

Huang, R. J., Hopkins J., & Nippold, M. A. (1997). Satisfaction with standardized language testing: A survey of speech-language pathologists. *Language, Speech, and Hearing Services in Schools, 28*(1), 12–29.

Jitendra, A. K., & Rohena-Diaz, E. (1996). Language assessment of students who are linguistically diverse: Why a discrete approach is not the answer. *The School Psychological Review, 25*(1).

Kayser, H. (1996). Cultural/linguistic variation in the United States and its implication for assessment and intervention in speech-language pathology: An epilogue. *Language, Speech, and Hearing Services in Schools, 27*, 385–387.

Keith, R. (1986). *SCAN: A screening test for auditory processing disorders.* San Antonio, TX: The Psychological Corporation.

Kratcoski, A. M. (1998). Guidelines for using portfolios in assessment and evaluation. *Language, Speech, and Hearing Services in Schools, 29*(1), 3–10.

Lewis, P. (1997). Applying research. *ASHA, 39*(2), 50–51.

Lichtenstein, R. (1984). *Preschool screening: Identifying young children with developmental and educational problems.* Orlando: Grune and Stratton.

Lidz, C. (1996). Dynamic assessment: The model, its relevance as a non-biased approach, and its application to Latino American preschool children. *Language, Speech, and Hearing Services in Schools, 27*, 367–372.

Lubinski, R. F. (1994). *Professional issues in speech-language pathology and audiology: A textbook.* San Diego, CA: Singular.

Management, M. C. f. H. A. a. (2000). Fact sheet. Logan: Utah State University.

Maremore, R. C., Densmore, A. E., & Harman, D. R. (2001). *Assessment and treatment of school-age language disorders: A resource manual.* San Diego, CA: Singular-Thomson Learning.

Meisels, S. C. (1990). *Who should be served? Identifying children in need of early intervention. Handbook of early childhood intervention.* Cambridge, MA: University Press.

Meyer, S. (1998). *Survival guide for the beginning speech-language clinician.* Aspen.

Meyer, S. M. (1993). *Survival guide for the beginning speech-language clinician.* Aspen.

Miller, L. (1993). First step: Screening test for evaluating preschoolers. San Antonio, TX: The Psychological Corporation Harcourt Brace Jovanovich, Inc.

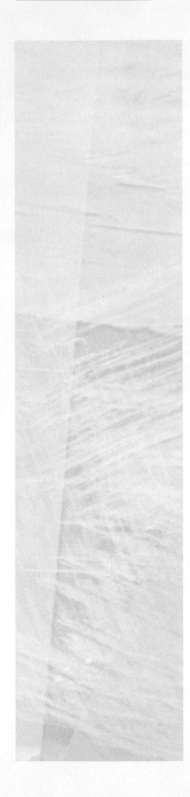

Morgan, D., & Guilford, A. (1984). *Adolescent language screening test (ALST)*.Tampa, FL: University of South Florida.

Mutti, M, Sterling, H., & Spalding, N. (1978). *Quick neurological screening test, revised edition.* Novato, CA: Academic Therapy.

Nelson, N. W. (1993). *Childhood language disorders in context: Infancy through adolescence.* Bellevue, WA: Merril Press.

Paul, R. (1995). *Language disorders from infancy through adolescence: Assessment & intervention.* St. Louis: Mosby.

Pellegrini, A. D. (1996). *Observing children in their natural worlds.* Mahwah, NJ: Lawrence Erlbaum Associates.

Peterson, H. A. (1994). *Appraisal and diagnosis of speech and language disorders.* Upper Saddle River, NJ: Prentice-Hall, Inc.

Semiel, E., Wiig, E., & Secord, W. (1995). *Clinical Evaluation of Language Fundamentals 3rd Edition (CELF-3).* San Antonio, TX: The Psychological Corporation, Harcourt, Brace & Company.

Shames, G. H., Wiig, E., & Secord, W. A. (1998). *Human communication disorders: An introduction.* Boston: Allyn and Bacon.

Spivak, L. G. (Ed.). (1998). *Universal newborn hearing screening.* New York: Thieme Medical Publishers.

Stockman, I. J.(1996). The promises and pitfalls of language sample analysis as an assessment tool for linguistic minority children. *Language, Speech, and Hearing Services in Schools, 27*(4), 355–366.

Toronto, A. (1973). *Screening test of Spanish grammar.* Evanston, IL: Northwestern University Press.

Westby, C., Stevens, D. M., & Oetter, P. (1996). A performance/competence model of observational assessment. *Language, Speech, and Hearing Services in Schools, 27,* 144–152.

Wyatt, T. (1977). Developing a culturally sensitive preschool screening tool. *ASHA, 39*(2), 50–51.

Yoshinaga-Itano, C., Sedey, A. L., Coulter, D. K., & Mehl, A. L. (1998). Language of early- and later-identified children with hearing loss. *Pediatrics, 102,* 1161–1171.

CHAPTER 13

Intervention

Key Concepts

◾

Intervention, as applied to the field of speech-language pathology, is used to describe what is done to facilitate changes in the speech and language behaviors of individuals with communication challenges.

◾

Successful intervention is based on an individualized program and ongoing assessment.

◾

Intervention results in the individual being able to use the forms and functions targeted in the intervention to communicate more effectively.

◾

The service delivery models (one on one, group, consultation) may vary across settings, but the overall goal of intervention, related to improvement in communication abilities, remains the same.

◾

Current trends in intervention focus on individualized, family-centered, culturally competent, team-based practices that are seated in improving the ability of individuals to independently use their speech and language abilities to communicate and learn.

Overview

◾

Review of Service Delivery Models Across Settings

◾

Current Trends in Intervention

◾

Practical Considerations in Supporting Your SLP

◾

Two Sample Snapshots of Intervention Approaches and Techniques

◾

Key Components of the Intervention Process

◾

Basic Principles for Guiding Behavior and Facilitating Social Interactions

◾

Enhancing Effectiveness in Intervention

Key Concepts continued

Ways to support and assist your SLP center on activities that involve appropriate preparation, implementation of SLP-designed intervention programs, and documentation of progress.

■

There are a wide variety of intervention approaches and techniques, but those used must fit the individual needs of the person receiving services.

■

Basic principles of guiding behavior and facilitating social interactions are keys to successful intervention.

■

Self-reflection regarding your skills will enhance your abilities to effectively implement intervention programs.

INTRODUCTION

Schiefelbusch (1983, p. 15) defines intervention in speech-language pathology as "an act of assistance." This means what is done to facilitate improved performance in targeted language goals and objectives in the intervention process. Goals and objectives are based on individualized needs determined through initial assessment and are modified based on ongoing assessment of progress. Thus intervention must link to assessment. It has been described by Weiss (1997, p. 275) as the "use of instructional contexts designed to facilitate speech and language abilities." The approach used may differ in terms of who is involved in the intervention, where the intervention takes place, and the degree of structure imposed on the individual in the instructional context.

It is important to note that the goal of intervention is to "make itself obsolete." The objective of any intervention program is to foster independence and new learning. This leads to "eliminate its rationale for existence by demonstrating that the individual is ready for dismissal" (Bernstein & Tiegerman-Farber, 1997 p. 75). This is a critical concept. Your SLP will determine when and how much intervention is needed and what role you will play as an SLPA. For example, a child with cerebral palsy who can use his communication device proficiently to communicate his ideas and formulate

his thoughts has demonstrated his ability to access his learning curriculum in school. He may be ready for dismissal from therapy. The aim is for the patient, client, or student to learn strategies that facilitate new learning. Once the ability to self-monitor or self-correct is established, the individual can extend new learning without the clinician's input.

Let us consider another example that involves intensive voice treatment in which the individual learns to monitor or "calibrate" his voice level output or intensity through instruction in sessions and practice with a handheld electronic device. Vocal intensity has been documented to be a critical factor in the intelligibility of speech, especially for patients with Parkinson's disease. Given the progressive nature of this disorder and its impact on speech intelligibility, it is important for patients to practice increasing and maintaining a "loud voice." The Lee Silverman Voice Treatment Program (Ramig, Countryman, O'Brien, Hoehn, & Thompson, 1996) has developed an intensive treatment protocol (approximately 16 sessions) that teaches the individual how to maintain his voice quality and affect his intelligibility through practice. This treatment focuses on increased loudness of productions. If patients can incorporate these skills into daily activities, they have been found to sustain gains realized through generalization to everyday communicative interactions. They have thus become independent of the provider of services. They may not need continued intensive programming if they are able to sustain changes realized through treatment.

It is a very different story for a young child in a preschool setting who has been identified with specific language impairment. Because language learning is a developmental process, intervention can close the gap between current functioning level and age-appropriate indicators for language use. However, because early language difficulties are predictive of later learning disabilities (Catts & Kamhi, 1997; Dickenson & Tabors, 2001; Fey, 1998), there is no guarantee that the student will be able to continue to bridge the gap on his own. This is especially true as language learning becomes more **decontextualized**. Decontextualization happens when there is no longer a context provided such as when older students are asked to read from a text book without pictures or explanations that help them understand the

material. Demands for vocabulary knowledge increase. As students become older, the concepts they are expected to understand become more abstract. Expectations regarding ability to complete more difficult academic work increase. This is why we see students in our public school system continue to need related services in language and learning abilities. Their language disorder becomes a learning disability that continues to affect academic performance and appropriate access to the regular curriculum. Language-based disorders may interfere with development of reading skills (Catts & Kahmi, 1999; Paul, 2001) and have the potential to be a problem of longstanding for the students themselves, their families, school personnel and the SLP and other related service personnel charged with teaching them.

The vast majority of SLPs (89.3 %) serve children with language disorders. (American Speech-Language-Hearing Association [ASHA]. 1999 Omnibus Survey). This statistic helps document why language interventions are needed in public school systems. It is not surprising that language and communication challenges occur in a significant number of the population, and those identified in early childhood are documented to continue to be part of the social, academic, and communicative life of the school-age student. Speech and language disorders are also associated with many medical issues that may be present at birth such as a cleft lip and palate, cerebral palsy, deafness. Disorders can occur throughout the lifespan of an individual such as a stroke, brain injury, an acquired hearing loss, or visual impairments. The underlying cause for many disorders such as stuttering has not been conclusively determined, yet research continues in this area. Communication is a part of everyday life, and impairment of this ability will most likely compromise learning, function, and the quality of life in some respect. Disorders have been traditionally categorized in terms of their impact on speech or language, although many individuals present with challenges in both areas. Disorders may be described as mild, moderate, or severe. Incidence figures vary anywhere from 10% to 22% of the population. This means that one in five individuals may experience a speech or language problem that affect his communication abilities at some point in his life. Thus speech and language services are very much needed by a significant

number of individuals who are identified as having speech-language or hearing disorders. The length, intensity, and types of intervention may vary significantly across populations, but the need for services will continue.

REVIEW OF SERVICE DELIVERY MODELS ACROSS SETTINGS

Intervention programs may look very different, depending on the individual needs of the patient, client, or student; the setting for service delivery; and the type of intervention provided. Service delivery models in school settings may include:

- Self-Contained Classrooms
- "Pullout" Services: Individual or Group
- Classroom-Based/ Integrative Service Delivery
- Collaborative Consultation
- Parent Support Programs and In-Service Education

Self-Contained Classrooms

In the school setting, you may see a continuum of service delivery models used by your SLP. **Self-contained classrooms** are sometimes used to group those children with similar disabilities and may be considered the **least restrictive environment (LRE)** for children who cannot function well or benefit from their education in a regular classroom setting. Self-contained classrooms may be staffed with special education teachers. Sometimes SLPs work intensively or coteach in these programs to meet the individualized needs of students in collaboration with the special education teacher. With the advent of greater attempts toward "full inclusion" of children in their least restrictive setting (LRE), many self-contained or what has also been termed "segregated programs" have been eliminated or reduced in number. This is consistent with the legislative intent of IDEA as explained in Chapter 11. If you work with this model, you will most likely work along side of your SLP with a small number of children with significant impairments in speech and language. Many advocates for full inclusion object to this type of programming on principle and question why these students are segregated for the greater part of their day in separate classroom environments.

A SELF-CONTAINED CLASSROOM

The Choice Program is a self-contained classroom-based program for students who are described as having significantly limited intellectual capacity (SLIC) or are described as having severe profound disabilities. These students often perform at significantly low levels on IQ tests as administered by psychologists and are described as "mentally retarded" or "overall **developmentally delayed.**" They are primarily segregated in smaller size classrooms with a resource teacher or special educator to receive intensive services and a separate curriculum. The SLP will often work with this team to provide services focused on functional communication.

Pullout

Many SLPs in public school settings continue to use a traditional **pullout** model of service delivery. They may schedule students to leave their regular classroom to receive individual therapy sessions once a week for 20 minutes to up to several times per week. They may pull out students from the regular classroom to work in small groups. Again, groupings may be based on types of communication challenge experienced by the students such as articulation problems or language-based reading problems associated with identified phonological deficits. Individual therapy sessions are sometimes reserved for the children who have more significant challenges. However, there are concerns regarding pullout in that it singles out a child for having a problem. Teachers and parents may be concerned about stigmatizing a student as different. They may also be concerned about removing the student from a context in which he can learn and practice his language in context-based routines. They may express the opinion that teaching skills out of context in a contrived setting may work against generalization of new learning unless steps to ensure generalization are implemented in a systematic way.

SIDELIGHT: *Brenda's Story*

Brenda's IEP stipulated that she be seen for speech-language therapy two times a week for 20 minutes to work on objectives related to her speech. Her SLP wanted to provide pullout services once a week individually and then include her in a follow-up group session with her SLPA for practice one other time a week for 20 minutes. Consultation to the classroom teacher regarding monitoring of "transfer" of specific targeted objectives was also provided. Although "pullout" services were the common practice in this school, her parents questioned why 20 minutes twice a week was the recommended level for service. They questioned how less than an hour of attention per week could result in changes in her speech.

Small Group Work

Group work is increasing given the impact from the number of children who are identified who can benefit from services. This is influenced by the shortage of appropriately qualified SLPs to provide services. A significant number of SLPs are concerned about increasing caseloads as numbers of identified students increase. Many SLPs attempt to manage their overall workload by providing services through a combination of models so they can serve more students. The **itinerant** SLP or traveling SLP who serves children in several schools may have a caseload of 50 students. ASHA has been concerned with this issue, because caseloads are reportedly much higher in several areas of the country. This compromises both the intensity and quality of services that can be provided. Several school districts are initiating models that require an SLP to provide service only in one site or building, so that time and focus on teaming and collaboration can be provided. Caseload size is thus kept low and enables the SLP to provide the services needed. However, the caseload size of an SLP working in the schools will often vary, depending on the types of services provided and the severity of needs of the students served. SLPs in the schools are often "generalists" and must be ready to serve students presenting with a wide range of disabilities. Caseloads may include children with autism, augmentative alternative communication (AAC) needs, students who are deaf or hard of hearing, or students with speech disorders such as stuttering, developmental articulation problems, or motor speech

issues such as dyspraxia, or dysarthria, and any student with a language-based learning disability or language problem that interferes with academic achievement. This may include students with cognitive impairments associated with mental retardation, head injury, or other developmental disabilities that include speech and language delays or disorders. Given increased demands for services from the SLP, a well-trained SLPA can prove invaluable to maintain the quality of service delivery provided to students in this setting.

Classroom-Based Services

Classroom based services, sometimes termed **integrative therapy**, allow SLPs to focus on students' needs within the context of their everyday routines and learning activities. Many SLPs will provide services within this context to reach an increased number of students as well as to make therapy more meaningful and relevant. Most often this model implies a team approach with the classroom teacher and other related service personnel who may be involved in providing intervention. A team approach is needed so that service providers are not working at cross-purposes from the classroom teacher and that the involvement of another adult is not seen as a distraction. This model of service delivery is often seen in preschool and kindergarten settings, because speech and language intervention is so easily integrated into the children's daily routines and activities. This model of service delivery may occur more often, given current trends for team-based services that are culturally relevant and "naturalistic" in nature. These trends are further described in other sections of this chapter. According to Bernstein & Tiegerman-Farber (1997, p. 280), this model is based on an appreciation for the social foundations of language development and the contextual support that is needed for students to integrate new learning.

Collaborative Consultation

Collaborative consultation is a term that demands definition. It is used to describe a continuum of activities between the regular classroom teacher and the SLP (Marvin, 1990). It is

often the strategy used to implement classroom-based service. Collaboration has been frequently defined as an "unnatural act committed by nonconsenting adults." Although intended as humor, this speaks of the effort and energy necessary for collaborative work to succeed. It takes time and energy to make collaborative plans and implement the plans as developed. Given the current atmosphere of pressure for increased productivity and effective utilization of resources, it is often difficult to set aside the time necessary to make this happen. Consultation has also been defined as "if I had known what was involved, I would have done it myself." This is obviously a play on words based on the time and energy needed to get all the people involved in a student's program "on the same page." It means time for meetings, individualized education plan (IEP) staffings, phone calls, or other means of communication with teachers and other specialists. This may be difficult to schedule or set up for the many people involved.

Again, consultation is a term that can carry many meanings. In this context, a model of consultant as "expert," an outsider coming in to tell the teacher what to do, has been replaced with a concept of reciprocal information sharing. This newer model recognizes the SLP and the teacher are on equal footing and need to work together to brainstorm creative and innovative ways to integrate speech and language goals into the existing curriculum for a particular student. SLPs may spend time observing the student in the classroom, studying the classroom curriculum, and giving suggestions for using the classroom as a language learning environment. Prelock (2000) discusses the ways a consultation model can be implemented. Activities may involve assessment, goal setting, planning, and implementation of intervention for students with identified communication problems as well as for students at risk. Such strategies as simply providing information in written form, collaboratively planning with the teacher, or working directly with students to demonstrate a strategy or model of interaction, can be implemented depending on what the teacher wants and is ready to receive. Marvin (1990), notes that within this model, the classroom teacher serves as the primary interventionist for the child with language and learning disorders. It

can be helpful if there is a third person to observe and record desired behaviors or collect data relevant to the specific student receiving this form of intervention. In some situations, the SLPA may take on the responsibility to be the third person in this scenario. The SLPA may also assist the SLP in supporting the classroom teacher by preparing materials, monitoring individual work, supporting and directly assisting students when needed, or implementing other strategies for data collection.

Parent Support Programs and In-service Education

Parent support programs and in-service education programs may take the form of workshops that provide family members, teachers, or other professionals with the information they need to facilitate changes in speech and language behaviors. The goal is to provide the information about strategies that can work at home or in everyday routines, activities, and places. These types of programs are increasing, especially in early care and education settings. Oftentimes the message is one of prevention. Programs deal with strategies that family members can use at home to facilitate the child's language learning and prevent the severity or the occurrence of later academic or communication issues. Specific programs designed for early intervention and prevention can be used by the trained SLP to support parents' education and learning. Workshop formats are sometimes used to foster parent-to-parent sharing and interaction. Interactive storybook reading strategies (Whitehurst et al., 1988, 1994), focus on parent interaction skills during storybook reading. These types of interactions have proven successful in increasing the oral language abilities as well as literacy learning activities of children with and without disabilities. The SLPA has a role to play in preparing materials and activities that can make a difference. An SLP may bring parents or other providers together to explore prevention or intervention activities that facilitate goals and objectives for individual students as a way of promoting generalization of targeted behaviors. SLPAs may work with their supervising SLP to prepare for and implement these workshops or in-

service trainings, depending on the audience and goals to be achieved.

Hospital or Agency Programs

Parallel delivery of service models might be seen in other settings, depending on the types of communication disorders seen or the focus on population served. For example, in a hospital setting, service may be provided in **acute care units** where the service provided involves screening and ongoing assessment and short-term intervention for the child or adult with stroke, traumatic injury, or other medically related condition. The SLP may serve on an inpatient rehabilitation team in this setting and work with other medically related disciplines (PT, OT, psychology, social work, physicians) to provide rehabilitative intervention to individuals, children or adults, who have suffered head injury, strokes, or other medically related problems. Specific to the hospital setting is the neonatal intensive care unit (NICU) for newborns and infants or the intensive care unit (ICU) for older patients who have suffered traumatic injury or medical problems. SLPs may or may not be involved in providing services to patients needing intensive care often related to critical medical conditions. However, if the SLP is involved, then the SLPA may play a role in preparation of materials or documentation of services to these patients. SLPAs may be more involved in the care of those patients seen in outpatient services or clinics. In these programs the individual is coming back to the hospital, often for traditional individual or group speech-language services. The SLPA may be asked to provide several practice sessions supplemental to individual sessions that the SLP schedules with the individual on an outpatient basis. The SLPA would support the implementation of these programs given the delegation of intervention activities according to the treatment plan designed by the supervising SLP.

Home Health Services

Home health services may also be a service delivery model used by the SLP. Again, depending on the nature of the disorder and treatment goals and objectives, the SLPA may be

involved in providing individual sessions to a designated patient or in preparing materials as needed for this service. If services are provided in the home on a follow-up basis, adequate on-site supervision can be a barrier to the delegation of intervention follow-through activities to the SLPA.

Skilled Nursing Facility (SNF)

The SLPA may also work with an SLP in a **skilled nursing facility (SNF)**, which is a service available for long-term care of patients who are not ready for discharge. Because of related medical conditions, these patients need extended care and nursing support in a full-service facility. Service from the SLP may focus on dysphagia or swallowing and feeding issues as well as functional communication. Although the SLPA cannot participate in swallowing or feeding activities given the ASHA delineated scope of responsibilities and the ASHA Code of Ethics (2001), they may work with the SLP to develop adaptations of modifications of the environment to support functional communication in daily routines. They may implement programs with care providers that enhance abilities and systems for communication of desires, needs, and concerns.

Rehabilitation Center

As noted in previous chapters, the SLPA may also be employed in a rehabilitation center or agency that provides services to adults following traumatic illness or injuries. The service delivery models used will most likely be individual or small group sessions and family education or support programs and in-service training. It is also important to mention that SLPAs may be employed as support personnel in a variety of other settings such as private preschools or special schools focused on appropriate programming for individuals with a specific challenge such as substance abuse or psychiatric or emotional disorders, brain injury, or learning disabilities. SLPAs may also be employed in private practices or agencies that provide individual or group outpatient service to a wide range of children and adults with communication challenges. You may therefore be able to find a setting as an

SLPA that enables you to work with a wide variety of individuals with a wide variety of challenges that affect their speech and language. This is one of the reasons why this position is so interesting.

CURRENT TRENDS IN INTERVENTION

Individualized Programs

Individualization is key to successful intervention. It implies a connection or link with assessment that determines the individual's overall pattern of abilities and includes a focus on strengths and needs in terms of speech, language, and literacy. It speaks of the issue of responsive practices that fit or match the individual profile and needs of the patient, client, or student. For example, it can be said with some assurance that no one child with autism is like any other. This implies that no one therapy approach or program can meet the needs of all individuals with a specific type of problem. One size does not fit all. There are certainly commonalities, but each intervention program must be specifically designed to match the needs of the individual receiving services.

Family-Centered Practice

Principles of family-centered care or practices have been reviewed in Chapter 4 of this text and are considered to be a critical component of intervention service to individuals with communication challenges. Family members' values, concerns, and priorities are respected, and their input is considered to be integral to intervention planning and implementation. Many programs, especially in early intervention, are designed to enhance communication interactions between caregiver and child (see Figure 13-1). There is also a trend to focus more intentionally on communication partner training for adults with speech and language problems secondary to aphasia or head injury or training of communication partners for individuals with AAC needs.

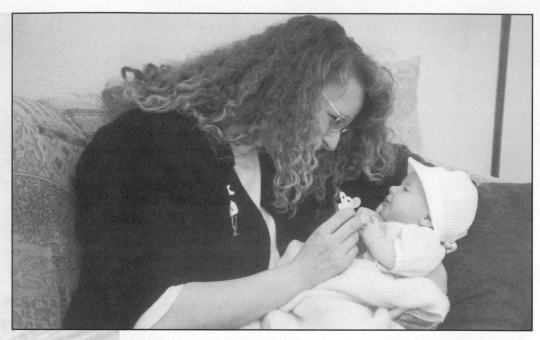

Figure 13-1 A natural environment with focus on parent-child interaction

Natural Environments

Consistent with the focus on inclusion of family members in all phases of intervention is the value placed on community-based services and supports. Early intervention in the **natural environment** is mandated by IDEA (1997) for infants and toddlers, birth to 3 years old and their families. The law defines natural environments as those places the child and family would be but for the fact they have an identified disability. Community-based intervention programs for adults will follow the same pattern with a focus on integration and practice of specific goals and objectives in daily routines, activities, and places. These programs intend to enhance functional communication and generalization of outcomes in a meaningful context. Intervention may be integrated into trips to the store, small group outings to a restaurant, writing process groups at the library, or other activities. This allows participants to practice generalization of communication function in real-life situations.

NATURAL ENVIRONMENT INTERVENTION PROGRAMS

Natural environment intervention programs can include:

- Home-based intervention
- Intervention in community-based activities and settings in which a given family typically participates (swim class, gymnastics, horseback riding, playgrounds, parks, hiking, etc.)
- Intervention in early care and education settings such as childcare homes or centers
- Parent and family groups and other community educational opportunities

Team-Based Intervention

As noted and discussed in Chapter 5 of this text, there is also the trend for team-based or **integrative therapy** services. The SLP and SLPA work with providers from other disciplines to develop and implement comprehensive intervention plans in meaningful contexts. Intervention programs require the expertise of many professionals to provide quality care and eliminate fragmentation of services provided. The family is increasingly considered to be a partner and integral team member in effecting change for the individual receiving service, whether in the school setting, the NICU, or the rehabilitation unit. Teams of professionals are evolving their practice to include more intentional focus on collaboration and teaming, integrated services, and comprehensive management of the individual with challenges.

This type of intervention is consistent with the current trend or value of full inclusion of individuals with disabilities into all phases and aspects of community life. In schools, students with disabilities must be placed in the LRE, meaning in their home school or regular classroom. They can only be placed in more restrictive programs, if they are determined to need such placements, because they cannot receive full benefits from accessing the regular curriculum. This is also true of younger children covered under Part C of IDEA, which stipulates children must receive intervention in the

"natural environment." This holds unless a more specialized setting, such as a hospital or outpatient clinic, is needed based on their disability as determined through the IFSP process. The value of full inclusion reflects the idea that everyone belongs, including individuals with disabilities. Formally, individuals with disabilities were frequently institutionalized or segregated from the rest of society. Over time, mainstreaming happened so that individuals with disabilities were "let in" to public schools and participate in nonacademic activities such as recess, art, or music. Eventually the concept of full inclusion evolved and greater numbers of students with disabilities were educated in regular classrooms. Full inclusion implies a sense of "belonging" from the beginning and thus focuses on interventions as integral to everyday routines, activities, and places with emphasis on full community participation.

Cultural Competence

Cultural competence also fits with the concept of full inclusion in that "all means all." It also goes beyond equal access and opportunity to include a focus on respect and celebration of diverse languages, values, and differences. It implies a willingness to listen and learn from families and representatives of cultures different from our own and a commitment to try, understand, accept, and resolve cultural conflicts when they interfere with intervention practices and programs. Chapter 6 in this text reviews several strategies that reflect a commitment to develop cultural competence in intervention practices. The SLPA can enhance intervention supports and services by developing culturally competent and responsive attitudes and practices that support the SLP in intervention.

Technology

Current advances in technology have changed the face of intervention for many individuals with communication challenges. Examples include:

- Augmentative alternative communication devices, including both "low tech" and "high tech" dedicated devices with computer interface capability and peripheral software to enhance language learning and communication

- Improved amplification with digital, programmable hearing aids
- Computer-enhanced learning programs to facilitate language and literacy learning as depicted in Figure 13-2
- Educational software such as interactive storybooks, writing workshop
- Computer programs and technological equipment that enhance assessment and documentation such as the visipitch and videostroboscopy
- Cochlear implants for hard-of-hearing individuals
- Peripheral software to enhance access to computers such as touch screens and switches
- Other assistive devices and equipment

Technology continues to change and the challenge is to keep up with innovations and advances in available equip-

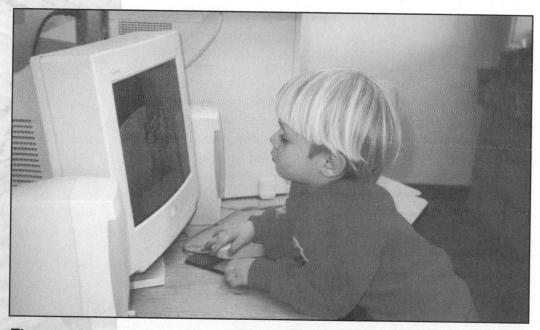

Figure 13-2 Technology facilitates interest and practice

ment and software. The SLPA has a potentially important role in enhancing access and implementation of intervention with computer-enhanced learning programs. These often encourage intensive practice of targeted goals and objectives. Having the support of an SLPA who has the technological "know how," interest, and ability to "troubleshoot" and maintain equipment, including computers, computer software, and programming of dedicated communication devices, will prove invaluable. It will enable the supervising SLP to spend more time in direct service delivery, assessment, or designing intervention programs and result in improved access of the individual to equipment and technology as a support to the intervention program.

The term augmentative alternative communication (AAC) refers to communication methods used by nonspeaking individuals and includes:

- Use of sign language
- Gesture
- Facial expressions and eye gaze
- Use of alphabet or picture symbol boards or systems
- An increasing number of sophisticated computer systems with synthesized speech and access options

AAC is now integrated into the mainstream of communication options for individuals with severe speech impairments so you will see these devices or methods being used across many settings that serve individuals with severe speech impairments. There has been an explosion in the past several years in AAC products and available related access devices. AAC has emerged as an area of specialization in speech-language pathology given the rapid advances in the field and the supportive legislation of the Technology Act and the Americans With Disabilities Act (ADA) described in Chapter 8. If you are particularly interested in learning about AAC applications, obtain a copy of a comprehensive text such as the *Handbook of Augmentative and Alternative Communication* by Glennon and DeCoste (1997) or attend a conference that focuses on hands-on applications of assistive technology such as Closing the Gap or the California State University Northridge (CSUN) Conference. Many states have rich resources developed given funding from the

Technology Act and hold statewide conferences and provide services and supports such as bank loans and instructional workshops to consumers and service providers. Continuing education will help you learn more about this topic. SLPAs might consider AAC or assistive technology as a potential area of specialization. It requires additional specific training regarding available systems, operational procedures, and use of these systems in a communication and learning context. Much of this information can be self-taught by observing AAC specialists, attending conferences focused on AAC training, and interacting with product representatives to learn the specifics of particular devices, their unique features, and programming strategies. Again, your knowledge of operational system features, maintenance of equipment, and programming capabilities of specific devices will prove invaluable to the SLP serving nonspeaking populations. AAC has also been frequently used on a temporary basis as a language learning strategy. Young children or adults find many of the techniques or equipment useful in functional communication situations and the technology is effective in facilitating efforts to learn or regain speech and language.

Peer Support

Peer-mediated learning or peer support is a recent trend in intervention that is receiving increased attention. The use of peers to support full inclusion has been an ongoing practice in many public schools and community programs. It has long been recognized that inclusion in a normalized situation helps the individual with a disability to develop or regain critical communication skills. This is true of young preschool children who interact with typically developing peers, as well as older adults who benefit from a peer coach or model in communicative interactions. The more intentional use of peers to enhance sociocommunicative interactions is being systematically investigated to look at the efficacy of such an approach. Peer coaching or mediation is used as an intervention strategy with many individuals with communication challenges, but has received more recent attention in programs designed to facilitate language learning in children with autism. Specific social skills' training has become part of many inclusive programs that have children with disabilities. Another example includes children who are deaf or hard of hearing. Peer support and modeling naturally happen in the context of an articulation group of inclusive preschool program and has been shown to impart significant benefits to both the individual with disabilities as well as the typically developing peers (Figure 13-3).

The current trends taking place in the profession and in health care and education combine with options for service delivery models to create innovative ways of providing services to individuals with communication challenges across settings. There are also counteracting realities such as reduced budgets, strains on existing resources, and shortages of appropriately trained personnel, especially from linguistically diverse populations. The intensive focus on standards and high-stakes testing in public schools sometimes acts as a detriment to putting energy and resources into intervention. Productivity pressures, health care reform, increased paperwork, and third-party reimbursement issues are also contributing factors to low morale among health care

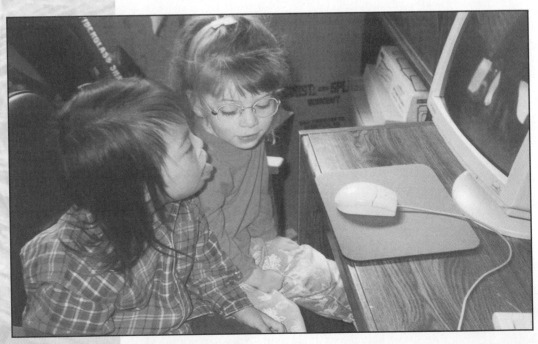

Figure 13-3 Peer support

providers and school personnel. As an SLPA, you will work with your supervising SLP to counteract any negative interference from these factors on quality of services provided.

PRACTICAL CONSIDERATIONS IN SUPPORTING YOUR SLP

Preparation is a key factor in supporting your SLP in extending services to individuals with communication challenges. There are several things to consider as you prepare for a session with an individual receiving services, including:

- Meeting ahead of time with your SLP to discuss individual objectives and treatment plans

- Preparing and organizing materials and checking any equipment that might be used

- Setting up the "environment" consistent with considerations of space, comfort, and age-appropriate materials

- "Picking up the individual" for the session consistent with the procedures specific to the setting

- Obtaining and recording SLP-specified baseline data

- Being prepared with specific treatment protocol, IEP, or lesson plan

- Being prepared with method of recording responses and documenting progress

- Communicating questions and concerns to your supervising SLP

During the session, you will be expected to implement the lesson or treatment plan as outlined by your supervising SLP and

- Develop and maintain rapport with those you serve

- Implement the designated treatment protocol in a specific sequence as designed by your SLP

- Provide clear directions and instructions that are age appropriate and match the individual's level of comprehension or understanding

- Maintain on-task behaviors
- Use specific feedback and reinforcement strategies that are consistent, discriminating, and meaningful to the individual
- Apply knowledge of learning theory or guidelines for guidance of behavior as needed
- Support social communicative interactions and generalization of behaviors and performance across contexts and situations
- Monitor and record progress toward goals

After intervention sessions there are many follow-up tasks to be completed including:

- Recording session summary notes
- Tabulating responses and calculating percentages
- Refiling materials and putting away equipment after checking it is in good working order
- Participating in monitoring generalization through on-line observations and collecting data in other contexts
- Completing session evaluations or reimbursement forms and filing information as needed if necessary or required
- Communicating questions and concerns to your supervising SLP

There are many tasks and activities that your supervising SLP will delegate to you. It is important to be clear about what is expected and to seek help and assistance as necessary to ensure quality of service delivery.

TWO SAMPLE SNAPSHOTS OF INTERVENTION APPROACHES AND TECHNIQUES

Specific intervention approaches are often tied to a basic philosophical framework or theoretical perspective. For example, there is a recent trend to return to basic principles of learning theory in the applied behavioral analysis (ABA)

approach currently receiving widespread attention for use with children described as autistic or falling on the pervasive developmental delay spectrum of disorders. ABA programs derive from a behavioral model that focuses on direct intervention in the form of carefully planned and systematic stimuli that elicit a response followed by often strict reinforcement schedules that are applied to increase the frequency of the targeted response or behavior. An example would be of a trainer-oriented approach (Fey, 1986) in which the trainer structures and controls all aspects of the situation from which behaviors are targeted to types of stimuli presented and type and schedule of reinforces used. The ABA approach is based on task analysis of a target behavior, with careful attention to the step-by-step sequence that must be implemented in order to learn the new behavior, practice it, and then generalize it to communication situations beyond those presented in intervention. One rendition of a strict behavioral approach is what is referred to as the Lovas method, which was initially developed and introduced by Ivar Lovas (1987). The intervention begins with shaping a targeted behavior by systematically introducing graded stimuli followed by contingent and tangible reinforcement of the desired behavior. Concerns of critics of this directive treatment procedure are centered on the teaching or shaping of specific performance skills out of context and thus issues of whether the behavior demonstrated in a somewhat artificial and controlled situation will generalize or become habituated. More recent applications of an ABA approach continue to be characterized by a comprehensive analysis of the steps needed to shape a behavior but the context of eliciting the targeted behavior are more natural or routine as are the reinforcement type and schedule applied. ABA has been written about by many authors and currently has a journal specifically dedicated to publishing articles dealing with adaptations and applications of this approach. The critical factors of task analysis, direct teaching, drill and practice, structure, intensity, and consistency are key in understanding how this approach is implemented. You can read more about approaches that use these principles as they apply to children described as autistic in the *Journal of the Association of Persons With Severe Handicaps* (1999).

In contrast, there is also a recent surge of attention to more "naturalistic" approaches to speech and language intervention. Naturalistic approaches are based on the premise that children learn language within the context of everyday routines, activities, and places. These approaches are consistent with the current focus on intervention in natural environments as referenced in IDEA reauthorization for the birth to 3 population. Naturalistic approaches involve working with individuals in settings and during activities where they would ordinarily be if they did not have a handicapping condition (Dunst & Bruder, 2001). Even though this approach has been most recently emphasized in the early childhood literature, the basic principles extend to intervention programs with adults and children alike. It is considered critically important to practice new skills in "context" regardless of the age of the individual you are working with.

As you learn about different approaches in your class work and practica you will see that most vary along a continuum from direct to indirect, from highly directive to less directive. All approaches to intervention target specific speech and language behaviors that the individual, child, student or patient needs help with. Those in early childhood tend to focus on inclusive and natural environments (home, community-based programs, childcare centers, and preschools), wherein the parent or teacher is often considered a key agent for change. There are many early intervention programs that facilitate parents or teachers in their learning about how to encourage and enhance speech and language behaviors.

KEY COMPONENTS OF THE INTERVENTION PROCESS

There are several key components of the intervention process. Knowing the specific behaviors to be targeted during therapy, why you are doing specific tasks or collecting specific data in sessions, where and when the intervention should be taking place, and how you should be performing your duties as an SLPA are the integral pieces to the intervention process.

The What of Intervention

Regardless of the approach, there are basic tenets inherent in any learning or therapeutic situation. These could be listed as knowing the "what" or specific target behaviors you are working on. This will vary depending on the individual strengths needs of the person receiving services. This is why assessment is so important because all therapy or intervention must link to assessment in this way. You may be working with students to improve their articulation of specific sounds or with adults in their ability to name and access specific vocabulary. In another context, you may be facilitating and supporting children to use longer and more complex sentences or targeting a student's ability to distinguish minimal differences between sounds so he can decode what he reads. You may be asked to work with a group of adults to use their communication skills with others in a group or reduce their moment of stuttering by using specific talking strategies. The "what" will vary with each individual you work with and be dictated by the SLP's interpretation of assessment data as well as the particular goals and objectives that he determines will enhance the individual's communication ability. For a school-age student you will see these goals and objectives reflected on the IEP, and for a very young child, on the IFSP. The adults you work with also have very specific goals and objectives that your SLP will share with you so that you can implement appropriate intervention

The Why of Intervention

Your SLP will help you understand the "why" you are doing what you are doing in treatment sessions, and your ongoing data collection will help your SLP know when to shift gears and move on to "next steps" or abandon a specific approach because it is not effective. Your ability to follow the treatment plans established by your SLP and collect accurate data to determine change are critical to the intervention process. Your supervising SLP knows the why of intervention, but you need to practice skill development for the how.

The Where and When of Intervention

The "where and when" of intervention will vary according to the specific setting in which you are employed. For example, school-age students' eligible services will be seen as part of their schedule through school, although their families may also seek outside services in a clinic or private practice to supplement the IEP developed through their district. Again, young children may be seen at home, in childcare settings, or in community programs or clinics, depending on the preferences of the family and the focus of the approach being used. Many adults are seen on a weekly basis in private practices or hospital settings or clinics. Adults also often receive daily therapy as part of their residential rehabilitation program or hospitalization when recovering from a stroke or other incident. The timing, schedule, and setting for intervention will vary depending on the individual's situation and needs.

The How of Intervention

The "how" of therapy is what you need to be concentrating on as you develop your skills as an SLPA. How you engage young children in activities that are motivating, meaningful, age-appropriate and fun while still addressing the targeted objectives becomes an art. How you talk with individuals and use strategies such as wait time, open-ended questions, parallel talk, or self-talk can make a significant difference. How you provide specific feedback regarding their performance helps the individuals you work with to take the "next step" toward successful participation in the session or activity. These skills are critical when attempting to engage school-age students in "work" they may perceive as drudgery or "drill and kill." It is equally important to create age level interesting materials and activities with adults to engage them in the therapeutic process. Ways of presenting information that use "cueing strategies" to prompt appropriate responses and clear concise directions regarding a task may make the critical difference in how the patient or individual responds to the activities you have developed. Roth and Worthington (2001) provide additional reference points for

key strategies for use in intervention. They use terms like *direct* and *indirect modeling, shaping of successive approximations, prompts, fading expansion, negative practice,* and *target-specific feedback.* Direct modeling involves providing a specific example for the individual to imitate, whereas indirect modeling of a specific behavior is to expose the individual to numerous well-formed examples of the target behavior. Shaping a target involves breaking down the target into its smallest components and teaching it in an ascending sequence of difficulty. Prompts, either verbal or nonverbal, are used as cues to facilitate an individual's appropriate response. Fading refers to the reduction of cues as the individual maintains the desired response or behavior. Expansion involves using the target behavior in a more mature or complex context. Sometimes negative practice may be used to have the individual intentionally produce an error to contrast the error with the appropriate response. This may increase an individual's ability to self-monitor his performance. As explained later, target-specific feedback that provides information regarding the accuracy of a response is needed. This type of feedback is different from more generalized feedback such as "good job" or "well done" or more general natural consequences such as being misunderstood.

Central to whatever you do as an activity within a therapeutic session is the concept of practice, practice, and more practice. You did not learn how to ride a bike without practice. You did not learn how to read without practice. Children will not improve their articulation abilities without practice. Practice in meaningful or contextual situations enhances the carryover of skills into everyday communication and language use. Another key concept regarding the "how" of intervention is feedback. You learn best and continue to use a new skill when you receive feedback on its usefulness. Your abilities as a keen observer of behavior will serve you well because you need to provide specific feedback to the individuals you work with regarding their performance. For example, a student is more likely to try again if he receives specific feedback that his answer or production of a certain sound was "very close" or "wow, you've got it, say it again." Individuals you work with need the feedback to know how they are doing in meeting their objective. Basic learning theory tells us we all perform better and more consistently when we experience success or receive reinforcement of our efforts. Both children and adults would more likely benefit from positive specific feedback such as "You almost have it, try again" versus "That's wrong" or "Yes, that is like the word you want to say" versus " No, that's not right."

Another way to frame intervention is to think about treatment as being a continuum involving phases of relearning or new learning. The first phase is often referred to as the establishment phase. This is when the focus of treatment is to facilitate the establishment of the target behavior. Focus may be on production or comprehension of a target in a very structured context (e.g., sound at syllable level, vocabulary meanings, and syntax structures in limited word combinations). This may involve having the individual perceive or identify the target and then produce the target, depending on the objective. Stabilization comes with the repeated practice and use of the target in a meaningful context. This framework may be most easily understood when you are working on intelligibility of speech production.

SPEECH SOUND TARGETS

Four methods commonly used to establish speech sound targets include:

■ Imitation: Present an auditory, visual, tactile, or kinesthetic model for the individual to identify and then imitate. Provide specific feedback regarding accuracy. " That's it. You've got it. It sounded just the same."

■ Contextual Utilization: Identify "can do" contexts in which the target is produced accurately. This leads to increased success and may help shape target responses. "I heard the sound when you said it in see. Let's try it in another word like same."

■ Phonetic Placement: Provide specific instruction regarding appropriate production with multimodality cues. "Place your tongue up behind your front teeth. Feel the air move."

■ Successive Approximation: Shape successive approximations by creating a series of responses that the individual can proceed through to gradually reach targets.

The second phase involves generalization of the target to new contexts. You reduce the cues needed as the individual produces the target behavior more independently. At the same time you may be introducing tasks that involve additional linguistic complexity and increased frequency of production. This may involve moving from syllables to words, phrases, sentences, story retelling, and then conversation. Because of your specificity of feedback the individual is better able to self-monitor their productions and self-correct any mistakes without your cues to remind them. As the target behavior becomes more automatic, you will hopefully see generalization of use in other settings and with other people. The third phase is called the maintenance phase. It is in this phase of intervention that the behavior becomes truly automatic, the individual is independent of your cues, and self-monitoring is high and the error rate is low. As you can see this frame for conceptualizing intervention phases is consistent with principles of basic learning theory (Bernthal & Bankson, 1998). You will refine the "how" of intervention as you observe your SLP and gain more experience with a variety of individuals and approaches. Remember that your supervising SLP can be an effective mentor in facilitating your skill and development as an SLPA.

BASIC PRINCIPLES FOR GUIDING BEHAVIOR AND FACILITATING SOCIAL INTERACTIONS

Behavior problems or resistance when working with individuals with communication disorders challenge many SLPs and SLPAs. These may look different depending on the age and abilities of the individual and may come up regardless of your work setting. Young children can easily get off task or try to avoid the activities you have prepared. Students in a school setting may be very self-conscious about their challenges or angry that they have to work so hard on learning a new behavior. They may display "behavioral outbursts" or impulsive behaviors that are associated with their disability. Young adults with head injuries may present very inappropri-

ate behaviors that need to be dealt with. Adults who are very frustrated or angry about their current situation may refuse to cooperate or participate in intervention activities. Appropriately dealing with anger, frustration, or other behaviors will be part of your responsibilities as an SLPA. However, resources and guidelines are available to help you navigate these challenges. The following thoughts came from a school-based SLP and have been somewhat modified as they apply to children, students, and adults.

It is important to remember that every school has a discipline policy and set of procedures when responding to behavioral issues. Talk with your supervisor about behaviors that are considered acceptable or unacceptable and what procedures you should follow for disciplinary referral. Know the rules ahead of time for handling challenging behaviors. Experienced SLPs and other professionals can help you implement a repertoire of teaching or management strategies designed to decrease undesirable behaviors. Regardless of your setting, if you feel unsafe for any reason, involve your supervisor or appropriate personnel as needed. In summary, it is important for you as an SLPA to identify the various factors that may be causing and maintaining an individual's use of inappropriate or challenging behavior because they can significantly interfere with success in therapy.

ENHANCING EFFECTIVENESS IN INTERVENTION

After you have gained experience in providing intervention services to a variety of individuals with very different challenges, you will learn that there is always more to learn. Susan Meyer (1998) writes about key challenges of successful intervention. She highlights several ideas introduced in this chapter such as use of verbal praise and encouragement; monitoring your own verbal and nonverbal models; presenting clear, precise, and concise directions; and providing response specific feedback. She talks about how guiding group interactions can also be challenging. Remember, the key to effective small group management is involvement and interest. Ongoing participation is critically important as

HELPFUL HINTS ABOUT GUIDING BEHAVIOR

- Prevent inappropriate behaviors by being prepared and organized. "When students have idle time…the potential for discipline problems increases exponentially."

- A positive attitude is catching. Let the individuals and families you work with see that you enjoy what you do. Be excited about therapy and about being with them.

- Meaningful and relevant activities help individuals "buy in" to what they are doing. Let individuals know why the task is important. Keep it simple. "We are playing this game so you can learn new words."

- Show respect to the individuals you work with. You will know that your efforts are working when students you work with say " excuse me," "thank you," "sorry," or "please" back to you.

- Set up clear behavioral expectations. Keep it simple. " First, you need to listen and then we can talk." "When you are here, you need to pay attention and complete the task. Then we can play that game." Be kind, confident, and firm.

- Make sure the individual understands what you have said. You may want the individual to repeat the expectations back to you or signal that they understand what you have said.

- Do not engage in a power struggle. Calmly state the "rule" or expectation and consequence.

- Giving second chances may be a mistake. Repeated "threats" to follow through with a consequence often do not help. You may want to call on your supervisor to help you de-escalate a situation before it gets to the point of "no return."

- Let it be over when it is over. Treat the Individual as a model student or patient. Be pleasant.

- Individuals will sometimes shut down if the task or activity goes on too long or if they have done it many times before. Monitor your pace and read your clients' cues.

- A lack of comprehension and fear of failure can sabotage the session you have planned. Be sure to provide clear instructions and be sensitive to the abilities of the individuals you are working with. Begin at a success level they can manage.

- Use humor and be willing to laugh, but remain the adult with children.

- Do not use sarcasm literally or through your tone of voice. Some individuals will not understand your intent. Preserve the dignity of each individual you work with.

- Make sure you are not consistently "testing" the individual. Provide time for mastery of new skills.

waiting for your turn in a group can take a very long time. This is certainly true for adults as well as children. It is all about how you set up a session to encourage multiple ways of interacting that facilitates successful participation. Developing your skills that enhance interactions with individuals as well as groups will come as you observe your SLP and others successfully engage young children, students, and adults in productive interactions. However, do not lose sight of the importance of what you do as well as how you do it. Knowing the goals and objectives, facilitating their attainment, and documenting change are critically important to the success of therapy (see Figure 13-4).

CONCLUSION

The magic of intervention is in the interaction. Your ability to use the skills and strategies introduced in this chapter will help you provide productive and successful services to children, students, clients, and patients. The skills you develop

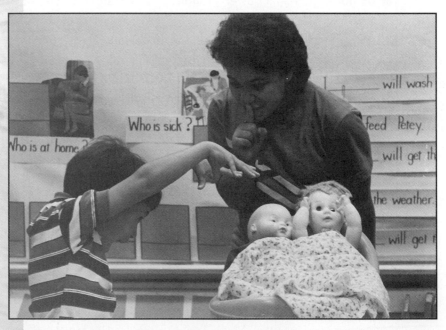

Figure 13-4 It's magic: Interaction is key!

over time will make a difference in the lives of individuals you work with as well as your own. This chapter has introduced you to several concepts, including the what, when, where, and how of intervention. There are many aspects to consider, including the role you play as facilitator regardless of setting and service delivery model used. Current trends such as the increasing use of technology and team-based services in intervention certainly creates new possibilities for enhancing the communication abilities of individuals with disabilities. Implementation of intervention programs may be as different as the number of individuals you work with. It is an exciting challenge and one you will meet with your supervising SLP.

DISCUSSION QUESTIONS

1. Compare and contrast the role of the SLP and SLPA in designing and implementing an intervention plan for an individual with communication challenges. What is critical for the SLPA to know and learn?

2. Discuss current trends in intervention (e.g., technology, full inclusion, etc.) and how they may affect how services are provided.

3. Explain how observation skills are critical in therapy.

4. What key strategies are critical for the SLPA to develop to enhance interactions during treatment sessions and why?

5. Discuss phases of intervention as referenced by Bernthal and Bankson (1998). How might they be implemented in small group work with five 8-year-old children with various articulation disorders?

SUGGESTED ACTIVITIES

1. Observe a language group or articulation therapy group session in a school or clinic setting. List the advantages for these students getting service as a group as opposed to individual therapy. What were

specific strategies used to maintain participation and involvement? Can you think of others that might have worked?

2. Observe individual or group therapy in a hospital or rehabilitation center. What strategies were successful in modifying communicative behavior or facilitating appropriate responses?

3. In small groups, review three different treatment plans for a young child, student in an elementary or middle school setting, and adult. Identify the goals and objectives. Brainstorm alternative activities and strategies that you might implement in a therapy session to address each objective. Set the stage by identifying the setting, service delivery model, tasks and activities you would use and the specific strategies that might be helpful to consider in eliciting targeted behaviors.

4. Videotape yourself in interaction with an individual with communication challenges. What specific strategies did you use to facilitate the individual's performance? What worked? How did you know?

REFERENCES

American Speech-Language-Hearing Association. (2001). *ASHA Code of Ethics*. Rockville, MD: Author..

American Speech-Language-Hearing Association. (2001). *Omnibus survey*. Retrieved March 2, 2001, from http://www.professional.asha.org

Andrews, M. L. (2002). *Voice treatment for children and adolescents*. Albany, NY: Delmar.

Bernstein, D., & Tiegerman-Farber, E. (1997). *Language and communication disorders in children*. Boston: Allyn & Bacon.

Bernthal, J., & Bankson, N. (1998) *Articulation and phonological disorders* (4th ed.). Boston: Allyn & Bacon.

Brown, F. & Bambara, L. (1999). Special series on intervention for young children with autism. *Journal of the Association for Persons with Severe Handicap, 24,* 130–244.

Catts, H. (1997). The early identification of language-based reading disabilities. *Language, Speech, and Hearing Services in the Schools, 28,* 86–89.

Catts, H., & Kamhi, A. (1999). *Language and reading disabilities*. Needham Heights, MA: Allyn & Bacon

Dickenson, D. K., & Tabors, O. (2001). *Beginning literacy with language.* Baltimore: Paul H. Brookes.

Dunst, C., & Bruder, M. B. (2001). Characteristics and consequences of everyday natural learning opportunities. *TECSE, 21,* 68–92.

Fey. M. (1986). *Language intervention with young children.* San Diego, CA: College-Hill Press.

Fey, M. (1998). Research to practice (and back again) in speech language intervention. *Topics in Language Disorders, 18,* 23–24.

Glennon S. L., & DeCoste D. C. (1997). *Handbook of augmentative and alternative communication.* San Diego, CA: Singular.

Lovas, O. I. (1987). Behavioral treatment and normal educational and intellectual functioning in young autistic children. *Journal of Consulting and Clinical Psychology, 55,* 3–9.

Lynch, E. W., & Hanson, M. J. (1992). *Developing cross-cultural competence.* Baltimore: Paul H. Brookes.

Marvin, C. (1990). Problems in school-based consultation and collaborative services: Defining the terms and improving the process. In W. Secord (Ed.), *Best practices in school speech-language pathology* (pp. 37–48). San Antonio, TX: Psychological Corporation, Harcourt Brace Jovanovich.

Meyer, S. M. (1998). *Survival guide for the beginning speech-language clinician.* Gaithersburg, MD: Aspen.

Paul, R. (2001). *Language disorders from infancy to adolescence* (2nd ed.). St. Louis: Mosby.

Prelock, P. (2000). An intervention focus for inclusionary practice. *Language, Speech, and Hearing Services in the Schools, 31,* 296–298.

Ramig, L., Countryman, S., O'Brien, C., Hoehn, M., & Thompson, L. (1996). Intensive speech treatment for patients with Parkinson's disease: Short and long-term comparison of two techniques. *American Academy of Neurology, 17,* 1496–1504.

Roth, F. P., & Worthington, C. K (1996). *Treatment resource manual for speech-language pathology.* San Diego, CA: Singular.

Schiefelbusch, R. (1983). Language intervention I children: What is it? In J. Miller, D. Yoder, & R. Schiefelbusch (Eds.), *Contemporary issues in language intervention* (ASHA Reports No. 12). Rockville, MD: American Speech-Language-Hearing Association.

Weiss, A. (1997). Planning language intervention for young children. In D. K. Bernstein & E. Tiegerman-Farber. *Language and communication disorders in children.* Boston: Allyn & Bacon.

Whitehurst, G. J., Falco, F., Lonigan, C. J., Fischel, J. E., Valdez-Menchaca, M. C., & Caulfield, M. (1988). Accelerating language development through picture book reading. *Developmental Psychology, 24,* 552–558.

Whitehurst, G. J., Falco, F., Lonigan, C. J., Fischel, J. E., Valdez-Menchaca, M. C., & Caulfield, M. (1994). Outcomes of an emergent literacy intervention in Head Start. *Journal of Educational Psychology, 84,* 541–556.

Whitehurst, G. J., Falco, F., Lonigan, C. J., Fischel, J. E., Valdez-Menchaca, M. C., & Caulfield, M. (1994). A picture book reading intervention in daycare and home for children from low-income families. *Developmental Psychology, 30,* 679–689.

Appendix A: Background Information and Criteria

American Speech-Language-Hearing Association (ASHA) Background Information and Criteria for the Registration of Speech-Language Pathology Assistants

(Effective January 1, 2003).

Approved by the Council on Professional Standards in Speech-Language-Pathology and Audiology, September 2000; revised April 2001.

Note: Reprinted by permission of the American Speech-Language-Hearing Association (http://www.asha.org).

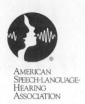

AMERICAN
SPEECH-LANGUAGE-
HEARING
ASSOCIATION

Background Information and Criteria for the Registration of Speech-Language Pathology Assistants

(Effective January 1, 2003)

Approved by the Council on Professional Standards in Speech-Language-Pathology and Audiology, September 2000

Background Information

In 1992, the Executive Board of the American Speech-Language Hearing Association (ASHA) appointed a Task Force on Support Personnel charged with reviewing issues related to support personnel and developing a position statement on their use. The position statement, supporting the establishment and credentialing of categories of support personnel in speech-language pathology, was passed by ASHA's Legislative Council in 1994 (LC 15-94).

The task force developed guidelines for one category of support personnel in speech-language pathologyóthe speech-language pathology assistant. These guidelines were approved by the Legislative Council (LC 1-95) with the provision that a strategic plan for their implementation be developed and brought forward to the LC.

A consensus panel consisting of representatives from ASHA, the ASHA Executive Board, ASHA's special interest divisions, and Allied and Related Professional Organizations was formed by resolution (EB 16-96) to develop the strategic plan. Consultants to the consensus panel included former members of ASHA's Task Force on Support Personnel, representatives of ASHA committees and boards, ASHA staff, and representatives of outside agencies.

In November 1996, on approval of the strategic plan, the Council on Professional Standards in Speech-Language Pathology and Audiology (Standards Council) was charged by the Legislative Council (LC) to develop and administer a credentialing process for speech-language pathology assistants. Although the 1996 Strategic Plan for Credentialing Speech-Language Pathology Assistants was approved by the LC as a model for developing these processes, the Standards Council was not required to follow precisely the guidelines offered by the consensus panel that developed the strategic plan.

This document describes the minimum criteria for the approval of individuals to become registered speech-language pathology assistants. The criteria are linked to the approval of technical training programs by the Council on Academic Accreditation in Audiology and Speech-Language Pathology (CAA) of the American Speech-Language-Hearing Association. The criteria include academic course work for assistants, clinical observations and field experiences, and workplace behaviors for performing assistant-level job responsibilities. The curriculum, job responsibilities, and workplace behaviors were developed on the basis of the speech-language pathology assistant scope of responsibilities established by ASHA in 1995 in the *Guidelines for the Training, Credentialing, Use and Supervision of Speech-Language Pathology Assistants* and on the results of ìA National Job Analysis of Speech-Language Pathology Assistantsî conducted in 1999 by the Educational Testing Service on behalf of the Standards Council and the CAA.

The curriculum guidelines were designed to provide technical training that leads to fulfillment of the specified job responsibilities, core technical skills, and workplace behaviors. Although the training program may attract individuals with a bachelor's degree in speech-language pathology, it is not designed as a pre-professional program. Individuals with a bachelor's degree do not automatically qualify to be registered assistants. They must obtain an associate-level degree, complete necessary course work, successfully pass field work assessments, and meet all other requirements.

Please note: Implementation language will be added in 2002 by ASHA's Council For Clinical Certification.

Refer to this document as: Background information and criteria for the registration of speech-language pathology assistants. (2002). *ASHA 2002 Desk Reference*, vol. 1, pp. 289ñ291.

Index terms: registration, speech-language pathology assistants, SLP assistant program, support personnel

Document type: Standards

Job Responsibilities for Speech-Language Pathology Assistants

Provided that the training, supervision, documentation, and planning are appropriate, the following tasks may be delegated to a speech-language pathology assistant:

a. assist the speech-language pathologist with speech-language and hearing screenings (without interpretation)

b. follow documented treatment plans or protocols developed by the supervising speech-language pathologist

c. document patient/client performance (e.g., tallying data for the speech-language pathologist to use; preparing charts, records, and graphs) and report this information to the supervising speech-language pathologist

d. assist the speech-language pathologist during assessment of patients/clients

e. assist with informal documentation as directed by the speech-language pathologist

f. assist with clerical duties such as preparing materials and scheduling activities as directed by the speech-language pathologist

g. perform checks and maintenance of equipment

h. support the supervising speech-language pathologist in research projects, in-service training and public relations programs

i. assist with departmental operations (scheduling, record keeping, safety/maintenance of supplies and equipment)

j. collect data for quality improvement

k. exhibit compliance with regulations, reimbursement requirements, and speech-language pathology assistant's job responsibilities

Activities Outside the Job Responsibilities for a Speech-Language Pathology Assistant

The speech-language pathology assistant:

a. may not perform standardized or nonstandardized diagnostic tests, formal or informal evaluations, or interpret test results

b. may not screen or diagnose patients/clients for feeding/swallowing disorders

c. may not participate in parent conferences, case conferences, or any interdisciplinary team without the presence of the supervising speech-language pathologist or other ASHA-certified speech-language pathologist designated by the supervising speech-language pathologist

d. may not provide patient/client or family counseling

e. may not write, develop, or modify a patient's/client's individualized treatment plan in any way

f. may not assist with patients/clients without following the individualized treatment plan prepared by the speech-language pathologist or without access to supervision

g. may not sign any formal documents (e.g., treatment plans, reimbursement forms, or reports; the assistant should sign or initial informal treatment notes for review and co-signature by the supervising speech-language pathologist)

h. may not select patients/clients for services

i. may not discharge a patient/client from services

j. may not disclose clinical or confidential information either orally or in writing to anyone other than the supervising speech-language pathologist

k. may not make referrals for additional service

l. may not counsel or consult with the patient/client, family, or others regarding the patient/client status or service

m. may not represent himself or herself as a speech-language pathologist

n. may not use a checklist or tabulate results of feeding or swallowing evaluations.

o. may not demonstrate swallowing strategies or precautions to patients, family or staff.

Workplace Behaviors

The SLP Assistant should demonstrate the ability to:

a. relate to clients/patients in a supportive manner

b. follow supervisor's instructions

c. maintain confidentiality and other appropriate workplace behaviors

d. communicate in oral and written forms

e. follow health and safety precautions

Reprinted by permission of the American Speech-Language-Hearing Association (http://www.asha.org).

Criteria for the Registration of Speech-Language Pathology Assistants

I. Degree

Applicants for registration must have an associate degree with a program of study designed to prepare the student to be a speech-language pathology assistant.

II. Program

Effective January 1, 2003, applicants for ASHA registration must have completed course work and field experiences in a technical training program for speech-language pathology assistants approved by the American Speech-Language-Hearing Association (ASHA).

Course work and fieldwork experience completed in an associate degree technical training program for speech-language pathology assistants prior to January 1, 2003, will be evaluated to determine whether the applicant meets all criteria for registration.

All applicants for registration must be referred for registration by the program director of the associate degree technical training program for speech-language pathology assistants where they have earned the degree and completed the field and course work requirements.

III. Course Work and Field Experiences

Applicants for registration must have earned 60 semester credit hours in a program of study that includes general education and the specific knowledge and skills for a speech-language pathology assistant. The training program will include clinical observation and a minimum of 100 clock hours of field experiences.

III-A. Curriculum Content

The curriculum must include 60 semester credit hours with the following content:

20–40 semester credit hours in general education

20–40 semester credit hours in technical content areas

a minimum of 100 clock hours of fieldwork experience(see Section III-B)

1. General education (20–40 semester credit hours)

   The general education sequence should include, but is not limited to, the following:

   a.   Oral and written communication

   b.   Mathematics

   c.   Computer applications

   d.   Social and natural sciences

2. Technical knowledge (20–40 semester credit hours)

   Course content must provide students with knowledge and skills to assume the job responsibilities and core technical skills for speech-language pathology assistants, and must include the following:

   a. overview of normal processes of communication

   b. overview of communication disorders

   c. instruction in assistant-level service delivery practices

   d. instruction in workplace behaviors

   e. cultural and linguistic factors in communication

   f. observation

   g. fieldwork experiences

III-B.   Fieldwork Experience

Applicants for registration must complete a minimum of 100 hours of supervised fieldwork experiences. The fieldwork must provide appropriate experiences for learning the job responsibilities and workplace behaviors of the speech-language pathology assistant. These experiences are not intended to develop independent practice.

1. Supervision

   Students engaging in fieldwork experience must be supervised by an ASHA-certified speech-language pathologist at least 50% of the time when engaged in patient/client contact.

2. Verification

   Applicants must obtain written verification from the training program that the fieldwork experience was successfully completed. This verification must include a description of the setting and assessment of technical proficiency.

Reprinted by permission of the American Speech-Language-Hearing Association (http://www.asha.org).

Appendix B: Knowledge and Skills for Supervisors

Knowledge and Skills for Supervisors of Speech-Language Pathology Assistants

Note. From American Speech-Language-Hearing Association. (2002). ASHA Supplement, in press. Reprinted by permission of the American Speech-Language-Hearing Association (http://www.asha.org).

AMERICAN
SPEECH-LANGUAGE-
HEARING
ASSOCIATION

Knowledge and Skills for Supervisors of Speech-Language Pathology Assistants

Working Group on Supervision of Speech-Language Pathology Assistants

This Knowledge and Skills document is an official statement of the American Speech-Language-Hearing Association (ASHA). The ASHA Scope of Practice (2001) includes providing supervision of speech-language pathology assistants (SLPAs) as one of a speech-language pathologist's professional roles. The ASHA Preferred Practice Patterns (1997) are statements that define universally applicable characteristics of practice, including those related to supervision. ASHA requires members who practice independently in speech-language pathology to hold the Certificate of Clinical Competence in Speech-Language Pathology. ASHA members and certificate holders must abide by the ASHA Code of Ethics (1994), which includes Principle of Ethics II Rule B: iIndividuals shall engage in only those aspects of the profession that are within their competence, considering their level of education, training, and experience;î and Rule D: iIndividuals shall delegate the provision of clinical services only to: (1) persons who hold the appropriate Certificate of Clinical Competence; (2) persons in the education or certification process who are appropriately supervised by an individual who holds the appropriate Certificate of Clinical Competence; or (3) assistants, technicians, or support personnel who are adequately supervised by an individual who holds the appropriate Certificate of Clinical Competence.

This document was prepared by the Working Group on Supervision of Speech-Language Pathology Assistants, composed of representatives from the Steering Committee of ASHAís Special Interest Division 11: Administration and Supervision (Elizabeth McCrea, chair; Laura Billetdeaux, Judy Brasseur, Deborah Carlson, Leisha Eiten, Anita Halper, and Wren Newman); other speech-language pathologists with expertise in the supervision of assistants (Jeaṛne Mullins, Lisa OíConnor); and ASHA National Office staff

Reference this material as: American Speech-Language-Hearing Association. (2002). Knowledge and skills for supervisors of speech-language pathology assistants. *ASHA Supplement 22*, 113ñ118.

Index terms: Competencies, SLP assistants, speech-language pathology, supervision, support personnel

Document type: Practice guidelines and policies

in the clinical issues in speech-language pathology unit (Diane Paul-Brown, coordinator; Amy Knapp). The ASHA monitoring vice president was Alex P. Johnson.

Preamble

Dramatic changes have occurred over the last decade in the manner in which speech-language pathology services are delivered due to the challenges of health care finance reform, public school caseloads, scientific and technological advances, and an expanding scope of practice for members of the profession. As one response to these challenges, the professionís governing bodies now recognize the role of SLPAs who can support ASHA-certified speech-language pathologists (LC 1-95). Assistants are individuals who, following academic coursework, clinical practicum, credentialing, and perhaps voluntary registration by ASHA, can perform tasks prescribed, directed, and supervised by ASHA-certified speech-language pathologists (ASHA, 1996; ASHA 2000).

The use of credentialed and supervised SLPAs is one way to increase the frequency of services to clients while maintaining service quality and controlling cost. The decision to shift responsibility for some aspects of speech-language pathology service delivery to assistants should only be made by ASHA-certified speech-language pathologists and only when the quality of care to patients/clients will not be compromised. In addition to direct patient/client contact, SLPAs may also assist service delivery by preparing materials, performing clerical duties associated with program or case management, or working on other appropriate assignments that fall within their defined scope of responsibilities (ASHA, 1996). Whatever tasks are assigned to SLPAs, implicit in the decision to use them is the ethical commitment by the ASHA-certified speech-language pathologist to provide appropriate supervision in order to ensure quality of care. It must be clear to all parties involved that the use of an SLPA is not meant to replace the work of a speech-language pathologist but, rather, to effectively extend it.

Reprinted by permission of the American Speech-Language-Hearing Association (http://www.asha.org).

Using an SLPA as an interpreter/translator requires additional knowledge and skills that are not addressed in this document. ASHAís Multicultural Issues Board is developing guidelines to address this need.

Introduction

In 1985 the ASHA Legislative Council adopted the position statement Clinical Supervision in Speech-Language Pathology and Audiology (ASHA, 1985). This document formally recognized the importance of the supervisory process in the clinical education of speech-language pathologists and audiologists as a fundamental mechanism to ensure quality service to clients. The position paper also outlined 13 tasks that are basic to effective clinical supervision and identified supervisor competencies that implement each task.

The importance of supervision in the competent and ethical use of SLPAs requires that the profession now identify and define the knowledge and skills necessary for supervisors of SLPAs. This document identifies the knowledge and skills that are consistent with the 13 tasks of supervision identified in the 1985 position statement, as well as those tasks identified in the ASHA Guidelines for the Training, Credentialing, Use, and Supervision of Speech-Language Pathology Assistants (ASHA, 1996). These tasks make it clear that the ASHA-certified supervisor retains legal and ethical responsibility for all aspects of case management and service delivery while at the same time helping assistants refine their skills within their scope of responsibilities and assigned tasks.

Role of the Supervisor

Direct and indirect supervision of SLPAs by speech-language pathologists expands the speech-language pathologistsí role as a service provider to include responsibility for the work of support personnel (ASHA, 1996). This broadened role demands that members of the profession who might supervise SLPAs understand the complexity of the supervisory process and be prepared to meet its challenges. The knowledge and skills delineated in this document are the first steps in that preparation.

Terminology

Clinical Supervision: Clinical supervision refers to the tasks and skills of clinical teaching related to the interaction between the client and the service provider.

Direct Supervision: Direct supervision means onsite, in-view observation and guidance by the speech-language pathologist while an assigned activity is performed by support personnel.

Indirect Supervision: Indirect supervision means those activities other than direct observation and guidance conducted by a speech-language pathologist. These may include demonstrations, record review, review and evaluation of audio- or videotaped sessions, and/or interactive television.

Knowledge and Skills

Supervisors of SLPAs have the knowledge and skills to:

1. Select and assign appropriate patients/clients to the SLPA.

   Knowledge required:

   a. Understand the ASHA Guidelines for the Training, Credentialing, Use and Supervision of Speech-Language Pathology Assistants (ASHA, 1996), including:

   > ethical and legal responsibilities of the ASHA-certified speech-language pathologist
   >
   > scope of job responsibilities of the SLPA
   >
   > exclusive responsibilities of the ASHA-certified speech-language pathologist
   >
   > appropriate amount of direct and indirect supervision
   >
   > ratio of supervisors to SLPAs
   >
   > SLPA access to supervisor

   Skills required:

   a. Assess the patient/clientís disorder and concomitant needs in order to determine if use of an assistant is appropriate.

   b. Determine those tasks that the SLPA has the training and expertise to perform.

   c. Assign tasks to the SLPA that are within the scope of the SLPAís job responsibilities and are consistent with his/her knowledge and skill.

2. Determine the nature of supervision that is appropriate for each SLPA.

   Knowledge required:

   a. Understand supervisory processes and practices, including strategies for direct and indirect supervision.

   Skills required:

   a. Determine the amount of supervision required based on the needs of the client, the experience of the SLPA, the service delivery setting, the task assigned, and other pertinent factors.

Reprinted by permission of the American Speech-Language-Hearing Association (http://www.asha.org).

b. Design and implement supervisory procedures that ensure patient/client confidentiality and quality of care.

c. Determine when it is necessary to alter the amount and type of supervision in response to changes in client/patient status and/or service delivery models, use of equipment, or assigned tasks.

3. Establish and maintain an effective relationship with the SLPA.

Knowledge required:

a. Understand components of an effective supervisory relationship with the SLPA.

b. Understand the dynamics of various learning styles.

c. Understand diverse styles of interpersonal communication.

Skills required:

a. Facilitate the SLPAís understanding of assigned tasks and the supervisory process.

b. Accommodate a variety of learning styles in the supervision of the SLPA.

c. Use effective interpersonal communication skills to maximize communication effectiveness in the supervision of the SLPA.

d. Facilitate problem-solving of tasks assigned by the SLPA.

e. Maintain a professional and supportive relationship that allows for both supervisor and SLPA growth.

f. Interact with the SLPA in an objective manner.

g. Establish joint communications regarding expectations and responsibilities in assigned tasks and the supervisory process.

h. Evaluate the SLPA and the effectiveness of the supervisory process.

i. Guide the SLPA in developing appropriate interpersonal skills (e.g., collaborative teamwork and conflict resolution), with patients/clients, family members, staff, and others).

4. Direct the SLPA in following screening protocols:

Knowledge required:

a. Understand speech-language screening tools and protocols, including how to administer them and document the results.

Skills required:

a. Teach the SLPA to administer and score appropriately the assigned screening tools, including:

differentiation of correct versus incorrect responses

accurate completion of protocols

accurate collection/scoring of patient/client screening data

b. Direct the SLPA in managing assigned screening protocols and documentation.

Seek the supervisorís guidance if the administration of screening tools is in question

Report any difficulty encountered in screening

Schedule screenings

Organize screening tools

c. Assist the SLPA in accurately communicating screening results, without interpretation to the SLP, including descriptive behavioral observations that enhance the clarity of results.

5. Demonstrate for and participate with the SLPA in the clinical process.

Knowledge required:

a. Understand best practices in speech-language pathology, dynamics of patient/client-clinician relationships, clinical techniques, clinical materials and equipment, and behavioral management techniques.

Skills required:

a. Demonstrate best practices for the SLPA.

b. Demonstrate an effective client-clinician relationship.

c. Demonstrate a variety of clinical techniques.

d. Demonstrate the use of client-specific materials and equipment.

e. Instruct the SLPA in the performance of tasks as outlined and demonstrated by the speech-language pathologist and to implement activities that use procedures prescribed by the speech-language pathologist.

f. Assist the SLPA in developing skills to maintain patient/client on-task behavior.

g. Teach the SLPA how to provide appropriate feedback regarding the accuracy of the patient/client response.

h. Teach the SLPA to use feedback and reinforcement that is consistent, discriminating, and meaningful to the patient/client.

i. Instruct the SLPA in giving directions and instructions that are clear, concise, and appropriate to the patient/clientís age and level of understanding.

Reprinted by permission of the American Speech-Language-Hearing Association (http://www.asha.org).

j. Instruct the SLPA in applying behavior management techniques and basic instructional strategies (e.g., asking questions, giving directions, providing positive reinforcement of desired behaviors) that are specific to the patient/client.

k. Teach the SLPA how to provide appropriate cuing strategies to assist the patient/client in approximating accurate responses.

6. Direct the SLPA in following individualized treatment plans that have been developed by the speech-language pathologist.

Knowledge required:

a. Understand communication disorders and the design of individualized treatment plans.

Skills required:

a. Instruct the SLPA in understanding a patient/clientís disorders and communication needs.

b. Develop an individualized treatment plan for each client for the SLPA to follow:

Direct the SLPA to execute clinical goals and objectives in the specified sequence

Instruct the SLPA in description and data collection to measure patient/client behavior change

Instruct the SLPA in documenting patient/client outcomes

c. Teach the SLPA how to describe patient/client progress.

7. Direct the SLPA in the maintenance of clinical records.

Knowledge required:

a. Understand clinical recordkeeping procedures.

b. Understand principles and procedures for maintaining client confidentiality.

Skills required:

a. Assist the SLPA in maintaining accurate clinical records.

b. Assist the SLPA to effectively document clinical interactions, including:

individual treatment plans and protocols

patient/client performance

other information on patient/client charts

c. Assist the SLPA in organizing records to facilitate easy retrieval of information concerning clinical interactions.

d. Assist the SLPA in following policies and procedures to protect the confidentiality of clinical records.

8. Interacts with the SLPA in planning and executing supervisory conferences.

Knowledge required:

a. Understand components of both the supervisory process and supervisory conferences.

b. Understand strategies for observation and analysis of supervisory conferences.

Skills required:

a. Establish a regular conference schedule.

b. Plan a supervisory conference agenda.

c. Involve the SLPA in a joint discussion of previously identified clinical or supervisory data or issues.

d. Adjust supervisory style and interact with the SLPA in a manner that facilitates the SLPAís self-exploration and problem-solving within assigned tasks.

e. Adjust supervisory conference content based on the SLPAís level of training and experience.

f. Encourage and maintain SLPA motivation for continuing self-growth and development of job skills.

g. Assist the SLPA in making commitments for changes in job skills.

9. Provide feedback to the SLPA regarding skills.

Knowledge required:

a. Understand the skill level of the SLPA.

b. Understand the tools used for evaluation of SLPA clinical skills.

c. Understand effective supervisory communication styles.

Skills required:

a. Develop and use clinical skill evaluation tools.

b. Assist the SLPA in the description and measurement of his/her progress and achievement of job skills.

c. Assist the SLPA in developing strategies for self-evaluation and documentation of job performance.

d. Use supervisory feedback to modify interactions with patients/clients.

10. Assist the SLPA in developing skills of verbal reporting and assigned informal written reporting to the SLP.

Knowledge required:

a. Understand standards and strategies for effective oral and written communication.

Reprinted by permission of the American Speech-Language-Hearing Association (http://www.asha.org).

Skills required:

a. Assist the SLPA in identifying appropriate information to be included in oral reports.

b. Teach the SLPA how to present verbal and written information in a logical, concise, and sequential manner.

c. Instruct the SLPA in the use of appropriate professional terminology.

11. Assist the SLPA in effectively selecting, preparing, and presenting treatment materials and organizing treatment environments.

Knowledge required:

a. Understand appropriate treatment materials for specific populations.

Skills required:

a. Assist the SLPA in choosing appropriate materials from an approved materials list to be used to implement the assigned treatment plan.

b. Assist the SLPA in effectively organizing the clinical setting to meet the needs of the client and obtain optimal patient/client performance.

c. Assist the SLPA in selecting materials that are age and culturally appropriate as well as motivating.

d. Assist the SLPA in efficiently preparing and selecting treatment materials in a timely manner.

12. Share information regarding ethical, legal, regulatory, and reimbursement aspects of professional practice.

Knowledge required:

a. Understand ethical, legal, regulatory, and reimbursement aspects of professional practice.

b. Understand the scope of practice in speech-language pathology.

Skills required:

a. Communicate professional codes of ethics and conduct (e.g., ASHA, state licensure boards, other professional legal bodies) to the SLPA.

b. Communicate an understanding of legal and regulatory requirements and their impact on the practice of the profession (e.g., licensure, IDEA, ADA, Medicare, Medicaid) to the SLPA.

c. Communicate an understanding of reimbursement policies and procedures of the work setting to the SLPA.

d. Communicate due process policies and procedures in the work setting to the SLPA.

e. Articulate clearly the speech-language pathologist's scope of practice and exclusive responsibilities of the SLPA.

13. Model and facilitate professional conduct.

Knowledge required:

a. Understand appropriate professional standards and conduct.

Skills required:

a. Assume ethical and legal responsibility for all patient/client care.

b. Analyze, evaluate, and modify own behavior.

c. Model ethical and legal conduct.

d. Meet and respect deadlines.

e. Provide current information regarding professional standards.

f. Assist the SLPA in demonstrating appropriate conduct, including

Respect/maintain confidentiality of patient/client information

Dress appropriately for the work setting

Use appropriate language for the work setting

Recognize own job limitations and perform within the boundaries of training and job responsibilities (e.g., refer the patient/client family and other professionals to the speech-language pathologist for any information regarding screening and treatment).

g. Assist the SLPA to effectively address patient/client attitudes and behaviors.

14. Direct the SLPA in the implementation of research procedures, in-service training, and public relations programs.

Knowledge required:

a. Understand research projects and their procedures, in-service training activities, and public relations programs.

Skills required:

a. Teach the SLPA how to complete assigned research tasks.

b. Teach the SLPA how to complete assigned in-service training responsibilities.

c. Teach the SLPA how to complete assigned public relation program activities.

Reprinted by permission of the American Speech-Language-Hearing Association (http://www.asha.org).

15. Train the SLPA to check and maintain equipment and to observe universal precautions.

   Knowledge required:

   a. Understand operational procedures for equipment, including performance checks and maintenance.

   b. Understand universal precautions policies and procedures.

   Skills required:

   a. Instruct the SLPA in maintaining and performing assigned checks of equipment.

   b. Assist the SLPA in the completion of universal precautions protocols.

16. Assist the SLPA in using appropriate language (oral and written) when interacting with patients/clients and others.

   Knowledge required:

   a. Understand appropriate oral and written language skills to use when interacting with patients/clients and others.

   Skills required:

   a. Model and instruct the SLPA with regard to the awareness of and sensitivity to cultural and linguistic needs of each client.

   b. Model and instruct the SLPA to adapt language according to the patient/clientís age, culture, and linguistic, cognitive, and educational level.

   c. Model and instruct the SLPA to be courteous and respectful at all times.

   d. Model and instruct the SLPA in maintaining appropriate pragmatic skills, such as eye contact, body language, facial expression, and conversational turn-taking, as well as topic initiation, maintenance, and closure.

17. Establish a system of accountability for document use and supervision of the SLPA.

   Knowledge required:

   a. Understand accountability systems for documentation of supervision of the SLPA.

   b. Understand supervision requirements for the SLPA.

   c. Understand due process rights and procedures.

   d. Understand conflict resolution strategies, including referral, as appropriate.

   Skills required:

   a. Document the type and amount of supervision provided to the SLPA.

   b. Develop conflict resolution strategies that protect due process of the SLPA and patient/client quality of care.

   c. Prepare summary reports regarding use of the SLPA, including accessibility of services to patients/clients, utilization cost-benefit analysis, and quality of service measures to administrators, patients/clients, and payers.

References

American Speech-Language-Hearing Association. (1985). Clinical supervision in speech-language pathology and audiology. *Asha, 27,* 57ñ60.

American Speech-Language-Hearing Association. (1988). Utilization and employment of speech-language pathology supportive personnel with underserved populations. *Asha, 30,* 55ñ56.

American Speech-Language-Hearing Association. (2001). *Code of ethics.* Rockville, MD: Author.

American Speech-Language-Hearing Association. (1996). Guidelines for the training, credentialing, use, and supervision of speech-language pathology assistants. *Asha, 38* (Suppl. 16), 21ñ34.

American Speech-Language-Hearing Association. (1997). Preferred practice patterns for the profession of speech-language pathology. *Asha, 38* (Suppl. 16), 21ñ34.

American Speech-Language-Hearing Association. (2000). *Council on Professional Standards in Speech-Language Pathology and Audiology: Background information and criteria for registration of speech-language pathology assistants.* Rockville, MD: Author.

American Speech-Language-Hearing Association. (2001). *Scope of practice in speech-language pathology.* Rockville, MD: Author.

Suggested Readings

Anderson, J. L. (1988). *The supervisory process in speech-language pathology and audiology.* Austin, TX: Pro-Ed.

Dowling, S. (2001). *Supervision: Strategies for successful outcomes and productivity.* Needham Heights, MA: Allyn & Bacon.

Hagler, P. & Macfarlane, L. (1997). *Collaborative service delivery by assistants and professionals* (rev. ed.). Edmonton, Alberta, Canada: Alberta Rehabilitation Coordinating Council.

Horton, A., Kander, M., Longhurst, T., & Paul-Brown, D. (1997). *Preparing and using speech-language pathology assistants.* Rockville, MD: American Speech-Language-Hearing Association.

Reprinted by permission of the American Speech-Language-Hearing Association (http://www.asha.org).

Appendix C: ASHA Code of Ethics

American Speech-Language-Hearing Association Code of Ethics

Note. From "Code of Ethics" (revised), by American Speech-Language-Hearing Association, 2001, ASHA Leader, 6(23), p. 2.Reprinted by permission of the American Speech-Language-Hearing Association (http://www.asha.org).

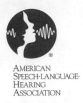

AMERICAN
SPEECH-LANGUAGE-
HEARING
ASSOCIATION

Code of Ethics

Last Revised November 16, 2001

Preamble

The preservation of the highest standards of integrity and ethical principles is vital to the responsible discharge of obligations in the professions of speech-language pathology and audiology. This Code of Ethics sets forth the fundamental principles and rules considered essential to this purpose.

Every individual who is (a) a member of the American Speech-Language-Hearing Association, whether certified or not, (b) a nonmember holding the Certificate of Clinical Competence from the Association, (c) an applicant for membership or certification, or (d) a Clinical Fellow seeking to fulfill standards for certification shall abide by this Code of Ethics.

Any action that violates the spirit and purpose of this Code shall be considered unethical. Failure to specify any particular responsibility or practice in this Code of Ethics shall not be construed as denial of the existence of such responsibilities or practices.

The fundamentals of ethical conduct are described by Principles of Ethics and by Rules of Ethics as they relate to responsibility to persons served, to the public, and to the professions of speech-language pathology and audiology.

Principles of Ethics, aspirational and inspirational in nature, form the underlying moral basis for the Code of Ethics. Individuals shall observe these principles as affirmative obligations under all conditions of professional activity.

Rules of Ethics are specific statements of minimally acceptable professional conduct or of prohibitions and are applicable to all individuals.

Reference this material as: American Speech-Language-Hearing Association. (2001, December 26). Code of ethics (revised). *ASHA Leader*, vol. 6 (23), p. 2.

Index terms: ASHA reference products, ethics (professional practice issues), ethics and related papers

Document type: Ethics and related documents

Principle of Ethics I

Individuals shall honor their responsibility to hold paramount the welfare of persons they serve professionally.

Rules of Ethics

A. Individuals shall provide all services competently.

B. Individuals shall use every resource, including referral when appropriate, to ensure that high-quality service is provided.

C. Individuals shall not discriminate in the delivery of professional services on the basis of race or ethnicity, gender, age, religion, national origin, sexual orientation, or disability.

D. Individuals shall not misrepresent the credentials of assistants, technicians, or support personnel and shall inform those they serve professionally of the name and professional credentials of persons providing services.

E. Individuals who hold the Certificates of Clinical Competence shall not delegate tasks that require the unique skills, knowledge, and judgment that are within the scope of their profession to assistants, technicians, support personnel, or any nonprofessionals over whom they have supervisory responsibility. An individual may delegate support services to assistants, technicians, support personnel, or any other persons only if those services are adequately supervised by an individual who holds the appropriate Certificate of Clinical Competence.

F. Individuals shall fully inform the persons they serve of the nature and possible effects of services rendered and products dispensed.

G. Individuals shall evaluate the effectiveness of services rendered and of products dispensed and shall provide services or dispense products only when benefit can reasonably be expected.

Reprinted by permission of the American Speech-Language-Hearing Association (http://www.asha.org).

H. Individuals shall not guarantee the results of any treatment or procedure, directly or by implication; however, they may make a reasonable statement of prognosis.

I. Individuals shall not provide clinical services solely by correspondence.

J. Individuals may practice by telecommunication (for example, telehealth/e-health), where not prohibited by law.

K. Individuals shall maintain adequate records of professional services rendered and products dispensed and shall allow access to these records when appropriately authorized.

L. Individuals shall not reveal, without authorization, any professional or personal information about the person served professionally, unless required by law to do so, or unless doing so is necessary to protect the welfare of the person or of the community.

M. Individuals shall not charge for services not rendered, nor shall they misrepresent,[1] in any fashion, services rendered or products dispensed.

N. Individuals shall use persons in research or as subjects of teaching demonstrations only with their informed consent.

O. Individuals whose professional services are adversely affected by substance abuse or other health-related conditions shall seek professional assistance and, where appropriate, withdraw from the affected areas of practice.

Principle of Ethics II

Individuals shall honor their responsibility to achieve and maintain the highest level of professional competence.

Rules of Ethics

A. Individuals shall engage in the provision of clinical services only when they hold the appropriate Certificate of Clinical Competence or when they are in the certification process and are supervised by an individual who holds the appropriate Certificate of Clinical Competence.

B. Individuals shall engage in only those aspects of the professions that are within the scope of their competence, considering their level of education, training, and experience.

C. Individuals shall continue their professional development throughout their careers.

D. Individuals shall delegate the provision of clinical services only to: (1) persons who hold the appropriate Certificate of Clinical Competence; (2) persons in the education or certification process who are appropriately supervised by an individual who holds the appropriate Certificate of Clinical Competence; or (3) assistants, technicians, or support personnel who are adequately supervised by an individual who holds the appropriate Certificate of Clinical Competence.

E. Individuals shall prohibit any of their professional staff from providing services that exceed the staff member's competence, considering the staff member's level of education, training, and experience.

F. Individuals shall ensure that all equipment used in the provision of services is in proper working order and is properly calibrated.

Principle of Ethics III

Individuals shall honor their responsibility to the public by promoting public understanding of the professions, by supporting the development of services designed to fulfill the unmet needs of the public, and by providing accurate information in all communications involving any aspect of the professions.

Rules of Ethics

A. Individuals shall not misrepresent their credentials, competence, education, training, or experience.

B. Individuals shall not participate in professional activities that constitute a conflict of interest.

C. Individuals shall refer those served professionally solely on the basis of the interest of those being referred and not on any personal financial interest.

D. Individuals shall not misrepresent diagnostic information, services rendered, or products dispensed or engage in any scheme or artifice to defraud in connection with obtaining payment or reimbursement for such services or products.

E. Individuals' statements to the public shall provide accurate information about the nature and management of communication disorders, about the professions, and about professional services.

---

[1] For purposes of this Code of Ethics, misrepresentation includes any untrue statements or statements that are likely to mislead. Misrepresentation also includes the failure to state any information that is material and that ought, in fairness, to be considered.

Reprinted by permission of the American Speech-Language-Hearing Association (http://www.asha.org).

F. Individualsí statements to the publicóadvertising, announcing, and marketing their professional services, reporting research results, and promoting productsóshall adhere to prevailing professional standards and shall not contain misrepresentations.

Principle of Ethics IV

Individuals shall honor their responsibilities to the professions and their relationships with colleagues, students, and members of allied professions. Individuals shall uphold the dignity and autonomy of the professions, maintain harmonious interprofessional and intraprofessional relationships, and accept the professionsí self-imposed standards.

Rules of Ethics

A. Individuals shall prohibit anyone under their supervision from engaging in any practice that violates the Code of Ethics.

B. Individuals shall not engage in dishonesty, fraud, deceit, misrepresentation, sexual harrassment, or any other form of conduct that adversely reflects on the professions or on the individualís fitness to serve persons professionally.

C. Individuals shall not engage in sexual activities with clients or students over whom they exercise professional authority.

D. Individuals shall assign credit only to those who have contributed to a publication, presentation, or product. Credit shall be assigned in proportion to the contribution and only with the contributorís consent.

E. Individuals shall reference the source when using other personsí ideas, research, presentations, or products in written, oral, or any other media presentation or summary.

F. Individualsí statements to colleagues about professional services, research results, and products shall adhere to prevailing professional standards and shall contain no misrepresentations.

G. Individuals shall not provide professional services without exercising independent professional judgment, regardless of referral source or prescription.

H. Individuals shall not discriminate in their relationships with colleagues, students, and members of allied professions on the basis of race or ethnicity, gender, age, religion, national origin, sexual orientation, or disability.

I. Individuals who have reason to believe that the Code of Ethics has been violated shall inform the Board of Ethics.

J. Individuals shall comply fully with the policies of the Board of Ethics in its consideration and adjudication of complaints of violations of the Code of Ethics.

Reprinted by permission of the American Speech-Language-Hearing Association (http://www.asha.org).

Appendix D: Protection of Rights

Protection of Rights of People Receiving Audiology or Speech-Language Pathology Services.

Note. From American Speech-Language-Hearing Association, January, 1994. ASHA, pp. 60-63. Reprinted by permission of the American Speech-Language-Hearing Association (http://www.asha.org).

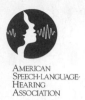

AMERICAN
SPEECH-LANGUAGE-
HEARING
ASSOCIATION

Protection of Rights of People Receiving Audiology or Speech-Language Pathology Services

Task Force on Protection of Clientsí Rights

This technical report was prepared by the American Speech-Language-Hearing Associationís Task Force on Protection of Clientsí Rights: Joseph A. Caniglia, Mary Pat Ciccariello, Charles C. Diggs (coordinator), Elizabeth Kennedy, Jean M. Lovrinic (1991-1993 vice president for governmental and social policies, monitoring vice president), and Seleria J. Williams. ASHAís Executive Board approved distribution of the report to members (EB 82B-93).

Introduction

In 1986, the Bylaws of the American Speech-Language-Hearing Association (ASHA) were amended (LC resolution 1-86) to include advocacy for ìthe rights and interests of persons with communication disordersî among ASHAís purposes (Article 2.1 [6]). However, no body of the Association was charged with determining what these rights include.

More recently, people with disabilities have awakened politically and begun to see the barriers to their full participation in society as a civil rights issue. Disability is no longer a source of shame or something to overcome to inspire others. This revolution in self-perception has led people with disabilities to assert and demand their rights. Passage and enactment of the Americans with Disabilities Act of 1992 is strong testimony to the power of such collective action by the community of people with disabilities, including people with speech, language, or hearing disabilities.

These forces of self-actualization are being exerted within society at the same time as the rights of consumers are being increasingly recognized by fed-eral legislators and regulators as well as by private accreditation bodies. The Individuals with Disabilities Education Act (formerly known as the Education of the Handicapped Act) asserts in Section 601(c) that ìIt is the purpose of this Act to assure thatÖthe rights of children with disabilities and their parents or guardians are protectedÖ.î The Omnibus Budget Reconciliation Act of 1990 requires that programs providing services funded by Medicare and Medicaid inform patients of their right to make their own health care decisions. The Health Care Financing Administrationís (HCFA) Survey Procedures and Interpretive Guidelines for intermediate Care Facilities for the Mentally Retarded specify that the ìindividual program plan must also include opportunities for client choice and self-management.î The accreditation manual for hospitals of the Joint Commission on Accreditation of Health-care Organizations (JCAHO) includes a section on patient rights. The outcome-based performance measures of The Accreditation Council on Services for People with Disabilities include sections on choice, rights, and dignity and respect.

Despite these trends and requirements, a model bill of rights for all persons who receive audiology or speech-language pathology services has not been developed by ASHA. The Guidelines for Meeting the Communication Needs of Persons With Severe Disabilities (1992), developed by the National Joint Committee for the Communicative Needs of Persons With Severe Disabilities and approved by ASHA, include a communication bill of rights for this population, and the Educational Rights for Children Who Are Deaf or Hard of Hearing developed by the Council of Organizational Representatives (COR), including an ASHA representative, identified rights for this particular population. However, neither of these documents are generalizable across the broad range of communication disabilities and possible settings of practice.

Reference this material as: American Speech-Language-Hearing Association. (1994, January). The protection of rights of people receiving audiology or speech-language pathology services. *Asha*, pp. 60-63.

Index terms: Client/patient rights, patient/client rights, model Bill of Rights, consumers

---

Reprinted by permission of the American Speech-Language-Hearing Association (http://www.asha.org).

While professional responsibility to persons served is inherent within ASHA's Code of Ethics, the Code by its very nature focuses on professional conduct and prohibitions. Clients' rights are implied but not explicit.

Therefore, ASHA's Executive Board formed a Task Force on the Protection of Clients' Rights in 1992 to develop a model bill of consumer rights that could be applied across communication disability types and practice settings. This bill was to be developed in consultation with ASHA's Council on Professional Ethics in Speech-Language Pathology and Audiology (COPE).

Process of Development of the Model Bill

To develop the model bill, the task force reviewed pertinent background materials, generated a series of draft documents, sought select peer review from ASHA members as well as from national consumer and parent groups, consulted with COPE, and seriously discussed all recommended changes prior to completing the model bill. This process is briefly described in the sections below.

Review of Background Materials

All members of the task force received review copies of the following documents:

- ï ASHA's Code of Ethics and Issues in Ethics statements (1992)
- ï ASHA's Standards for Professional Service Programs in Audiology and Speech-Language Pathology (1992)
- ï HCFA's Survey Procedures and Interpretive Guidelines for Intermediate Care Facilities for the Mentally Retarded (October 1988)
- ï A Communication Bill of Rights (from the 1992 Guidelines of the National Joint Committee for the Communicative Needs of Persons With Severe Disabilities)
- ï COR's Educational Rights (1992)
- ï The Patient Rights section from the 1993 JCAHO *Accreditation Manual for Hospitals* (together with an example of how one hospital protects patient rights)
- ï Outcome Based Performance Measures from The Accreditation Council for People with Disabilities (1992)
- ï A Client Bill of Rights (Flower, 1984)
- ï Aphasic Patient's Bill of Rights (Tanner, 1986)

Draft Documents

During its development of draft documents, the task force developed certain criteria for inclusion of rights within the model bill. To be included, a right had to:

- ï apply to both children and adults receiving services;
- ï apply to all settings of practice;
- ï apply to both audiology and speech-language pathology services;
- ï be understandable to consumers;
- ï reflect rights advocated by self-help/mutual aid groups concerned with communication disabilities;
- ï be realizable in the present.

The last criterion eliminated rights such as the right to access services regardless of ability to pay. Such a right does not exist today in other areas of health care delivery and should not be expected from recipients of audiology and speech-language pathology services in these settings.

Select Peer Review

After three conference call meetings of the task force, a draft of a model bill that met all the above criteria, along with detailed comments on each right, was sent to 51 ASHA members representing Association committees, related professional organizations (RPOs), and individuals with specific interest in this topic; to 89 consumer and parent groups; to 12 clients of task force members; and to 38 ASHA National Office staff. The documents were also discussed at a meeting of ASHA's Consumer Advisory Task Force.

A total of 67 comments were received: 28 from ASHA members (13 from committees, 10 from RPOs, 5 from individuals), 29 from consumers (28 groups and 1 individual), and 10 from National Office staff. Twenty-six (38.8%) of these responses endorsed the documents without recommending any changes. These responses were distributed equally between members and consumers.

Other commenters recommended adding new rights, expanding and/or clarifying existing rights; changing terminology used, including legal restrictions on some rights; and changing the order of presentation of some of the rights. Comments were distributed equally among all rights presented.

During two additional conference calls, the task force considered all comments seriously, discussed needed changes, and developed revised draft documents that were submitted to COPE. The task force coordinator met with COPE in late May 1993 and

Reprinted by permission of the American Speech-Language-Hearing Association (http://www.asha.org).

provided a written report of their comments to the task force. During a sixth conference call, all changes recommended by COPE were incorporated into the model bill.

The Model Bill

As the result of the above process, the following Model Bill of Rights for People Receiving Audiology or Speech-Language Pathology Services was developed.

Model Bill of Rights for People Receiving Audiology or Speech-Language Pathology Services

Clients as consumers receiving audiology or speech-language pathology services have:

1. THE RIGHT to be treated with dignity and respect;

2. THE RIGHT that services be provided without regard to race or ethnicity, gender, age, religion, national origin, sexual orientation, or disability;

3. THE RIGHT to know the name and professional qualifications of the person or persons providing services;

4. THE RIGHT to personal privacy and confidentiality of information to the extent permitted by law;

5. THE RIGHT to know, in advance, the fees for services, regardless of the method of payment;

6. THE RIGHT to receive a clear explanation of evaluation results, to be informed of potential or lack of potential for improvement, and to express their choices of goals and methods of service delivery;

7. THE RIGHT to accept or reject services to the extent permitted by law;

8. THE RIGHT that services be provided in a timely and competent manner, which includes referral to other appropriate professionals when necessary;

9. THE RIGHT to present concerns about services and to be informed of procedures for seeking their resolution;

10. THE RIGHT to accept or reject participation in teaching, research, or promotional activities;

11. THE RIGHT, to the extent permitted by law, to review information contained in their records, to receive explanation of record entries upon request, and to request correction of inaccurate records;

12. THE RIGHT to adequate notice of and reasons for discontinuation of services; an explanation of these reasons, in person, upon request; and referral to other providers if so requested.

These rights belong to the person or persons needing services. For sound legal or medical reasons, a family member, guardian, or legal representative may exercise these rights on the person's behalf.

Comments

During the process of developing the model bill of rights, certain comments were made about each of the rights. These comments are presented below to provide additional information about the rights:

1. THE RIGHT to be treated with dignity and respect.

Clients of audiology and speech-language pathology services are human beings.

Their communication ability may be reduced, and they may present sensory, perceptual, cognitive, or emotional complications. But, these consumers deserve the same dignity and respect that are given to people without a communication disability. This dignity and respect can be shown in many areas that include the manner of greeting and addressing clients; selection of materials appropriate to the consumer's age, gender, interest, cultural background, and disability; and acceptance of the client's unique, non-destructive personality characteristics.

2. THE RIGHT that services be provided without regard to race or ethnicity, gender, age, religion, national origin, sexual orientation, or disability.

Providers of speech, language, or hearing services must not discriminate in the delivery of professional services on the basis of race or ethnicity, gender, age, religion, national origin, sexual orientation, or disability. The inherent nature of a program or the expertise of providers may limit services available to consumers. Such practices can be nondiscriminatory if restrictions are applied uniformly to all potential clients.

3. THE RIGHT to know the name and professional qualifications of the person or persons providing services.

Professional qualifications include the service provider's national and state certification/licensure status as well as level of education, training, and experience. Professional qualifications do not include personal data such as home address, age, marital status, family composition, or sexual orientation.

Reprinted by permission of the American Speech-Language-Hearing Association (http://www.asha.org).

4. THE RIGHT to personal privacy and confidentiality of information to the extent permitted by law.

Personal privacy and confidentiality need to be preserved during screening, assessment, and intervention, provided that individual well-being is not at risk and disclosure is not required by law. A requirement of consumer permission prior to release of information promotes privacy and confidentiality.

Certain medical, legal, or educational situations may necessitate release without prior permission. The client has the right to explanation of these instances when they occur.

In other specific situations, medical or legal documentation may indicate that the person with the communication disability is not capable of releasing information. In such cases, a guardian or court-appointed representative may be given access to information that is deemed personal and confidential.

5. THE RIGHT to know, in advance, the fees for services, regardless of the method of payment.

Prior to receiving services, the consumer has the right to be advised of fees and provided written documentation when requested. To evaluate fees completely, clients need to know the length of any treatment sessions, the number of scheduled sessions per week, and whether individual and/or group sessions will be provided. It is also important that specific information on fees for missed or canceled appointments and fees for consultation be provided. The right to fee information exists whether payment is to be made directly by the consumer or by a third party.

6. THE RIGHT to receive a clear explanation of evaluation results, to be informed of potential or lack of potential for improvement, and to express their choices of goals and methods of service delivery.

The spirit of this right is to enable clients to become active participants in service delivery. Within a reasonable time after completion of an evaluation, consumers need to be informed of the results in a form and manner comprehensible to them. The use of highly technical terminology without a full explanation does not provide the understanding needed.

Inclusion of the client in the development of both the general approach to services and the individualized plan also promotes active participation in service delivery. Provider explanation of options that exist, including their advantages and disadvantages, and serious consideration of the consumer's preferences in determining goals and methods of service delivery likewise encourage active participation.

Whenever possible, the client is entitled to know the predicted outcome of proposed services that includes how effective services might be and how long they might take. Consumers are likewise entitled to know the reasons why services may not be recommended and any changes in their prognoses.

7. THE RIGHT to accept or reject services to the extent permitted by law.

In some unusual situations, certain legal edicts may supersede this right. An example would be participation in services as ordered by a family court judge. In other situations where medical or legal documentation indicates that the person needing services cannot understand their implication, a family member, guardian, or legal representative may exercise this right on the person's behalf.

8. THE RIGHT that services be provided in a timely and competent manner, which includes referral to other appropriate professionals when necessary.

The timeliness of initiating services may vary from setting to setting because of such factors as due process procedures required by law, medical concerns, state regulations, or third-party reimbursement policies and guidelines. The client has the right to ask about any delays in the initiation of services, receive an explanation, and be given other alternatives. Once services have started, they should be continuous and sufficient in number, frequency, and manner of delivery to meet established goals.

Consumers have the right to seek services from other audiologists or speech-language pathologists. In some situations, referral to professionals other than audiologists or speech-language pathologists is necessary for the client's welfare.

9. THE RIGHT to present concerns about services and to be informed of procedures for seeking their resolution.

Concerns about services need to be considered seriously and resolved as appropriate. When the service provider cannot resolve concerns, referral to other personnel within the facility who can provide further assistance is appropriate.

10. THE RIGHT to accept or reject participation in teaching, research, or promotional activities.

Participation in teaching, research, public relations, marketing, or other activities of the facility is completely voluntary and requires the informed consent of the consumer. The client needs to know the relevant features of the activity to the extent that such information could conceivably influence the decision to participate. When consumers perceive a penalty,

Reprinted by permission of the American Speech-Language-Hearing Association (http://www.asha.org).

real or implied, if they decline or withdraw from participation, then participation is not voluntary. Even if the activity is integral to service delivery, the consumer has the right to refuse participation. In such cases, clients have the right to know that alternatives exist within the same facility and within the community.

11. THE RIGHT, to the extent permitted by law, to review information contained in their records, to receive explanation of record entries upon request, and to request correction of inaccurate records.

Consumers have the right to request access to their records to the extent permitted by law and to receive explanation of record entries upon request. Also upon request, clients have the right to timely receipt of copies of these records. A reasonable fee may be charged for duplication and/or mailing.

Prompt, appropriate corrections to records are also part of this right. When disagreement about the accuracy of records exists, notation of the consumerís viewpoint as part of the records is appropriate.

12. THE RIGHT to adequate notice of and reasons for discontinuation of services; an explanation of these reasons, in person, upon request; and referral to other providers if so requested.

Services may be discontinued for many reasons. They include, but are not limited to, achievement of education/habilitation/rehabilitation potential, failure or inability to pay for services, irregular attendance, or lack of client motivation. Consumers are entitled to an explanation of these reasons, in person if so requested, so that they understand that the decision is neither arbitrary nor capricious and can make any necessary behavioral changes to improve future relationships with providers.

Sufficient notice that present services will be discontinued will facilitate the clientís arrangement for services from another provider or team, if so desired. A referral list of such providers is also helpful in this regard.

Use and Dissemination

The model bill was developed for voluntary use by programs offering audiology or speech-language pathology services. Its use can assist programs to meet the federal and accrediting body requirements discussed in the introduction. Even without such external pressures, distribution of this model bill to all persons receiving audiology or speech-language pathology services and its prominent display within a facility demonstrates a programís commitment to cli-

ents as consumers of professional services and its sensitivity to their needs. Such an atmosphere promotes client trust, confidence, and satisfaction and can contribute to efficacy of intervention. Use of the model bill implies a programís willingness to redress any abrogation of the rights via appropriate channels within the facility.

The task force recommends that the model bill of rights and the task forceís report be published in *Asha* to inform all ASHA members of their availability. The task force further recommends that the model bill and task force report be sent to the consumer and parent groups who received draft versions for comment. Finally, the task force recommends that both documents be sent to appropriate standards bodies of the Association so that the content of the model bill and the report of the task force can be considered for inclusion in future standards for clinical certification, ethics, academic program accreditation, and professional service program accreditation.

References

Accreditation Council on Services for People with Disabilities. (1992). *Outcome based performance measures, Field Review Edition*. Landover. MD: Author.

American Speech-Language-Hearing Association. (1992, March). Code of Ethics. *Asha* (Suppl. 9). pp. 1-2.

American Speech-Language-Hearing Association. (1992, March) Issues in Ethics. *Asha* (Suppl. 9), pp. 6-21.

Council of Organizational Representatives (1992). *Educational rights for children who are deaf or hard of hearing.* Presentation at the annual convention of the American Speech-Language-Hearing Association. San Antonio, by E. Cherow, R. R. Davila, D. Dickman, & S. Boney.

Council on Professional Standards. (1992. September). Standards for Professional Service Programs in Audiology and Speech-Language Pathology. *Asha*, pp. 63-70.

Flower, R.M. (1984). *Delivery of speech-language pathology and audiology services*. Baltimore: Williams & Wilkins, (p. 253).

Health Care Financing Administration. (1988, October). Survey procedures and interpretive guidelines for intermediate care facilities for the mentally retarded, *State operations manual: Provider certification*. Washington, DC: U.S. Government Printing Office, J-1-J-138.

Joint Commission on Accreditation of Healthcare Organizations. (1992). *Accreditation manual for hospitals, 1993*. Oakbrook Terrace, IL: Author, (pp. 105-107).

National Joint Committee for the Communicative Needs of Persons With Severe Disabilities (1992, March). Guidelines for meeting the communication needs of persons with severe disabilities. *Asha* (Suppl. 7), pp. 1-8.

Tanner, D.C. (1986). *Aphasic patientís bill of rights*. Tulsa, OK: Modern Education Corporation.

Reprinted by permission of the American Speech-Language-Hearing Association (http://www.asha.org).

Appendix E: Sample Individualized Education Program

Sample Individualized Education Program.

Form reprinted with permission from the Colorado Department of Education, Special Education Services Unit.

Administrative Unit Name	Date
Denver Public Schools - Eisenhower Elem	3	20	01

Hannah Richardson	1234	3	23	95
Legal Name of Child/Student	Child/Student ID	DOB

Individualized Education Program (IEP)
** Eligibility Meeting (Kindergarten to Age 14) **

Dates of Meetings *(Complete both dates)*

Dates of next Eligibility Meeting *(on or before)*	3/20/04 *(Month/Day/Year)*	Date of Next IEP review Meeting *(on or before)*	3/20/02 *(Month/Day/Year)*

Reason for Meeting *(Check one box only)*

☐ Initial   ☒ Triennial   ☐ Review *   * (required for change in disability, significant change in placement, or exit from special education program)

CHILD/STUDENT AND FAMILY INFORMATION

	Prior to Meeting	After Meeting
District of Residence (if BOCS)	Denver	Denver
Home School	Eisenhower	Eisenhower
School of Attendance	Eisenhower	Eisenhower
Unit/Facility of Attendance (if out of district)		
Primary Disability, if any	Preschool	Multiple
Secondary Disability, if any (optional)		
Primary Special Education Instructional Setting		

Grade Kinder   Age 6   Gender: ☐ Male   ☒ Female

Race/Ethnicity ☐ Native American   ☐ Asian/Pacific Islander   ☐ Black   ☐ Hispanic   ☒ White

Primary Language Parent Survey, date received: _____

Primary Language/Mode of Communication in the Home _____

Primary Language/Mode of Communication of the Child/Student _____

If the primary home language is other than English, then the child's/student's English language proficiency must be evaluated prior to the special education referral. It is recommended to also evaluate the child's/student's proficiency is his/her primary language.

Name of Instrument _____   Date _____

Proficiency Level	English	Primary Language
Listening Comprehension (all grades)		
Speaking (all grades)		
Reading (from 2nd grade on)		
Writing (from 2nd grade on)		
Composite score (if appropriate)		

Child/Student's Parent(s)	George and Kathy Richardson
Address	1212 Lilac Way
City/State/Zip	Denver, CO 80223
Telephone Number	303-424-1234 (h) 303-421-5678(w)
	Home Work Home Work

Is there an educational Surrogate parent?   Yes ☐   No ☒

MAY BE COMPLETED PRIOR TO THE MEETING.
Aug-2001   (5b) Page 1 of 10

Reprinted by permission of the Colorado Department of Education, Special Education Services Unit.

Hannah Richardson	1234	3/23/95
Legal Name of Child/Student	Child/Student ID	DOB

Participants in Meeting

THE FOLLOWING PARTICIPANTS MUST BE IN ATTENDANCE AT ALL ELIGIBILITY MEETINGS:

George Richardson
Child's/Student's Parent
(unless parent decided not to attend)

Kathy Richardson
Child's/Student's Parent
(unless parent decided not to attend)

Phil Gardner
Special Education Director or Designee

Mary McDuffie
Special Education Teacher/Provider

Sean Howard
General Education Teacher (if the child/student is
or may be participating in the general education
environment)

Student (if appropriate)

Julia Dominguez
Building Principal or Designee

OTHER EVALUATION PERSONNEL AND THOSE PROVIDING SERVICES TO THE CHILD/STUDENT

Tina Wilson
Speech/Language Specialist

Gert Rebel
School Nurse

Cassidy Lackey
Occupational Therapist

Chris Pates
Physical Therapist

Jennie Yantis
School Psychologist

Al Sadler
School Social Worker

Audiologist

School Counselor

Other (specify area represented)

Other (specify area represented)

THE FOLLOWING PERSONS WERE ALSO IN ATTENDANCE AT THE MEETING
NOTE: Include name of person knowledgeable about second language acquisition, if appropriate.
NOTE: Agency representative must be invited for possible out-of-district placement.
NOTE: A representative of a facility or private school the student attends must be invited.

NAME	AREA REPRESENTED

Aug-2001   (5b) Page 2 of 10

Reprinted by permission of the Colorado Department of Education, Special Education Services Unit.

Hannah Richardson	1234	3/23/95	3/10/01
Legal Name of Child/Student	Child/Student ID	DOB	Date of Meeting

Documentation of Evaluation Data and Present
Level of Educational Performance and Needs

◇ EDUCATIONAL ◇

How does this child/student perform within the general curriculum (content standards) and on age appropriate tasks and benchmarks?

Names or Types of Formal and Informal Evaluations Administered	Scores/Results	Dates Evaluations Administered	Names and Titles of Evaluators/Interpreters
Tera - Informal Testing	_1-2%_	_3/2/01_	_Mary Mc Duffie_

Language of Evaluation if Other than English _____

Record classroom observation by someone other than the classroom teacher for the child/student with a suspected perceptual/communicative disability:

Strengths: _Sweet, friendly girl who is always polite to peers and adults. Hannah tries very hard. She is more readily available to focus and learn. Knows 12 capitol letters, 10 lower case, a few sounds, shapes □, ♡, counts-13, writes to 4, knows all colors except black. Can sing ABC._

Needs: _Alt. pre-academic skills, extra time to respond, repeat question - give choice for answers._

◇ SOCIAL/EMOTIONAL/ADAPTIVE BEHAVIOR ◇

How does this child/student manage feelings and interact with others? How well does the child/student adapt to different environments, i.e., home, school, and community?

Names or Types of Formal and Informal Evaluations Administered	Scores/Results	Dates Evaluations Administered	Names and Titles of Evaluators/Interpreters
Vineland		_2/16/01_	_Al Sadler, MSW_
Interview w/ parent		_3/2/01_	
and student		_3/2/01_	

Language of Evaluation if Other than English _____

Record Adaptive Behavior for a child/student with suspected Significant Limited Intellectual Capacity:

Strengths: _Hannah is pleasant, kind and an eager learner at school. Her skills across all domains are inconsistant with areas of deficit followed by strengths. Typically, children's abilities follow a developmental trajectory but for Hannah she exhibits_

Needs: _peaks & valleys. Hannah's strengths are in the areas of daily living skills, spec.fically coping skills and play. Hannah has a few friendships. She manages feelings well. Enjoys social interaction_

Vineland - Communication 72 2-8, Socialization 84 3-8, Daily Living Skills 69 3-6, Motor 66 3-0 Composite 72 3-3 Age Equivalent

MAY BE DRAFTED PRIOR TO THE MEETING.
Aug-2001   (5b) Page 3 of 10

Reprinted by permission of the Colorado Department of Education, Special Education Services Unit.

Hannah Richardson	1234	3/23/95	3/20/01
Legal Name of Child/Student	Child/Student ID	DOB	Date of Meeting

Documentation of Evaluation Data and Present
Level of Educational Performance and Needs

◇ **PHYSICAL/MOTOR AND PHYSICAL HEALTH** ◇

How is the child's/student's vision, hearing, coordination, and general health?

Does the child/student have a medical diagnosis?   Yes ☒   No ☐

__Uterine stroke, right hemiparesis__   __Dr. Finkle, neurologist__
If yes, what is the diagnosis?   Name of physician making diagnosis:

If the child/student has a health problem, is there a health care plan?   Yes ☐   No ☒

If yes, what is the location of the plan? _____

	Right	Left		Right	Left
Vision Screening:	Wears glasses		Hearing Screening:	Pass	Pass

Names or Types of Formal and Informal Evaluations Administered	Scores/Results	Dates Evaluations Administered	Names and Titles of Evaluators/Interpreters
School Function Assessment	Classroom - 2 Playground/Recess - 2 Bathroom/Toileting - 4 Transitions 5	Transportation - 3 Mealtime/snack - 4	

Language of Evaluation if Other than English _____

Record health history and current health status and, when appropriate, fine, gross, and sensory motor skills.

Strengths: Overall health good. Tendon transfer surgery 1/01 on right wrist. Seeing finger movement. (8th surgery) Wears glasses - patching left eye half of awake time. Trying Ritalin for attention difficulties (2.5mg) 3 to 4 colds over the winter. Balance difficulties when around

Needs: many children. Needs constant supervision on playground.

◇ **COMMUNICATIVE** ◇

How does this child/student listen, understand language, and express him or herself?

	Names or Types of Formal and Informal Evaluations Administered	Scores/Results	Dates Evaluations Administered	Names and Titles of Evaluators/Interpreters	Severity Rating Scale
Articulation	Formal Observation	Noticable Errors	2/12/01	Tina Wilson	4
Fluency		Acceptable		MA CCC-SLP	2
Voice		Acceptable			2
Functional Language	Peabody Picture Vocab.	91SS 27%ile			3 social use of language
Language (elf Preschool	Receptive	95SS 37%ile			4
Language (elf Preschool	Expressive	73SS 4%ile			
Language of Evaluation if Other than English	NA	Total Lang. 82SS 12%ile		composite 4	

Strengths: Hannah has demonstrated significant growth in the development of her receptive language structures (vocabulary & concepts, sentence and word structures) clarity of Hannah's speech is negatively impacted by dyspraxia mainly affecting clarity of multisyllabic words and continuous speech. Patterns include deletion of final consonants & reduction of multisyllabic words.

Needs: Improve - Following directions, expressive word structures and sentence structures, word retrieval for expressive language/labeling.
  -Clarity of expressive speech
  -Sequencing for auditory processing and expressive language
  -Spontaneous verbal exchanges with peers in classroom

Reprinted by permission of the Colorado Department of Education, Special Education Services Unit.

Hannah Richardson	1234	3/23/95	3/20/01
Legal Name of Child/Student	Child/Student ID	DOB	Date of Meeting

Documentation of Evaluation Data and Present
Level of Educational Performance and Needs

◇ **COGNITIVE** ◇

How does the child/student think, problem solve, and learn within the environment?

Names or Types of Formal and Informal Evaluations Administered	Scores/Results	Dates Evaluations Administered	Names and Titles of Evaluators/Interpreters
Wechsler Preschool	Performance : 68	3/7/01	Jennie Yantis
and Primary Scale	Verbal : 66		Ed S
of Intelligence	Full Scale IQ: 64		

Language of Evaluation if Other than English

Strengths: Hannah was administered the WPPSI-R. During testing she was cooperative and good natured. She said she loved puzzles. For the motor activities, Hannah was unable to use her right hand, so performance score may be slightly depressed. Hannah also had trouble with word retrieval and retrival of ideas. When questions were repeated; however,

Needs: She was often able to come up with an answer. Hannah scored relatively well on one task requiring attention to detail, but little language. These scores may be depressed due to motor difficulties and language difficulties. Hannah could benefit from

Performance	Verbal
OA: 5	Inf : 7
GD: 3	Com : 5
BD: 4	Ar : 5
M 2 : 2	Voc : 3
P G : 8	Sim : 4
(AP: 2)	

◇ **TRANSITION/LIFE SKILLS** ◇ visual cues in instruction. DAS at TCH (5/00) Perform - 75

How prepared is the student to transition to each level of school. How does the student function in school, home, Verbal -68 community.

Names or Types of Formal and Informal Evaluations Administered	Scores/Results	Dates Evaluations Administered	Names and Titles of Evaluators/Interpreters
Informal			Mary McDuffie

Language of Evaluation if Other than English

Strengths: - friendly, outgoing, cooperative

- has mastered her way around building areas that she uses each week.

Needs: - support in specials / playground with other students

Additional concerns of the Parent(s) for enhancing the child's/student's education:

MAY BE DRAFTED PRIOR TO THE MEETING.
Aug-2001   (5b) Page 5 of 10

Reprinted by permission of the Colorado Department of Education, Special Education Services Unit.

Hannah Richardson	1234	3/23/95	3/20/01
Legal Name of Child/Student	Child/Student ID	DOB	Date of Meeting

Determination of Eligibility and Disability

Have sufficient and appropriate evaluations been completed, documented, and considered to determine the child's/student's current level of functioning, achievement, performance, and educational needs?

If no, obtain additional information and reconvene the meeting.

Yes ☑   No ☐

Can the child/student receive reasonable educational benefit from general education alone?

Yes ☐   No ☑

Is the child's/student's performance due to the lack of instruction in reading or math?

Yes ☐   No ☐

For the child/student whose primary language is other than English, is limited English acquisition the primary cause of the child's/student's learning problems?

If any response is yes, terminate the meeting.

Yes ☐   No ☐

If no, does the child/student have a disability as defined in the State Rules for the Administration of the Exceptional Children's Educational Act?

If no, terminate the meeting.

Yes ☑   No ☐

If the child/student has a disability, the disability is:
(If more than one disability is determined, the primary disability should be identified with a "1", the secondary disability with a "2".)

☐ Significant Limited Intellectual Capacity

☐ Significant Identifiable Emotional Disability

☐ Perceptual or Communicative Disability

☐ Hearing Disability (requires communication plan)

☐ Vision Disability (requires Literacy Modality plan)

☐ Speech/Language Disability

☐ Preschool Child with a Disability

Physical Disability:

☐ Traumatic Brain Injury

☐ Autism

☐ Other Physical Disability

Multiple Disabilities:

☐ Deaf-Blind (requires Communication and Literacy Modality plans)

☑ Multiple Disabilities with Cognitive Impairment

Complete the appropriate checklist for determination of each disability selected.

Reprinted by permission of the Colorado Department of Education, Special Education Services Unit.

Hannah Richardson	1234	3/23/95	3/20/01
Legal Name of Child/Student	Child/Student ID	DOB	Date of Meeting

Goals and Objectives

With the exception of the Initial IEP, the committee must review and document progress toward completion of the child's/student's previous goals and objectives prior to the development of new goals and objectives.

Annual Goal to be Measured by Achievement of Benchmarks (#   ): (Goals should reflect standards/key components/access skills)

Hannah will improve her communication skills for successful participation in verbal classroom situations as measured by the following objectives.

Short-term Instructional Objectives/Benchmarks	Criteria and Evaluation Procedures to be Used (i.e., formal/informal measures, observations, recorded data, work samples, etc.)	Schedule for Achievement of Objective		Progress (Not Evident, Not Yet Proficient, Proficient or Advanced) *	
		Beginning Date	Target Completion Date	Date	Proficiency
(# A) Hannah will retell a 3-4 step sequence story with picture cues and a 3-step sentence related to a familiar story without picture cues 80% when asked Baseline: Retells last step in a 3 sequence picture story	Informal Measures	3/20/01	3/20/02		
(# B) Expand pronoun structures (her, they, hers, them) as well as grammatical structures (is, are) and word structures (not), past tense endings, also (to) and (will) @ 80% accuracy Baseline: Has plural (s) & (ing) Articulation skills interfere		3/20/01	3/20/02		
(# C) Eliminate final consonant deletions in structured therapy for 4-5 word combinations & include /l/ & /r/ approximations in single words 2 and 3 word combinations when spontaneously labeling @ 80% accuracy Baseline: Final Cons. Deletions eliminated in 3 word structures Doesn't produce l or r in 3 word structures		3/20/01	3/20/02		
(# D)Increase verbal exchanges with peers to 3-4 exchanges in the classroom setting 1-2x per session Baseline: Presently 1 exchange		3/20/01	3/20/02		

* Not Evident: Skill/behavior rarely or never is demonstrated, even with sufficient prompts or cues.
No Yet Proficient: Skill/behavior is demonstrated inconsistently , even with frequent prompts or cues.
  Proficient: Skill/behavior is demonstrated consistently, over time with only occasional prompts or cues.
  Advanced: Skill/behavior is generalized (demonstrated in different settings or environments) and transferable (adapted to different contexts) with no prompts or cues.

Aug-2001   **(5a) PAGE 7 OF 10**

Reprinted by permission of the Colorado Department of Education, Special Education Services Unit.

Hannah Richardson	1234	3/23/95	3/20/01
Legal Name of Child/Student	Child/Student ID	DOB	Date of Meeting

Special Education and Related Services

Service Delivery:
Statement of specific services to be provided:

Special Education Services:	Service Coordinator #1	Other Service Providers			
		#2	#3	#4	#5
Type of Service Provider (assignment)	Resource	Sp/Lang	O.T	P.T	
Projected Beginning Date of Service	3/20/01	3/20/01	3/20/01	3/20/01	
Projected Ending Date of Service	3/20/02	3/20/02	3/20/02	3/20/02	

Hours of Special Education Services per Week by Service Provider					
Indirect (consultation)	1	.25	.25	.25	
Direct in General Classroom	8		.50-.75		
Direct Outside General Classroom	3	1		.5	
Total Hours by Provider	12	1.25	.75-1.5	.75	

Describe how parent(s) will be informed of the child's progress toward annual goals. How often will this occur?

Is the child eligible for services beyond the regular school year? Yes ☐ No ☒ ☐ To be determined by Date: _____
Documentation:

Does the child/student require:

Special Transportation? Yes ☐ No ☒

A Communication plan? (Required for a child/student with hearing disabilities) Yes ☐ No ☒

A Literacy Modality plan? (Required for a child/student with vision disabilities) Yes ☐ No ☒

A Behavior Support plan? (May be reviewed and modified throughout duration of the IEP) Yes ☐ No ☒

Assistive Technology services and/or devices? If yes, describe: Yes ☒ No ☐

Aug-2001   (5b) Page 8 of 10

Reprinted by permission of the Colorado Department of Education, Special Education Services Unit.

Hannah Richardson	1234	3/23/95	3/20/01
Legal Name of Child/Student	Child/Student ID	DOB	Date of Meeting

Accommodations/Modifications and Participation
in State and District Assessments

Accommodation/Modifications:

Describe the curricular and instructional accommodations/ modifications necessary for the child/student to participate in all activities related to the general education curriculum, considering the identified needs of the child/student. *(Consider language needs of the child/student and grade level content standards.)*

Extra time for Hannah to verbalize, modifications of length, quantity of assignments as needed, preferential seating, modification of equipment as needed

Check whether the child/student will participate in the CSAP or CSAP-Alternate for each content area(s) administered at the child/student's grade level. <u>Check all that apply</u>. *(If the CSAP-A is not available at the child/student's grade level, then a Body of Evidence must be documented below.)*

	CSAP	CSAP -A	CSAP -A Not available at grade Level
Reading and Writing	☐	☐	☒
Mathematics	☐	☐	☒
Science (8th Grade Only)	☐	☐	☐

List all standard accommodations to be used in the CSAP administration:

Check whether the child/student will participate in the District Assessment or the District Alternate for each content area(s) administered at the child/student's grade level. <u>Check all that apply</u>. *(If a child/student requires a district alternate, then a Body of Evidence must be documented below.)*

	District	District-Alternate
Reading/ Writing/ Language Arts	☐	☒
Mathematics	☐	☒
Other: _____	☐	☐
Other: _____	☐	☐

List district assessment accommodations:

Body of Evidence: If CSAP-A or district assessment is not available at the student's grade level, or the student requires a district alternate, a Body of Evidence must be provided. Check all forms of documentation that are being used for this student to document progress towards standards in any of the above content areas.

☒ Performance Assessments	☐ Personal Communications
☒ Structured Observation	☐ Student Self-Assessment
☒ Interviews and Record Reviews	☒ IEP Goals and Objectives
☒ Progress Reports	☐ Report Cards

Other (describe):

Reprinted by permission of the Colorado Department of Education, Special Education Services Unit.

Hannah Richardson	*1234*	*3/23/95*	*3/20/01*
Legal Name of Child/Student	Child/Student ID	DOB	Date of Meeting

Recommended Placement in the Least Restrictive Environment
(Special Education Instructional Setting)

Check all settings which were considered (first column) and all settings in which special
education and related services will be provided (second column).

Considered	**Selected**	**Considered**	**Selected**

* *Out of the entire school week, what percent of the time is the child/student receiving special education services.*

| Neighborhood/Home School | | Center School or District other than the Student's Home School | |

✷ GENERAL CLASSROOM, WITH SUPPORT FROM SPECIAL EDUCATION　　　　　**GENERAL CLASSROOM, WITH SUPPORT FROM SPECIAL EDUCATION**

Considered	Less than 21 percent of the time	Selected	Considered	Less than 21 percent of the time	Selected
[ ]	Less than 21 percent of the time	[ ]	[ ]	Less than 21 percent of the time	[ ]
[✓]	21 to 60 percent of the time	[ ]	[ ]	21 to 60 percent of the time	[ ]
[✓]	Greater than 60 percent of the time	[✓]	[ ]	Greater than 60 percent of the time	[ ]

OUTSIDE GENERAL CLASSROOM　　　　　**OUTSIDE GENERAL CLASSROOM**

[✓]	Less than 21 percent of the time	[✓]	[ ]	Less than 21 percent of the time	[ ]
[✓]	21 to 60 percent of the time	[ ]	[ ]	21 to 60 percent of the time	[ ]
[ ]	Greater than 60 percent of the time	[ ]	[ ]	Greater than 60 percent of the time	[ ]

Other Instructional Settings

[ ]	Home	[ ]	[ ]	Public School Separate Facility	[ ]
[ ]	Hospital	[ ]	[ ]	Private Separate School Facility	[ ]
[ ]	Community	[ ]	[ ]	Public Residential Facility	[ ]
[ ]	Administrative Unit Separate Facility	[ ]	[ ]	Private Residential Facility	[ ]
			[ ]	Correctional Facility	[ ]

Of those special education instructional settings selected place an asterisk (*) by the primary setting.

Provide justification for placement decision:

PARENTAL CONSENT (Required for Initial placement only)

I have been informed of (in my primary language) and understand my special education rights and procedural safeguards.　　　Yes [X]　No [ ]

Consent is given for my child/student to receive special education and related services.　　　Yes [X]　No [ ]

George Richardson	*3/20/01*
Signature of Parent(s)	Date
Kathy Richardson	*3/20/01*
Signature of Parent(s)	Date

If Appropriate, translation provided by:

Signature of Interpreter	Date

Aug-2001　　　　　**(5b) Page 10 of 10**

Reprinted by permission of the Colorado Department of Education, Special Education Services Unit.

Appendix F: Sample Individualized Family Service Plan

Sample Individualized Family Service Plan.

Note. Form reprinted with permission from Boulder County Early Childhood Connections.

Individualized Family Service Plan

Family Information

Child's Name: Clara Lieberman   Birthdate: 5/23/95   Age (in mos.): 27   Adjusted Age: NA   Date: 10/22/97

Parent(s) or Guardian(s) Donald and Rachel Lieberman   Initial Date of Referral: 9/96

Address: Boulder, CO   Phone: (h) 123-4567   (w)

Service Coordinator: Jeff Hanson   Phone: (303) 604-2654   Scheduled Review Date: 4/22/97

Important Friends and Relatives

- grandparents
- Maddy - neighbor girl
- church
- Uncle Mike and Aunt Lori

Helpful professionals and programs (i.e., doctor, child care providers, therapists, etc.)

- Child Learning Center
- Dr. Sara Kincade
- Play Center - Mary Jones
- Nurse Ruth
- Hospital Therapist

What does your child enjoy most or do best?

- playing with balls
- watching videos
- singing & movement
- playing with friends

What are your family's strengths and resources?

- supportive extended family
- church
- lots of love
- mother a speech pathologist

What are your family's priorities for the next few months?

- walking
- communication
- peer interactions
- getting off seizure medication

What are your concerns or questions regarding your child?

What are Clara's visual difficulties?
How much should we push the walker?

Child's School District: Boulder   Child's Social Security Number: 235-01-5678

Private Insurance Carrier Name (opt.): Colorado HMO   Name of Insured: Rick Lieberman   Group # 2568   Policy # 001-101

Medicaid Type: Medicaid #

Rev. 7/9/01

Reprinted by permission of Boulder County Early Childhood Connections.

LOOK WHAT I CAN DO!

for _____Clara_____

Movement, coordination, balance (Gross Motor Development)

Parent observations: Date 10/22/97

Clara stands on the couch to observe things going on. She is cruising along furniture and is very mobile. She is less fearful about moving and enjoys climbing stairs and is less resistant to being helped with her walker. She likes crawling into closed, tight spaces. She's pulling herself to a stand. She is bouncy and energetic.

Team members' observations: Date 10/20/97

More comfortable when you hold her hands. Not comfortable using walker independently. Prefers to scoot on her bottom. Pulls to stand through a half-kneel.

Use of hands and fingers, coordination, interacting with toys and objects (Fine Motor Development)

Parent observations: Date 10/15/97

Clara gestures with songs. She enjoys throwing balls. She likes her sand box filled with beans. She is good at putting things away.

Team members' observations: Date 10/20/97

Her fine motor skills have improved. She responds well to verbal cues to use her hands, especially her left. She can pass objects from hand to hand. Clara does not like her hands forcefully manipulated.

Rev. 7/9/01

Reprinted by permission of Boulder County Early Childhood Connections.

LOOK WHAT I CAN DO!

for: _Clara_

Verbal, nonverbal, understanding, oral motor (Communication)
Parent observations: Date _10/22/97_

Understands most everything. Very social. Good at communicating her needs with vocalizations and gestures. Likes talking on the phone. Starting to point to where she wants to go.

Team members' observations: Date _10/15/97_

Engaging. Using more vowels. Can put 3 words together. She does a lot of jabbering and clicking her tongue. Interested in the pictures on her augmentative communication device.

Dressing, feeding, potty training, taking care of own needs (Self Help/ Adaptive Behavior)
Parent observations: Date _10/22/97_

Clara eats and sleeps well. Starting to use a regular cup instead of a sippy cup. She doesn't like her hair brushed or washed.

Team members' observations: Date _10/15/97_

She enjoys snack at preschool. In diapers - not showing interest in potty training. Uses a fork effectively. Can take her socks off.

Rev. 7/9/01

Reprinted by permission of Boulder County Early Childhood Connections.

LOOK WHAT I CAN DO!

for: _Clara_

Child Assessment/IFSP

Page 3 of 5

Personality, interaction with friends, family members and others, likes and dislikes, (Social-Emotional Development)

Parent observations: Date _10/22/97_

Happy, easy-going. She enjoys attention, performing, and be the center of things. Clara really likes babies and the other children. She likes to be in control of her situation. She notices an infant carrier a mile away.

Team members' observations: Date _10/5/97_

She is very affectionate, caring and nurturing. Switching activities is sometimes difficult for her. She has a good sense of humor.

Play, attention, problem solving (Cognitive Development)

Parent observations: Date _10/22/97_

Loves to play babies-acts out 2 to 3 step play sequences (feed doll, burp doll, rock doll). She enjoys watching television. Interested in books. She loves to explore and figure things out.

Team members' observations: Date _10/17/97_

Clara's attention span has increased. Does not enjoy puzzles. She is doing 2-step visual imitation. Parallel play with peers. Enjoys water table.

Rev. 7/9/01

Reprinted by permission of Boulder County Early Childhood Connections.

Individualized Family Service Plan

for: _Clara_

Child Assessment/IFSP

Page 4 of 5

Your child's health:

Generally healthy or in the hospital/clinic frequently?   Date _10/10/97_

Frequent colds. No more ear infections after placement of PE tubes. Recent EEG - discussing getting off seizure medications (Phenobarbitol and Dilantin). Planning heel cord release and removal of extra bones in big toes.

Are there any health concerns that should be considered in planning services and supports (precautions, equipment needs such as ventilator, suction, inhaler, medications, allergies)?

Allergic to peanuts.

Do you have any concerns about your child's hearing or vision?

Yes - possible cortical vision impairment. Vision seems to vary day to day. Comfort with walker - visually related?

Date(s) and location(s) of last hearing/vision screenings?

Hearing - Boulder Hearing Assoc. 9/1/97
Vision - Play Center 7/28/97

Rev. 7/9/01

Reprinted by permission of Boulder County Early Childhood Connections.

Individualized Family Service Plan

for _Clara_

Statement of Eligibility

Page 5 of 5

Age _27_   Adjusted Age _NA_

Eligible for Part C under the Individuals with Disabilities Education Act (IDEA) due to:

✓ Medical Condition:

Name of Condition _Uterine Stroke_   Documented by: _Dr. Finkle_

✓ Developmental Delay:

Eligibility Certified by (name and title) (A minimum of 2 disciplines is required to confirm eligibility.):

1) _Mara Smith_ _Educator_   2) _Mindy Seguin_ _Psychologist_

   Name   Discipline   Name   Discipline

Domain	Evaluator	Source of Information/Date			Age Levels, %ile, SD or informal results	Areas of Delay
		Parent Report	Observation	Other Sources		
Social/Emotional	Ping Wa	✓	✓	Transdisciplinary Play-Based Assessment	Parent requested these not be reported	
Adaptive Behavior	Ping Wa	✓	✓			
Cognitive	Jack Smith	✓	✓			
Gross Motor	Janet Scott	✓	✓			✓
Fine Motor	Janet Scott	✓	✓			✓
Feeding/Oral-Motor	Sheila Jackson	✓	✓			
Expressive Communication	Sheila Jackson	✓	✓			✓
Receptive Communication	Sheila Jackson	✓	✓			
Hearing		✓				
Vision	Norah	✓				
Health	Snellcheck	✓				✓

Rev. 7/9/01

Reprinted by permission of Boulder County Early Childhood Connections.

Individualized Family Service Plan

for _Clara_   **Signatures**

Date: _10/22/97_

Family Acknowledgement.

I have had an opportunity to participate fully in the development of the IFSP and am informed about the available resources, services and supports.

Yes ☑ No ☐ Comments: _____

Donald Lieberman 10/22/97   _Rachel Lieberman_ 10/22/97
Signature of parent/guardian   Date   Signature of parent/guardian   Date

IFSP Participants: The following individuals participated in the development of the IFSP.

Service Coordinator: _Ping Wa_   Address: _Boulder, CO_   Phone: _____

Other: _____   Role: _Social Worker_   Phone: _____

Address: _____

Other: _Jackson Mstr_   Role: _Psychologist_   Phone: _____

Address: _____

Other: _Shelia Jackson_   Role: _Speech Language Pathologist_   Phone: _____

Address: _____

Other: _Noah Snillchock_   Role: _Nurse_   Phone: _____

Address: _____

Other: _____   Role: _____   Phone: _____

Address: _____

Other: _____   Role: _____   Phone: _____

Address: _____

Please send copies of this IFSP to:

Name: _Dr. Kincannon_   Address: _Denver, CO_   Initial: _RL_

Name: _Child Learning Center_   Address: _Boulder, CO_   Initial: _RL_

Name: _____   Address: _____   Initial: _____

Reason for Conference: ☐ Interim IFSP   ☐ Initial IFSP   ☑ 6 Month Review   ☐ Annual IFSP

Interim plan because: _____   Other: _____

Rev. 7/9/01

Reprinted by permission of Boulder County Early Childhood Connections.

Appendix G: Educational Rights of Parents

An Explanation of Procedural Safeguards
Available to Parents of Children With Disabilities
(August 1999).

Note: Reprinted by permission of the Colorado Department of
Education, Special Education Services Unit.

INTRODUCTION

Described in this pamphlet are parent educational rights
required under federal and state special education rules and
regulations. It is important that you, as a parent, understand
your rights in special education relating to your child.

School staff are available to assist you in understanding
these rights and are available on request to provide you with
any further explanation. If needed, the school will provide an
interpreter or translation to help assure that you understand.

FREE APPROPRIATE PUBLIC EDUCATION

You have a right to participate in meetings with respect to
the:

- identification,
- evaluation,
- eligibility,
- Individualized Education Program (IEP),

- placement, and
- the provision of a free appropriate public education (FAPE) for your child.

Your child's general education teacher should be involved with the IEP development.

An eligible child with a disability has a right to receive a free appropriate education that is outlined as an Individualized Education Program. The IEP is meant to address your child's unique needs.

Termination of FAPE

A student's right to FAPE under special education law ends at the end of the semester in which the student turns 21, or when the student has graduated with a regular high school diploma or GED. A student's right to FAPE is not terminated by any other kind of graduation or completion certificate.

A student's right to FAPE under special education law would also end if the IEP team determines that special education services are no longer needed. If a parent does not agree that their son or daughter should graduate with a regular high school diploma, or that their son or daughter no longer needs special education services, they are entitled to procedural due process to resolve the disagreement.

PRIOR NOTICE TO PARENTS

The school will notify you by letter if they are proposing to change or refuse to change your child's special education program. The notice must be easily understandable. You must also receive notice of special education meetings about your child within a reasonable time so you can attend.

The school district must provide you with written prior notice before each time it proposes or refuses to initiate or change the identification, evaluation, or educational placement of your child or the provision of a free appropriate public education to your child.

The notice must include:

1. a full explanation of all the procedural safeguards and state complaint procedures available to you in your native language;

2. a description of the action proposed or refused by the school district;

3. an explanation of why the school district proposes or refuses to take the action;

4. a description of any other options the school district considered and the reasons why those options were rejected;

5. a description of each evaluation procedure, test, record, or report the school district used as a basis for the proposed or refused action;

6. a description of any other factors which are relevant to the school's proposal or refusal;

7. a statement that you, as a parent of a child with a disability, have protection under the procedural safeguards of special education law, and the means by which a copy of the procedural safeguards can be obtained; and

8. sources for you to contact to obtain assistance in understanding the provisions of special education.

If you need assistance in understanding any of the procedural safeguards, or anything else relating to your child's education, please contact the Director of Special Education of your local school district.

A copy of the procedural safeguards will be provided to you at a minimum:

- upon the initial referral for evaluation,
- upon each notification of an IEP meeting,
- upon re-evaluation of your child, and
- upon receipt by the school district of a request for a due process hearing.

The procedural safeguards notice must be written in your native language or other mode of communication, unless it is clearly not feasible to do so, and written in an easily understandable manner. The school district must make sure that you understand your special education rights,

ensure that this will be translated to you if necessary, and document their process of providing you these rights.

PARENT CONSENT

Your written permission is required before your child is initially evaluated, re-evaluated, and placed in special education.

The school must obtain your informed consent before conducting a pre-placement evaluation, initial placement, and re-evaluation of your child in a program providing special education and related services. However, in cases of re-evaluation, the school district does not have to have your consent if it can demonstrate that it has taken reasonable measures to obtain your consent and you failed to respond. The school district may require your consent for other services and activities.

Your consent is not required before reviewing the existing data as part of an evaluation or a re-evaluation; or before giving a test or other evaluation that is given to all children unless, before they give a test or evaluation, they have asked for consent from all parents.

Information regarding consent will be written in your native language or other mode of communication. You should understand:

- the reason written consent is being asked,
- that giving your consent is voluntary, and
- that you can revoke your consent at any time. (If you revoke your consent, that revocation is not retroactive [i.e., it does not negate an action that has occurred after the consent was given and before the consent was revoked]).

Your consent should identify any records to be released, to whom they will be released, and for what purpose they will be released. Giving your written consent also means that you understanding and agree that the school will perform the activities for which you have given your consent.

If you refuse consent for initial evaluation or a re-evaluation, the school district may continue to seek an evaluation by using due process hearing procedures. Pending any

due process hearing decision, your child would remain in his or her present educational placement, unless you and the school district agree otherwise. A school district may not use your refusal to consent to one service or activity to deny you or your child any other service, benefit, or activity of the school district, except as may be required by special education law. Also, you have a right to appeal the decision of a due process hearing officer.

INDEPENDENT EDUCATIONAL EVALUATION

If you disagree with the school's evaluation of your child, you can request an independent evaluation, conducted by someone not employed by your school district.

If you disagree with an evaluation obtained by your school district, you have the right to obtain an independent educational evaluation of your child at public expense, unless the school can show its evaluation is sufficient. An independent educational evaluation is an evaluation conducted by a qualified examiner who is not employed by the school district. The school district will provide, upon your request, information about where an independent educational evaluation may be obtained.

Your school district may initiate a due process hearing to show that the school district's evaluation is sufficient. If it is determined, by decision of a hearing officer, that the evaluation is appropriate, you still have the right to an independent educational evaluation, but not at public expense.

If you request an independent educational evaluation, the school district may ask why you object to the public evaluation. However, the school district cannot require an explanation from you, and the school district may not unreasonably delay either providing the independent education evaluation at public expense, or initiating a due process hearing to defend their evaluation.

If you obtained an independent educational evaluation at private expense, the results of the evaluation must be considered by the evaluation and/or planning team in any decision made with respect to the provision of a free appropriate

public education for your child, and may be presented as evidence at a due process hearing regarding your child.

If a hearing officer requests an independent educational evaluation as part of a hearing, the cost of the evaluation must be at public expense.

Whenever an independent evaluation is at public expense, the criteria under which the evaluation is obtained, including the location of the evaluation and the qualification of the examiner, must be the same as the criteria which the school district uses when it initiates an evaluation, to the extent those criteria are consistent with your right to an independent educational evaluation. A school district may not impose additional conditions or timelines related to obtaining an independent evaluation at public expense.

EDUCATIONAL SURROGATE PARENTS

Some children do not have parents who can advocate for them in the special education process. An educational surrogate parent is someone appointed to represent the child at special education meetings.

Each school district shall have a method for determining whether a child needs an educational surrogate parent and shall ensure that an individual is assigned, through the Colorado Department of Education, to act as an educational surrogate parent for a child whenever the parents of a child are not known and/or the school district cannot, after reasonable efforts, locate the parents, or if parental rights have been terminated for that child.

The person assigned as the educational surrogate parent shall not be an employee of the state education agency, school district, or any other agency that is involved in the education or care of the child.

The educational surrogate parent may represent the child in all matters relating to the identification, evaluation, and educational placement of the child, including the provision of a free appropriate public education.

TRANSFER OF RIGHTS AT AGE OF MAJORITY

When a student reaches 21, or become emancipated, all special education rights transfer from the parent to the student.

All rights of parents under special education law transfer to the student when the student reaches the age of majority under state law (21 in Colorado), or earlier if the student is emancipated. These rights include, but are not limited to: consent for evaluation or re-evaluation, decisions about services and placement, and rights to special education due process procedures.

The school district must notify the student and the parent of the transfer of rights. Beginning at least one year before the student reaches the age of majority, the student's IEP must include a statement that the student has been informed of his or her rights, under IDEA, that will transfer to the student on reaching the age of majority.

STUDENT RECORDS

You have the right to see or request copies of your child's school records. If you disagree with items in the records, you can ask if they can be changed or removed.

Access to Records

The Family Educational Rights and Privacy Act (FERPA) give rights to parents regarding their children's education records. These rights transfer to a student, or a former student, who is attending any school beyond the high school level, or who has reached age 18. Schools may still provide access to records to the parents of a student who is 18 and a dependent.

Your school district must permit you to inspect and review any education records relating to your child with respect to the identification, evaluation, and educational placement of your child, and the provision of a free appropriate public education to your child. The school district must

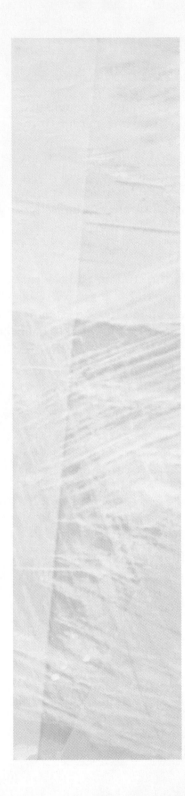

comply with your request without unnecessary delay, and before any meeting regarding an IEP, or any hearing relating to the identification, evaluation, or educational placement of your child, or the provision of a free appropriate education to your child, and in no case more than 45 days after your request has been made.

Your rights to inspect and review education records under this section includes:

- the right to a response from the school, or other participant agency, to reasonable requests for explanations and interpretations of the records;

- your right to have your representative inspect and review the records; and

- your right to request that the school district provide copies of the records containing the information if failure to provide those copies would effectively prevent you from exercising your right to inspect and review the records.

The school may presume that you have authority to inspect and review records relating to your child unless the school district has been advised that you do not have the authority under applicable state law governing such matters as guardianship, separation, and divorce.

If any education record includes information on more than one child, you have the right to inspect and review the information relating to your child or to be informed of that specific information.

The school district must provide you, on request, a list of the types and locations of education records collected, maintained, or used by the school district.

Fees for Searching, Retrieving, and Copying Records

The school may not charge a fee to search for or to retrieve information in your child's educational records, but may charge a fee for copies of records which are made for parents if the fee does not effectively prevent the parents from exercising their right to inspect and review those records.

Record of Access

The school must keep a record of those persons or organizations obtaining access to your child's educational records, including the name of the person or organization, the date access was given, and the purpose for which the person or organization was authorized to use the records. The school does not have to keep a record of access by eligible parents or students, or authorized school employees.

Amendment of Records at Parent's Request

If you believe that information in your child's education record is inaccurate, misleading or violates the privacy rights, or other rights of your child, you may request the school district to amend the information. The school district must decide whether to amend the information within a reasonable period of time or receipt of your request. If the school district decides to refuse to amend the information, it must inform you of the refusal and of your right to a hearing.

The school district shall provide an opportunity for a hearing (under the Family Educational Rights and Privacy Act) to challenge the information in the education records to ensure that the information is not inaccurate, misleading, or otherwise in violation of the privacy rights, or other rights of the student.

If, as a result of the hearing, the school district decides that the information is inaccurate, misleading, or otherwise in violation of the privacy rights, or other rights of the student, it must amend the information and inform you in writing of the amendment.

If, as a result of the hearing, the school district decides that the information is not inaccurate, misleading, or otherwise in violation of the privacy rights, or other rights of your child, it must inform you of the right to place in the records a statement commenting on the information or giving any reasons for disagreeing with the decision of the school. Any explanation placed in the student's records must be maintained by the school as part of the records of the student as

long as the record or contested portion is kept by the school. If the records of the student or the contested portion is disclosed by the school district to any person or organization, the explanation must also be disclosed to the person or organization.

DISCIPLINE

Discipline is an important part of learning. The IEP Team, including the parent, needs to determine appropriate disciplinary procedures for students with disabilities.

Discipline issues relating to students with disabilities are extensive. Additional information can be obtained from your school administrator or IEP Team.

A free appropriate public education must be made available to all eligible children with disabilities, including children with disabilities who have been removed from school (e.g., suspended or expelled) for more than a total of ten school days in a given year.

1. After a total of 10 school days:
   The IEP team must meet to:
   - Develop a plan for conducting a functional behavioral assessment.
   - Develop a plan for completing a behavior intervention plan, including appropriate behavior interventions to address that behavior, or to review and modify an existing behavior plan.
   - Determine whether the child is receiving an appropriate education.
   - Additionally, a manifestation determination to decide whether there is a relationship between your child's disability and the behavior may need to be conducted.

2. If as the result of the manifestation determination, the IEP team, including the parent, agree either that:
   A. Services were not appropriate or if the behavior was a manifestation of your child's disability, then,

- your child may not be removed (expelled or suspended) for more than 10 days unless one of the following circumstances applies:
  - your child was in possession of drugs or weapons, or
  - it is determined that he/she is substantially likely to injure him/herself or others (see items 6 and 7); or
- **B.** Your child's behavior was not a manifestation of his/her disability, then,
  - your child may be disciplined in the same manner as a child without a disability would be disciplined, and
  - the school district must continue providing a free appropriate public education for your child.
3. If you disagree with the determination that your child's behavior was not a manifestation of his/her disability or with any decision regarding placement, then you may request a hearing (an expedited hearing shall be arranged under these circumstances).
4. At any time, any member of the IEP team can request an IEP meeting to be held to revise the behavior intervention plan. If requested, the meeting must take place.
5. If your child has been suspended or expelled for more than 10 days or has been placed in an alternative educational setting, the school district must ensure that your child has access to the general curriculum and be provided services and modifications described in his/her current IEP.
6. The IEP team, including the parent, may decide that your child should be placed in an interim alternative educational setting for up to 45 days if your child:
   - brings a weapon to school or a school function,

- is in possession of or using illegal drugs, and/or
- sells or solicits the sale of a controlled substance while at school or a school function.

7. If the school district believes that your child's behavior is substantially likely to result in injury to himself or herself, the school district may ask a hearing officer to conduct an expedited hearing to consider a change of educational placement. The hearing officer must consider the following factors:

1. the likelihood that maintaining the current placement will result in injury to your child or others;

2. the appropriateness of the child's current placement;

3. whether the school district has made reasonable efforts to minimize the risk of harm in your child's current placement, including the use of supplementary aids and services; and

4. the interim alternative educational setting that is proposed by the school personnel.

The school district may report a crime committed by your child with a disability to appropriate authorities. Law enforcement officers and officers of the court will use federal and state laws to determine appropriate actions. Copies of the special education and disciplinary records of your child will be provided to the appropriate authorities to the extent permitted by the Family Educational Rights and Privacy Act.

MEDIATION

You might disagree with the special education testing, services or placement for your child. You can try to resolve your disagreements by requesting mediation, which is a free service. A mediator is a neutral person, not employed by the school district, who assists you and the school in resolving differences. You may also request a due process hearing. Please have the school explain the process before you make a final decision.

There might be times when you and the school district disagree on important issues regarding your child's education. If agreement cannot be reached, you have the right to request an impartial mediator to help you and the school reach a mutually agreeable solution.

- Both you and the school district must agree to mediation.

- Mediation is conducted by a qualified, impartial mediator, who is trained in effective mediation techniques.

- Mediation is a service that is available to you at no cost, and at a minimum must be available to you when you request a due process hearing.

- Mediation cannot be used to delay or deny your right to a due process hearing or deny any other rights afforded under special education law.

- Each session in the mediation process shall be scheduled in a timely manner and shall be held at a location that is convenient to the parties in the dispute.

- Any agreement reached by the parties in the dispute in the mediation process shall be set forth in a written mediation agreement.

- Discussions during mediation are confidential and may not be used as evidence in subsequent due process hearings or civil proceedings.

- Parties to mediation may be required to sign a confidentiality pledge before the mediation process begins.

STATE COMPLAINT PROCEDURES

If you feel the school district/agency is violating special education requirements for your child, you can file a written complaint with the Colorado Department of Education to resolve the problem.

You have a right to file a written complaint with the Colorado Department of Education if you feel the school district or agency has violated a specific requirement of special education law.

The complaint must be filed in writing with the Colorado Department of Education, Federal Complaints Officer, explaining the alleged violations. The Federal Complaints Officer will have 60 calendar days after the complaint is filed to:

1. give the school district or agency an opportunity to respond to the allegations;

2. give the parent an opportunity to submit additional information about the allegations;

3. carry out an independent on-site investigation, if the Federal Complaints Officer determines that an on-site investigation is necessary;

4. review all relevant information and made an independent determination of whether a violation of special education law has occurred;

5. issue a written decision to the school district or agency and the parents of the findings, including reasons for the final decision.

The school district is obligated to implement the final decision.

The address for filing a Federal Complaint is:
Federal Complaints Officer
Colorado Department of Education
201 East Colfax, 3rd floor
Denver, CO 80203

Before filing a Federal Complaint it is advisable to call the Federal Complaints Officer at 303-866-6685.

IMPARTIAL DUE PROCESS HEARING

If an agreement cannot be reached between you and the school district, you may request a due process hearing. The hearing will be conducted by an impartial hearing offi-

cer. As a parent involved in the hearing you must be given certain rights, including the right to an appeal.

You or the school district may initiate a due process hearing regarding the school's proposal or refusal to initiate or change the identification, evaluation, or educational placement of your child or the provision of a free appropriate public education to your child.

Before a hearing is initiated, you or your attorney should provide written notice (which will remain confidential), to the school district, providing the following information:

1. name of your child;
2. address of residence of your child;
3. name of the school your child is attending;
4. description of the problem(s) relating to the proposed or refused initiation or change, including related facts; and
5. a proposed resolution of the problem to the extent known and available to you.

The school district will have a form available for you to use to file the written notice. The school district may not deny you your right to a hearing for failure to provide the notice required.

The written request for a hearing should be submitted to the Director of Special education of your school district. The school district must then immediately inform the Colorado Department of Education of your request for a hearing.

When a hearing is initiated the school district shall inform you of the availability of mediation. The school district must also inform you of any free or low-cost legal or other relevant services available in the area if you or the school initiate a due process hearing. The school should also provide this information to you whenever you request it.

The hearing will be conducted by an impartial hearing officer obtained through the Colorado Department of Education. The Department maintains a list of hearing officers and statements of their qualifications. Three hearing officers' names, selected by rotation, are provided to the parent(s) and the school district and by process of elimination

both parties participate in the determination of a hearing officer.

The hearing cannot be conducted by an employee of the Colorado Department of Education or school district involved with the education or care of your child, or by any person having a personal or professional interest which would conflict with his or her objectivity in the hearing.

The hearing officer should reach a decision within 45 days of your request for a hearing, unless the hearing officer determines that more time is needed.

The decision made in a due process hearing is final unless there is an appeal.

Expedited Due Process Hearings

The Colorado Department of Education will arrange for an expedited hearing, if requested by a parent or school district, in any case where you disagree with issues of placement of your child into an interim alternative placement or in cases where you disagree with a determination that your child's behavior was not a manifestation of his/her disability.

Due Process Hearing Rights

Any party to a hearing or an appeal of a hearing decision has the right to:

1. be accompanied and advised by counsel, and by individuals with special knowledge or training with respect to the problems of children with disabilities;

2. present evidence and confront, cross-examine, and compel the attendance of witnesses;

3. prohibit the introduction of any evidence at the hearing that has not been disclosed to that party at least five (5) days before the hearing;

4. obtain a written or electronic verbatim record of the hearing; and

5. obtain a copy of written or electronic findings of fact and decisions. (After deleting any personally identifiable information, the Colorado

Department of Education will transmit those findings and decisions to the State advisory panel and make them available to the public.)

At least five (5) business days before a hearing, each party must disclose to all other parties all evaluations completed by that date, and any recommendations based on any evaluations that the party intends to use at the hearing. A hearing officer may bar any party that fails to comply with this disclosure rule from introducing the relevant evaluation or recommendation at the hearing unless the other party consents to its introduction.

As parents, you must be given the right to have your child present at the hearing, and the right to open the hearing to the public. Each hearing must be conducted at a time and place, which is reasonably convenient to you and your child.

The record of the hearing and the findings and hearing decision must be provided to you at no cost.

Administrative Appeal of a Due Process Hearing: Impartial Review

A party may appeal to the Division of Administrative Hearings within 30 days after receipt of the impartial hearing officer's decision.

If there is an appeal, an administrative law judge shall conduct an impartial review of the hearing and shall:

1. examine the entire hearing record;

2. ensure that the procedures at the hearing were consistent with the requirements of due process;

3. seek additional evidence if necessary (if a hearing is held to receive additional evidence, the hearing rights described above apply);

4. afford the parties an opportunity for oral or written argument, or both, at the discretion of the administrative law judge, at a time and place reasonably convenient to the parties;

5. make a final and independent decision on completion of the review and mail such to all parties

within 30 days of the filing or mailing of the notice of appeal; and

6. give a copy of written or electronic findings and the decision to the parties. (After deleting any personally identifiable information, the Colorado Department of Education will transmit those findings and decisions to the State advisory panel and make them available to the public.)

The administrative law judge may grant specific extensions of any of the timelines. The decision made by the administrative law judge is final, unless a party brings a civil action.

Civil Action

Any party has the right to bring a civil action in State or Federal Court. The action may be brought in any State Court of competent jurisdiction or in a U.S. District Court, without regard to the amount in controversy. In any action brought under this section, a Court shall receive the records of the administrative proceedings, hear additional evidence at the request of a party, and, basing its decision on the preponderance of the evidence, shall grant the relief that the Court determines to be appropriate.

Child's Status During Proceedings

Pending any administrative or judicial proceeding, unless you and the school district agree otherwise, your child must remain in his or her present educational placement. However, if the child was placed in an interim alternative educational placement, then the child would remain in the alternative placement pending the decision of the hearing officer, or until the expiration of the time for which the student was removed, whichever comes first (unless the parent and the school district agree to another placement). If the school personnel maintain that it is dangerous for the child to be in the current placement (placement prior to removal to the interim alternative educational setting), pending a due process proceeding, the school district may request an expedited due process hearing.

If a hearing involves an application for initial admission to public school, your child, with your consent, must be placed in the public school program until the completion of all the proceedings.

Award of Attorney's Fees

If any action or proceeding discussed above, the Court, in its discretion, may award reasonable attorney's fees as part of the cost to the parents or guardians or a child or youth with disabilities who is the prevailing party. However, neither due process hearing officers, nor the federal complaints officer, may award attorney's fees.

Attorney fees may not be awarded for any meeting of the IEP Team unless such a meeting is convened as a result of an administrative proceeding or judicial action.

PRIVATE SCHOOL PLACEMENT

If the parents of a child with a disability enroll their child in a private school without the consent of the school district, a court or due process hearing officer may require the school district to reimburse the parents for the cost of that enrollment *only* if the court or hearing officer finds the school district has not made a free appropriate public education available to the child, prior to enrollment, *and* that the private placement is appropriate.

Appendix H: Child and Elder Abuse

SIGNS OF CHILD ABUSE

The following signs of child abuse may indicate that abuse is occurring according to Prevent Child Abuse America (http://www.preventchildabuse.org), National Clearinghouse on Child Abuse and Neglect Information (http://www.colib.com), and Child Abuse Prevention Network (http://www.child-abuse.com). Remember that physical abuse signs may be seen on the child's physical body, whereas evidence of the other types of abuse are more behavioral. Behavioral signs may occur by themselves or may accompany physical indicators.

Behavior changes in a child indicating abuse include:

- Shows sudden changes in behavior or school performance
- Has not received help for physical or medical problems brought to the parents' attention
- Has learning problems that cannot be attributed to specific physical or psychological causes.
- Is always watchful as though preparing for something bad to happen
- Lacks adult supervision
- Is overly compliant, an overachiever, or too responsible
- Comes to school early, stays late, and does not want to go home

Behavior in an adult indicating possible abuse to a child include:

- Appears to be indifferent to the child. Shows little concern for the child and does not respond to the school's requests for information, conferences, or home visits

- Denies the existence of or blames the child
- Wants others to use harsh physical discipline if the child misbehaves
- Sees the child as entirely bad, worthless, or burdensome
- Demands perfection from the child
- Seems apathetic or depressed
- Behaves irrationally or in a bizarre manner

Signs of Physical Abuse

Physical abuse includes any nonaccidental physical injury caused by the child's caretaker. It may happen one time or repeated times. Even though the injury is not an accident, the adult may not have intended to hurt the child. Harsh physical discipline may occur when an adult is frustrated or angry and strikes, shakes. or throws a child. Some forms of physical abuse are intentional such as burns, bites, cuts, twists limbs, or otherwise harms a child.

Young children are very active and frequently fall down and bump into things. Their injuries tend to be to their elbows, noses, foreheads, and other bony areas. Bruises and marks on the soft tissue of the face, back, neck, bottom, arms, thighs, ankles, backs of legs, or genitals are likely to be caused by physical abuse. Head injury is the most common cause of child abuse related deaths (National Clearinghouse on Child Abuse and Neglect Information, p. 4).

Signs of a child who is suffering from physical abuse include:

- Unexplained burns, bites, bruises, broken bones, or a black eye
- Fading bruises or other marks noticeable after an absence from school. Bruises change color as they fade (red to blue to black-purple to green tint (dark) to pale green or yellow)
- Appearing frightened of the parents and protests or cries when it is time to go home from school
- Shrinking at the approach of adults or ducking when someone makes a quick move

- Difficulty playing or difficulty concentrating in school
- Reports injury by a parent or another adult caregiver

Signs of Neglect

Child neglect is characterized by failure to provide for the child's basic needs. Neglect may be physical (not enough food or not adequate clothing for cold weather), medical (refusal to seek medical attention when it is obvious the child needs it), educational (failure to enroll a child older than 7 years old in school), or emotional (chronic or extreme spouse abuse in the child's presence). Severe neglect often results in death, especially when the child is very young. Although physical abuse tends to be sporadic, neglect is ongoing. Neglect can also occur in childcare settings such as when children are left in their cribs most of the day and not provided stimulation outside of their crib.

When looking at neglect, you tend to see patterns. You will need to ask yourself: Do they occur frequently, almost everyday, periodically over weekends or vacations, or around a particular event in the child's life? Indicators a child is suffering from neglect include:

- Frequent absences from school
- Begging or stealing food or money from classmates
- Lacking necessary medical or dental care, immunizations, or glasses
- Consistently dirty and has severe body odor
- Lacking sufficient clothing for the weather
- Difficulty learning to talk
- Overly friendly to strangers
- Thinking and speaking badly of himself
- Abuse of alcohol or other drugs
- States there is no one at home to provide care

Signs of Sexual Abuse

Sexual abuse is considered anything from inappropriate touching to intercourse, rape, and exploitation through pros-

titution or pornography. Usually a perpetrator is an adult, but it can be someone under 18 who is in a position of authority over the child. For example, a 14-year-old camp counselor who inappropriately touches a 5-year-old in his care is engaging in sexual abuse. Both boys and girls are vulnerable to sexual abuse, but boys are less likely to report it. Usually the abuser threatens to hurt the child or his family if he tells about the abuse. The abuser also knows how to manipulate children, promising them gifts or attention in exchange for playing sex games. Indicators that a child is suffering from sexual abuse include:

- Difficulty walking or sitting
- Suddenly refuses to change for gym to participate in physical activities
- Becomes secretive and stops talking about home life
- Has difficulty sleeping
- Suddenly finds physical contact frightening
- Demonstrates bizarre, sophisticated, or unusual sexual knowledge or behavior
- Becomes pregnant or contracts a venereal disease, especially if under the age of 14
- Runs away
- Reports sexual abuse by a parent or another adult caregiver

Signs of Emotional Abuse

Emotional abuse includes blaming, belittling, or rejecting a child, consistently treating siblings differently, and showing continual lack of concern by the caretaker for the child's welfare. It can also include bizarre behavior or cruel forms of punishment (locking a child in the closet). This type of abuse is difficult to detect and prove. The effects of mental injury which may include delays in physical development, speech or other disorders, rocking motions, or odd reactions to people in authority, are more difficult to detect than bruises and broken bones. Some of the effects may not show up for years.

Behaviors of the emotionally abused are similar to those of emotionally disturbed children. To help distinguish

between them, you may watch how the parents interact with the child. The parents of emotionally disturbed children demonstrate concern and pursue treatment for the child. The parents of emotionally abused children often blame their child for the problems, refuse offers of help, and do not seek help.

Emotional abuse usually occurs along with physical or sexual abuse. Emotional abuse always accompanies physical abuse, but emotional abuse may not be accompanied by physical abuse.

Indicators that a child is suffering from emotional abuse include:

- Shows extremes in behavior, such as overly compliant or demanding behavior, extreme passivity, or aggression
- Is either inappropriately adult (parenting other children) or inappropriately childlike (frequent rocking or head banging)
- Is delayed in physical or emotional development
- Has attempted suicide
- Reports lack of attachment to the parent

SIGNS OF ELDER ABUSE

The signs and symptoms of elder abuse are described next. Unlike child abuse, elder abuse can involve finances. The information was taken from the following Web sites: Clearinghouse on Abuse and Neglect of the Elderly (http://www.elderabusecenter.org), Elder Abuse Prevention (http://www.oaktrees.org), National Elder Abuse Incidence Study (http://www.aoa.dhhs.gov/abuse/report/default.htm), Elderly Place (http://www.geocities.com/~elderly-place), and Administration on Aging (http://www.aoa and http://www.ElderAbusefyi.com)

Physical Abuse

Physical abuse occurs when a person is touched in an inappropriate way, such as hitting, punching, kicking, slapping,

and pushing. Physical abuse usually leaves marks such as bite marks, bruises, welts, and burn marks. Marks usually are found on the arms, wrists, face, neck, and abdominal area.

Indicators of physical abuse in elders include:

- Cuts, lacerations, welt marks
- Burn marks
- Hair loss or hemorrhaging below the scalp from someone grabbing or pulling hair
- Sores on the body, open wounds
- Changes in weight
- Poor skin conditions
- Unexplained injuries such as fractures and breaks
- Bruises, scratches, bite marks, fingerprints, black eyes, broken fingernails
- Over- or undermedicated

Behavioral changes in an individual suffering from elder abuse include:

- Depression or withdrawal from family and friends
- Mood swings, changes in behavior
- May seem frightened, teary eyed

The abuser may refuse to take the elder to the doctor or let others see him alone. The explanations for the injuries are inconsistent with the symptoms. The abuser may even have bite or scratch marks because the elder is fighting back.

Sexual Abuse

Sexual abuse is sexual contact made without consent. When an elder is not able to make decisions about consensual sex, it is rape.

Indicators that an individual is suffering from sexual abuse include:

- Bruises, cuts, or soreness around the breast or genital area
- Clothes with blood or tear marks
- Difficulty walking or sitting

Behavior changes indicating an individual is suffering from sexual abuse include:

- Withdrawal from family and friends
- Flinching at movements
- Frightened of the opposite gender

The abuser may not let family and friends around the elder, and the explanations do not match the indicators of abuse.

Emotional/Psychological Abuse

Abuse that occurs when a person is demeaning to another person is called emotional/psychological abuse. The abuser may treat the elder like a child or call him names, and the elder may talk negetively about himself. This type of abuse may be in the form of words or actions designed to humiliate, intimidate, confuse, or frighten an elderly person.

Indicators of emotional/psychological abuse include:

- Emotionally upset, disturbed
- Nervous behavior, repeated actions
- Negative attitude, agitation, anger
- Rocking, sucking, biting

Behavioral changes indicating emotional/psychological abuse include:

- Withdrawal, depression, or denial
- Helplessness
- Hesitation to talk openly
- Confusion or disorientation
- Fear, withdrawl, depression

The abuser talks down to the elder and calls the elder hurtful names. The abuser may also withdraw the elder from family and friends.

Financial Abuse

Financial abuse occurs when an individual is taken advantage of financially. This may include stealing money, lying

about the elder needing certain care, or cashing the elder's checks without permission.

Indicators of financial abuse include:

- Withholding money and cashing checks without permission
- Signature does not match the elder's, or the elder cannot write
- Personal belongings begin to disappear
- Misuse of power of attorney
- Not providing needed services for the elder
- Not taking the elder to the doctor
- Unusual items charged on the elder's credit card

Behavior changes indicating financial abuse include:

- Requests that funds be transferred
- Abrupt changes on a will
- Unsure of where all his money has gone
- Unable to pay bills or buy clothes or other necessities
- Elder withdraws a lot of money at the same time or within the same week

The abuser suddenly has money. Family members appear out of nowhere to gain access to the elder's money. The abuser may also forge the elder's signature on accounts.

Neglect and Abandonment

Neglect and abandonment happen when an elder is not being properly cared for (bathed, fed, and medicated) or when he is being ignored.

Indicators of neglect and abandonment include:

- Untreated sores, rashes, or lice
- Malnutrition/dehydration
- Unsanitary living conditions
- Health is not being cared for
- Dirty bed and linens
- Inadequate clothing

Behavior changes indicating neglect and abandonment include:

- Strong odor from lack of hygiene
- Obvious weight changes
- Bed sores
- Begs for food
- Needs medical and dental care

The abuser provides unclean living conditions and will not allow family and friends in the home. The abuser may leave the elder alone when the elder needs care.

REFERENCES

National Clearinghouse on Child Abuse and Neglect Information
  http://www.colib.com

Glossary

Acquired Immune Deficiency Syndrome (AIDS)—A virus that interferes with the body's immune system, allowing it to become vulnerable to life-threatening illnesses.

acute care unit—The unit or department of a hospital that deals with patients with medically related illness that requires close monitoring owing to its recent and serious nature.

American Sign Language (ASL)—A gesture-based language system.

American Speech-Language-Hearing Association (ASHA)—The national association for professionals such as speech-language pathologists, audiologists, and speech, language and hearing scientists.

Americans with Disabilities Act (ADA)—The law that prohibits discrimination by employers, government agencies, and public accommodations against people with disabilities.

anecdotal record—A record or description of a specific event.

aphasia—The loss of the ability to speak as a result of brain injury or trauma.

articulation—The movement of the mouth and tongue that shapes sound into speech.

ASHA Code of Ethics—ASHA's professional code for ethical behavior for SLPs and SLPAs.

assessment—a process for determining an individual's speech and language strengths and weaknesses.

augmentative alternative communication—Method of communicating that is based on symbols or gestures rather than speech.

bloodborne pathogen—Disease that is spread through blood.

Cardiopulmonary resuscitation (CPR)—A process of restoring a heartbeat and breathing.

Cardiovascular accident (CVA)—Commonly called a stroke.

case history—A form that an individual or a family member fills out to give detailed information about a child's development or the history of a problem.

case manager—An individual who gathers all the information that relates to an individual with a disability and coordinates services for that individual.

center-based program—An intervention program that is provided at a center—a school, health center, or private office.

checklist—A list of items that may be checked off when they are observed.

child-centered service—A type of intervention program that focuses solely on the child with disabilities.

Child Find—A group of professionals who screen and evaluate preschool children to determine if a child is eligible for special education services.

communication skills—The ability to use language to receive and express information and emotion.

confidentiality—The act of keeping personal information about the individuals you serve in strict privacy.

culture—The attitudes, values, customs, and language that form an identifiable pattern or heritage.

decontextualized—Out of context. The absence of a context or concrete visual cues, pictures, or explanations that would enhance comprehension of material or information.

development—The process of growth and learning during which a child acquires skills and abilities.

developmental delay—Development that is slower than normal.

developmental disability—A condition that prevents a person from developing normally.

developmental milestones—A developmental goal that acts as a measurement of developmental progress over time, such as an infant rolling over between 2 and 4 months of age.

diary record—A day-to-day record of events.

discharge—A term commonly used to document the decision to terminate services or release a patient from a hospital or residential institution.

disease—Illness.

Down syndrome—A syndrome identified at birth related to chromosomal abnormalities that is associated with physical and developmental disabilities.

due process hearing—Part of the procedures established to protect the rights of parents and children with disabilities during disputes under the IDEA. These are hearings before an impar-

tial person to resolve disputes related to the identification, evaluation, placement, and services by a child's educational agency.

dysphagia—Swallowing disorders associated with structural or functional abnormalities of the swallowing mechanisms that affect feeding.

early intervention—Providing therapies and other specialized services to minimize the effects of conditions that can delay early development for children from birth to 5 years of age.

ethics—Critical reflections about morality and rational analysis of it. Study of how we make judgments of right and wrong.

evaluation—The process of determining the developmental level of a child. Evaluations are used to determine if a child needs educational services, as well as to determine what types of services he needs. The evaluation consists of a services of tests covering all areas of development.

event sampling—Observing a specified number of events.

expressive language—The ability to use gestures, words, and written symbols to communicate.

family-centered practice or care—A type of intervention program that focuses on the child and his or her family as a whole.

frequency count—Counting how many times something occurs.

G-tube—A tube that goes into the stomach from which an individual receives nutrients.

home health—A model of service delivery that treats the patient in his or her home.

human immunodeficiency virus (HIV)—A virus that affects an individual's immune system and may cause AIDS.

immune system—The body's ability to fight off disease.

inclusion The practice of having children with disabilities attend the same school and classes they would attend if they did not have a disability.

individualized education plan (IEP)—A written report that details the special education program to be provided a child aged 3 and older with a disability.

individualized family service plan (IFSP)—A written report that details the early intervention services to be provided to a child, from birth to three years of age with a disability.

Individualized habilitation plan (IHP)—A written report that sets forth the services needed to enable a person with a disability to learn to work productively.

Individuals with Disabilities Education Act (IDEA)—This law establishes the right of children with disabilities to a ìfree appropriate public education.î

integrative therapy—A service delivery model that usually includes a minimum of two therapists working together or addressing more than one objective within a therapeutic activity.

intelligibility—The degree that an individual's speech is understood by others.

interdisciplinary team—A team that is made up of many different disciplines that work as a group, not as separate experts.

itinerant—A delivery of service model that demands the SLP serve children in more than one school on his or her caseload.

language—The expression and understanding of human communication.

language comprehension—The process of understanding language.

language sample—A sample of an individual's language skills in a natural environment.

latex—A milky liquid in certain plants and trees. It is the basis of rubber.

learning disability—A disorder that manifests itself in a discrepancy between ability and academic achievement. They do not stem from mental retardation, sensory impairments, emotional problems, or lack of opportunity to learn.

least restrictive environment (LRE)—The requirement under the IDEA that children with disabilities receiving special education must be made a part of a regular school to the fullest extent possible. Included in the law as a way of ending the traditional practice of isolating children with disabilities.

mainstream—A term for the practice of involving children with disabilities in regular school and preschool environments.

managed care—Organized system of health care services in which financing, clinical services, and management are combined.

mean length of utterance (MLU)—Average number of morphemes per utterance.

Medicaid—A federal program that offers medical assistance to people who are entitled to receive supplementary security income.

Medicare—A federal program that provides payments for medical care to people who are receiving social security payments.

morpheme—The smallest unit of meaning in a language, typically root words, but also all prefixes and suffixes in a language.

multidisciplinary team—A team made up of many different disciplines (speech-language, OT, PT, teacher, etc.) that function as separate experts.

narrative—A story or description of actual or fictional events.

narrative description—A method of transcribing a language sample where everything is documented in a stream of information.

natural environment—Refers to the places, activities, and routines an individual would be involved with but for the fact he or she has a disability.

nebulizer treatment—A mist form of medication that is breathed in and given to an individual who has asthma.

neonatal intensive care unit (NICU)—A medical setting dedicated to the care of premature or medically compromised newborns.

neurodevelopmental—Refers to the neurologic system as it relates to the development of the human organism.

neuromuscular—Pertaining to the system of neurologic innervations of muscles.

observation—the act of watching or noticing or the act of noting and recording.

occupational therapist (OT)—A therapist who specializes in improving the development and relearning of fine motor and adaptive skills (dressing, eating, etc.).

on task—Behavior that is appropriate and relevant to the activity or task to be accomplished.

outpatient—An individual who receives services routinely after being released from a medical facility such as a hospital.

overreferrals—When a screener is too sensitive and identifies individuals who do not need further assessment.

patient—An individual receiving services by an SLOP in a hospital or nursing home or medically related facility.

Parkinson's disease—A progressive, degenerative, neurologic disease resulting from nigrostriatal dopamine deficiency with resulting associated disorders of speech.

Part C of IDEA—The provisions in IDEA that make early intervention services available to infants and toddlers with disabilities.

perseveration—The continuation of a response (words, actions) when it is no longer appropriate.

phoneme—A sound; the smallest unit of speech.

phonetics—The study of perception and production of speech sound.

phonology—The sound system of a language and the way the sounds are combined.

physical therapist (PT)—A therapist who works with individuals to help them overcome physical problems such as low muscle tone or weak muscles. They tend to work on gross motor skills needed in activities such as walking, hopping, or riding a bike.

Pierre Robin sequence—A syndrome with physical features that may include cleft palate and associated problems with feeding or other medical complications.

portfolio—A collection or work, teacher's notes or comments, pictures, or products to document a person's skills or development.

pragmatics—The study of language use independent of language structure.

problem-oriented record (POR)—A medical record for an individual organized according to areas of difficulty or illness.

progress note—A description or summary of what occurred during a therapy session.

protection and advocacy (P & A)—A nationwide system providing legal services for families of children with disabilities.

public accommodation—A place, such as a school, restaurant, or theater, generally open to the public. The ADA prohibits discrimination against people with disabilities by public accommodations.

Public Law 94-142—The Education for All Handicapped Children Act of 1975, which provides for a ìfree appropriate public educationî for children with disabilities. Its name was changed to the Individuals with Disabilities Education Act (IDEA).

Public Law 99-457—The law that established early intervention services for infants, birth to 3 years, with disabilities. This law is now Part H of IDEA.

pullout—A term used to describe a service delivery model that demands the individual be removed from regularly scheduled activities such as pullout from the classroom for therapies.

range of motion—Refers to the normal range or distance of a movement pattern.

receptive language—The ability to understand spoken or written communication as well as gestures.

referral—Sending an individual to another professional with a specific specialty.

registration—A credentialing process that documents certain standards of education or experience have been met.

regression—The loss of developmental skills.

related services—Transportation and other developmental, corrective, or supportive services needed to enable a child to benefit from a special education program. Under the IDEA, a child is entitled to receive these services as part of his special education program.

resistance—An individual's ability to fight off disease.

sample size—The number of utterances required for a language sample.

sampling—The process of taking out a few to look at the whole.

screener—An examination tool used to screen whether an individual needs further assesment.

screening—A process of testing to determine if an individual needs further speech-language evaluation.

Section 504 of the Rehabilitation Act—A federal law that prohibits discrimination on the basis of disability in programs receiving federal funds.

self-contained classroom—Refers to a grouping of students with disabilities based on the fact they have a certain type of severity of disability.

semantics—The study of language content.

service coordinator—An individual who helps an individual family obtain and organize services for himself, their child, or family member.

sharp—A sharp object like a needle used in a health care setting.

skilled nursing facility (SNF)—A unit of a hospital or other agency that serves patients who require skilled nursing care given the severity of dysfunction.

SOAP notes—A format for documentation of subjective, objective, assessment, and planning observations and comments regarding a patient's status, often used in a hospital setting.

social security disability insurance (SSDI)—A federal disability insurance system to provide financial assistance to qualified people with disabilities.

special education—The term commonly used to refer to the education of children with disabilities; it includes instruction individually designed to help children with disabilities learn.

speech-language therapist or pathologist—A therapist trained to work with people to improve their speech and receptive and expressive language skills.

stimulable—When an individual is able to produce a sound after cuing or short training when they were unable before.

stroke—See CVA.

student—Students seen in a school-based setting.

supplemental security income (SSI)—A federal public assistance program for qualified people with disabilities.

supported employment—Employment for people with disabilities that includes some assistance, such as a job coach.

syntax—The study of language forms; rules and principles for combining grammatical elements and words into utterances and sentences.

tactile defensiveness—A commonly used term by OTs to describe a person's difficulty in integrating sensations perceived through touch.

therapy—Treatment of speech and language difficulties.

time sampling—Observing at specified intervals of time.

transcription—A written form of an individual's speech, language, or interaction with another individual.

transdisciplinary team—A team that works together in a collaborative way but it is made up of different disciplines.

transfers—A position change for an individual who needs assistance moving from one position to another with physical assistance.

triennial review—A review of an IEP that occurs every 3 years. The student will be retested at this time to redetermine eligibility for special education.

type token ratio (TTR)—A measure of vocabulary diversity obtained by dividing the number of different words in a sample of 50 utterances by the total number of words.

underreferrals—When a screener is not sensitive and passes over individuals who should have been identified as needing further assessment.

unit record—A medical file for an individual.

universal precautions—Precautions developed by the Centers for Disease Control and Prevention to limit transmission of diseases spread through the blood.

vocational training—Training for specific job skills.

worldview—An individual's set of subjective values that are derived from religious background, cultural heritage, and personal experiences.

Index